Advanced Paediatric Life Support

SEVENTH EDITION

Advanced Paediatric Life Support

A Practical Approach to Emergencies

SEVENTH EDITION

Advanced Life Support Group

EDITED BY

Stephanie Smith

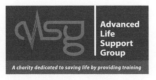

WILEY Blackwell

Registered Offices
John Wiley & Sons, Inc., 111 River Street, Hoboken, NJ 07030, USA
John Wiley & Sons Ltd, The Atrium, Southern Gate, Chichester, West Sussex, PO19 8SQ, UK

For details of our global editorial offices, customer services, and more information about Wiley products visit us at www.wiley.com.

Wiley also publishes its books in a variety of electronic formats and by print-on-demand. Some content that appears in standard print versions of this book may not be available in other formats.

Library of Congress Cataloging-in-Publication Data applied for

Paperback ISBN: 9781119716136

Printed and bound in Great Britain by Bell and Bain Ltd, Glasgow

Cover Design: Wiley
Cover Image: © Russell Ashworth

Set in 10/12 Montserrat by Straive, Pondicherry, India

Contents

Contributors to seventh edition

Working group chair

Stephanie Smith BM BS FRCPCH, Honorary Emergency Paediatric Consultant, Nottingham Children's Hospital, Nottingham, UK

Associate editors

The seriously ill child

Andrew Baldock FRCA FFICM, Consultant Paediatric Anaesthetist and Intensivist, Southampton Children's Hospital, Southampton, UK

Els Duval MD PhD, Clinical Head Pediatric Intensive Care Unit, University Hospital Antwerp, Edegem, Belgium

Jacquie Schutz MBBS FRACP DipObs, Paediatric Emergency Physician, Paediatric Emergency, Department Women's and Children's Hospital, Adelaide, South Australia

The seriously injured child

Alan Charters RGN RSCN RNT DHealthSci MAEd BSc(Hons) PgDip(Ed), Consultant Practitioner, Paediatric Emergency Care, Portsmouth, UK

Bimal Mehta MBChB BSc FRCPCH FRCEM, Consultant in Paediatric Emergency Medicine, Alder Hey Children's Hospital NHS Foundation Trust, Liverpool, UK

Life support

Jason Acworth MBBS FRACP (PEM), Paediatric Emergency Physician, Queensland Children's Hospital; Clinical Professor, Faculty of Medicine, University of Queensland, Australia

Marijke van Eerd MSc BSc RN RN(Child) PGCE, Paediatric Advanced Clinical Practitioner, Children and Young People's Emergency Department, Nottingham University Hospitals NHS Trust, Nottingham, UK

Appendices

Peter Davis MRCP(UK) FRCPCH FFICM, Consultant in Paediatric Critical Care Medicine, Bristol Royal Hospital for Children, University Hospitals Bristol and Weston NHS Foundation Trust, Bristol, UK

Esyld Watson MBBCH FCEM FAcadMEd PgDip(Med Ed), Consultant in Paediatric and Adult Emergency Medicine Prince Charles Hospital, Merthyr Tydfil, Wales

Contributors to chapters

James Armstrong BSc BMBS FRCA, Consultant in Paediatric Anaesthesia, Nottingham University Hospitals NHS Trust, Nottingham

Dave Bramley FRCSEd(A&E) FRCEM FIMCRCSEd, Consultant in Emergency Medicine and Pre-Hosptial Emergency Medicine, South Tyneside and Sunderland NHS Foundation Trust; Chief Medical Officer for the Great North Air Ambulance Service

Andrea Burgess FRCS-ORLHNS, Consultant Paediatric ENT Surgeon, Southampton Children's Hospital, Southampton

Jonathan Davies MB BChir MA DCH FRCA, Consultant Paediatric Anaesthetist, Nottingham University Hospitals NHS Trust, Nottingham

Joe Fawke MBCHB FRPCH, Consultant in Neonatal Medicine, University Hospitals Leicester NHS Trust; National Course Director, RCUK Newborn Life Support (NLS) and Advanced Resuscitation of the Newborn Infant Courses; ILCOR NLS Task Force Member; Head of East Midlands School of Paediatrics

Chris FitzSimmons FRCEM, Consultant in Paediatric Emergency Medicine, Sheffield Children's Hospital NHS Foundation Trust, Sheffield

Julie Grice MRCPCH, Consultant in Paediatric Emergency Medicine, Alder Hey Children's Hospital NHS Foundation Trust, Liverpool

Michael J. Griksaitis MBBS(Hons) MSc MRCPCH FFICM, Consultant Paediatric Intensivist, Southampton Children's Hospital; Honorary Senior Clinical Lecturer, Faculty of Medicine, University of Southampton, Southampton

Rachel Harwood MRCS PhD, Registrar in Paediatric Surgery, Alder Hey Children's Hospital NHS Foundation Trust; Honorary Clinical Fellow, University of Liverpool, LIverpool

Dan B. Hawcutt BSc(Hons) MBChB(Hons) MD MRCPCH, Reader in Paediatric Clinical Pharmacology, University of Liverpool; Honorary Consultant, Alder Hey Children's Hospital; Director of NIHR, Alder Hey Clinical Research Facility

Giles Haythornthwaite MRCPCH, Paediatric Emergency Medicine Consultant; Clinical Director for Medical Specialties, Bristol Royal Children's Hospital; Clinical Lead for Paediatric Trauma, Southwest Operational Delivery Network, Bristol

Richard Hollander MD, Consultant in Pediatric Critical Care, Beatrix Children's Hospital, University Medical Centre Groningen, the Netherlands

Hasnaa Ismail-Koch DM FRCS-ORLHNS, Consultant Paediatric ENT Surgeon, Southampton Children's Hospital

Musa Kaleem MBBS MRCPCH FRCR, Consultant Paediatric Radiologist, Alder Hey Children's NHS Foundation Trust, Liverpool

Angela Lee MBE PgDip Bsc(Hons) RGN RSCN, Nurse Consultant Paediatric Trauma and Orthopaedics, Royal Berkshire NHS Foundation Trust, Reading

Chris Moran MD FRCS, National Clinical Director for Trauma, NHS-England and NHS-Improvement; Professor of Orthopaedic Trauma Surgery, Nottingham University Hospital; Honorary Colonel, 144 Parachute Squadron, 16 Medical Regiment

Clare O'Connell MB BCh BAO FRCEM, Consultant in Emergency Medicine and Paediatric Emergency Medicine, North Cumbria Intergrated Care Trust

Ahmed Osman MSc MRCPCH FHEA, Consultant Paediatric Intensivist, Southampton Children's Hospital, Southampton

Paul Reavley MBChB FRCEM FRCS (A&E)Ed MRCGP DipMedTox, Paediatric Emergency Medicine Consultant, Bristol Royal Hospital for Children, Bristol

Martin Samuels MD FRCPCH, Consultant Respiratory Paediatrician, Staffordshire Children's Hospital and Great Ormond Street Hospital, London

Nandini Sen DTM&H FRCEM, Consultant in Emergency Medicine, Manchester University NHS Foundation Trust, Manchester

Andrew Simpson FRCS(Ed) FRCEM MClinEd DCH, Consultant in Emergency and Paediatric Emergency Medicine, North Tees and Hartlepool NHS Foundation Trust

Edward Snelson MRCPCH, Consultant Paediatric Emergency Medicine, Clinical Lead, Children's Emergency Department, Norfolk and Norwich University Hospital, Norwich

Eleanor Sproson FRCS, Consultant Paediatric ENT Surgeon, Queen Alexandra Hospital, Portsmouth

Sarah Stibbards FRCEM BSc(Hons), Clinical Director, Major Trauma and Consultant Paediatric Emergency Medicine, Alder Hey Children's Hospital NHS Foundation Trust, Liverpool

Neil Thompson BSc BMedSci BM BS RCPCH, Consultant in Paediatric Emergency Medicine, Imperial College Healthcare NHS Trust, London, UK

Robert Tinnion RCPCH MD, Consultant Neonatologist, Royal Victoria Infirmary, Newcastle Hospitals NHS Foundation Trust, Newcastle

Paul Turner BM BCh FRCPCH PhD, Clinical Reader and Honorary Consultant in Paediatric Allergy and Clinical Immunology, Imperial College London; Chairperson, Anaphylaxis Committee, World Allergy Organization

Jamie Vassallo PgCert DipIMC PhD, Emergency Medicine and Pre Hospital Emergency Medicine Registrar, Post Doctoral Research Fellow, Academic Department of Military Emergency Medicine

Julian White AM MB BS MD FACTM, Consultant Clinical Toxinologist and Unit Head, Toxinology Department, Women's and Children's Hospital, North Adelaide; Clinical Academic, Discipline of Paediatrics, Medical School, University of Adelaide, Australia

Andrea Whitney MRCP, Consultant Paediatric Neurologist, Southampton Children's Hospital, Southampton

Sarah Wood Paediatric and Neonatal Surgical Consultant, TPD and Governance Lead, Alder Hey Childrens Hospital NHS Foundation Trust, Liverpool

Bogdana S. Zoica MD, Paediatric Critical Care Consultant, King's College Hospital, London

Contributors to the status epilepticus algorithm

Richard Appleton Alder Hey Children's Hospital NHS Foundation Trust, Liverpool

Melody Bacon Royal London Hospital, Barts Health NHS Trust, London

Harish Bangalore Great Ormond Street Hospital, London

Celia Brand Royal Hospital for Children and Young People, NHS Lothian, Edinburgh

Juliet Browning University Hospitals Dorset, Poole, Dorset

Richard Chin University of Edinburgh; Royal Hospital for Children and Young People, NHS Lothian, Edinburgh

Susana Saranga Estevan Addenbrooke's Hospital, Cambridge

Satvinder Mahal Great Ormond Street Hospital, London

Kirsten McHale Royal Alexandra Children's Hospital, University Hospitals Sussex NHS Foundation Trust, Brighton

Ailsa McLellan Royal Hospital for Children and Young People, NHS Lothian, Edinburgh

Nicola Milne Epilepsy Scotland, Glasgow

Suresh Pujar Great Ormond Street Hospital, London

Tekki Rao Luton and Dunstable University Hospital, Luton

Steven Short Scottish Ambulance Service, Edinburgh

Stephen Warriner Portsmouth Hospitals University Trust, Portsmouth

Michael Yoong Royal London Hospital, Barts Health NHS Trust, London

Foreword

It hardly seems possible that it is 30 years ago that I sat down as an overconfident senior registrar and wrote the preface for the Advanced Paediatric Life Support manual. Now, three decades later: older, even balder, definitely less overconfident and most probably a little bit wiser, I have been given the opportunity to reflect on the evolution of the APLS manual and the APLS course by writing the Foreword to this - the seventh edition.

Believe it or not, at the time it was first published, APLS was a disruptive intervention. By that I mean that it challenged the status quo and sought to change the very fundamentals of emergency paediatric practice. At the most basic level it implied quite bluntly that the old Oslerian paradigm of history, examination, differential diagnosis, investigation and treatment was not fit for purpose in an emergency situation. Rather the new concept of primary assessment and resuscitation followed by secondary assessment and emergency treatment was advocated. To make matters worse it went on to derive, publish and teach a set, algorithmic approach to many clinical problems that had traditionally been managed by physician choice. As an example, I can well remember the conversations we, the editors, had about the algorithm for the management of status epilepticus. We finally constructed an APLS status epilepticus treatment algorithm from the wisps of published evidence and filled in the gaps with our best guesses. Our logic was that forearmed with an algorithm any trained practitioner could manage the situation to the point of arrival of an expert. This approach upset a number of established clinicians who felt that, as practitioners of the art of medicine, they could craft personalised treatment only by having free choice, and that anything that interfered with that free choice was bad for patients. Over the next 6 editions of APLS these arguments have abated and, indeed, the algorithms themselves are often now owned and regularly updated by expert sub-speciality groups. The smell of paraldehyde and the need for glass syringes has become history, and debates continue as evidence based medicine evolves.

Most practitioners who deal with paediatric emergencies nowadays will never have known anything other than the 'APLS approach' to emergency care, and that is the true success of the disruption the manual and course started all those years ago. There are, of course, dangers in becoming the new normal, in particular it is easy to rest on the laurels of success. Avoiding complacency is important and is why this latest (seventh) edition is as important as the first edition was all those years ago. The current APLS working group and the book editors are at the peak of their careers and are wholly committed to keeping the content and teaching of APLS at the very cutting edge of current practice. Knowing the energy they bring as the current custodians of APLS is why I have no hesitation in recommending this new edition to you. It will serve you, and sick and injured children, well.

Kevin Mackway-Jones
Manchester, 2023

Preface to first edition

Advanced Paediatric Life Support: The Practical Approach was written to improve the emergency care of children, and has been developed by a number of paediatricians, paediatric surgeons, emergency physicians and anaesthetists from several UK centres. It is the core text for the APLS (UK) course, and will also be of value to medical and allied personnel unable to attend the course. It is designed to include all the common emergencies, and also covers a number of less common diagnoses that are amenable to good initial treatment. The remit is the first hour of care, because it is during this time that the subsequent course of the child is set.

The book is divided into six parts. Part I introduces the subject by discussing the causes of childhood emergencies, the reasons why children need to be treated differently and the ways in which a seriously ill child can be recognised quickly. Part II deals with the techniques of life support. Both basic and advanced techniques are covered, and there is a separate section on resuscitation of the newborn. Part III deals with children who present with serious illness. Shock is dealt with in detail, because recognition and treatment can be particularly difficult. Cardiac and respiratory emergencies, and coma and convulsions, are also discussed. Part IV concentrates on the child who has been seriously injured. Injury is the most common cause of death in the 1–14-year age group and the importance of this topic cannot be overemphasised. Part V gives practical guidance on performing the procedures mentioned elsewhere in the text. Finally, Part VI (the appendices) deals with other areas of importance.

Emergencies in children generate a great deal of anxiety – in the child, the parents and in the medical and nursing staff who deal with them. We hope that this book will shed some light on the subject of paediatric emergency care, and that it will raise the standard of paediatric life support. An understanding of the contents will allow doctors, nurses and paramedics dealing with seriously ill and injured children to approach their care with confidence.

Kevin Mackway-Jones
Elizabeth Molyneux
Barbara Phillips
Susan Wieteska
Editorial Board
1993

Preface to seventh edition

The Advanced Paediatric Life Support (APLS) course is now delivered in 76 centres across the United Kingdom and 17 centres on every continent across the world. This amazing achievement is due to the small, dedicated team based at the Advanced Life Support Group (ALSG) in Manchester and to the thousands of trained instructors from many disciplines, who give their time and expertise so generously. Thank you all.

This manual (the seventh in the last 30 years) supports the APLS and Paediatric Life Support (PLS) courses, as well as being used as a gold standard for acute paediatric clinical practice. It builds on the contributions from previous authors whose names can be found on the ALSG website. Thank you to them and to all those who have worked so hard to produce this edition.

This manual has been updated throughout. There is an increased emphasis on preparation for effective team working to improve patient safety. The seriously ill child section has been restructured to consolidate information into chapters reflecting the ABCDE approach.

Evolving techniques such as point of care ultrasound (POCUS) are included in several chapters, and POCUS is described in more detail in an excellent appendix at the end of the manual. APLS does not specifically teach this skill, rather we acknowledge its place in many aspects of emergency management and care.

The entire manual has been updated in line with the 2021 International Liaison Committee on Resuscitation (ILCOR) guidelines as well as with consensus best practice. The international nature of APLS means the manual is written to reflect different cultures and clinical practices wherever possible.

Additional and detailed information for those who wish to take their learning further is included in the 10 appendices. **This information is not essential knowledge for all** but we hope will be interesting reading for many.

Since the sixth edition of APLS there has been the worldwide COVID-19 pandemic which had an impact on the way courses were delivered as well as the timescale for this edition of the manual. It is essential that we incorporate the lessons learned from this experience into delivery of both healthcare and the way it is taught.

Stephanie Smith
May 2023

Acknowledgements

A great many people have put a lot of hard work into the production of this book, and the accompanying Advanced Paediatric Life Support course. The editors would like to thank all the contributors for their efforts and all the APLS instructors who took the time to send us their comments on the earlier editions.

We are greatly indebted to Kirsten Baxter and Kate Denning for their exceptional hard work and dedication towards this publication; their encouragement and guidance throughout the process has been gratefully received.

We would like to express our special thanks to Ayşe Mehta for producing the excellent line drawings, Jason Acworth and Children's Health Queensland for the new photographs that illustrate the text and Catherine Giaquinto for designing the new algorithms for this edition.

For the cover image, thank you to Russell Ashworth and his son Noah Ashworth, Chloe Donaldson, Manivannan Manoharan, Julia Maxted, Angela Armitage and Nila Prince.

We would also like to thank Laura May for kindly allowing adaptation of the UHCW NHS Trust Paediatric TRAUMATIC list. Rowan Pritchard Jones and Michael Watts for allowing images from the Mersey Burns App. Michael J. Griksaitis and Bogdana Zoica for the POCUS chapter and figures. Jamie Vassallo for the PTCA algorithm. Marijke van Eerd for the Paediatric Major Trauma and analgesia calculation chart. Ross Smith on behalf of the Child and Young Person's Advance Care Plan. Tim Nutbeam and Ron Daniels on behalf of the UK Sepsis Trust. The Status Epilepticus Guidelines development group.

For the shared use of their images, illustrations, tables and algorithms, we would like to thank:

Alder Hey Radiology Department Teaching Library
ASIA – American Spinal Injury Association
Bristol Royal Hospital for Children and RTIC Severn
British Society for Paediatric Endocrinology and Diabetes
British Thoracic Society/Scottish Intercollegiate Guidelines Network
Children's Health Queensland
National Tracheostomy Safety Project: Paediatric Working Party
Northern Neonatal Network
Resuscitation Council UK
Royal College Paediatrics and Child Health and Harlow Printing
Safeguard Medical Technologies
Teleflex Medical Australia and New Zealand
Victorian Department of Health

ALSG gratefully acknowledge the support of the Royal College of Paediatrics and Child Health (UK). The Specialist Groups of the RCPCH agreed to advise on the clinical content of chapters relevant to their specialism. ALSG wish to thank the following:

Association of Paediatric Emergency Medicine

Anastasia Alcock FRCPCH DTM&H DRCOG PgDIP, Paediatric Emergency Medicine Consultant, Evelina London

Jane Bayreuther FRCPCH, Consultant in Paediatric Emergency Medicine, Southampton. On behalf of APEM

Charlotte Clements BSc(Hons) MBChB MRCPCH MSc PGCert (Darzi), Consultant Paediatrician, Clinical Lead for the Paediatric Emergency Department, North Middlesex University Hospital NHS Trust; Secretary, Association of Paediatric Emergency Medicine

Miki Lazner MBChB MMSc (Child Health) FRCPCH, Paediatric Emergency Medicine Consultant, Clinical Lead Paediatric Trauma, University Hospitals Sussex NHS Foundation Trust; Paediatric Lead, Sussex Trauma Network; Guidelines Representative and Executive Committee Member, Association of Paediatric Emergency Medicine (APEM)

Michael Malley MA MBBS MRCPCH DTMH, Consultant in Paediatric Emergency Medicine, Bristol Royal Hospital for Children

Rachael Mitchell MRCPCH MA (Cantab), Consultant in Paediatric Emergency Medicine, Kings College Hospital NHS Foundation Trust

British Association General Paediatrics

Christine Brittain RCPCH, Sub-speciality PEM, Acute Paediatric Consultant, PAU Lead, Musgrove Park Hospital Somerset Foundation Trust

British Association of Perinatal Medicine

Hannah Shore MBChB MRCPCH MD, Consultant Neonatologist, Lead Clinician for Leeds Centre for Newborn Care

Tim J. van Hasselt MBChB BMedSc MRCPCH, Neonatal sub-specialty trainee, West Midlands, NIHR Doctoral Research Fellow, University of Leicester

British Paediatric Allergy, Immunity and Infection Group

Alasdair Bamford MBBS FRCPCH DTM+H PhD, Consultant and Specialty Lead in Paediatric Infectious Diseases, Great Ormond Street Hospital for Children NHS Foundation Trust; Honorary Associate Professor, UCL GOSH Institute of Child Health; British Paediatric Allergy Infection and Immunity Group (BPAIIG) secretary

Enitan Carrol MBChB MD DTMH FRCPCH, Professor and Honorary Consultant in Paediatric Immunology and Infectious Diseases, University of Liverpool and Alder Hey Children's NHS Foundation Trust

Saul Faust MBBS PhD FRCPCH OBE, Professor and Honorary Consultant in Paediatric Immunology and Infectious Diseases, University of Southampton and University Hospital Southampton NHS Foundation Trust

Paul Turner BM BCh FRCPCH PhD, Clinical Reader and Honorary Consultant in Paediatric Allergy and Clinical Immunology, Imperial College London; Chairperson of Anaphylaxis Committee, World Allergy Organization

Elizabeth Whittaker MB BAO BCh MRCPCH DTM&H PhD, Consultant in Paediatric Infectious Diseases; Clinical Lead in Paediatric Infectious Diseases, Imperial College Healthcare NHS Trust, London; Senior Clinical Lecturer in Paediatric Infectious Diseases, Imperial College London; Convenor for British Paediatric Allergy Immunity and Infectious Diseases Group (BPAIIG)

British Paediatric Respiratory Society

Elise Weir MBChB MRCPCH PGCert Child Health, Consultant in Paediatric Respiratory Medicine, Royal Hospital for Children, Glasgow

British Society of Paediatric Radiology – trauma imaging

Judith Foster MB ChB(Hons) FRCR, Consultant Paediatric Radiologist, University Hospitals Plymouth; Paediatric Trauma Lead for British Society of Paediatric Radiology

Child Protection Special Interest Group

David Lewis MBBS MSc(Paeds) MRCP FRCPCH, Consultant Community Paediatrician and Designated Doctor for Child Protection (Herefordshire and Worcestershire ICB); Chair of the Child Protection Specialist Interest Group (affiliated to the Royal College of Paediatrics and Child Health)

Paediatric Critical Care Society

David Finn MBBS MRPCH MSc, Paediatric Intensive Care Consultant, Leeds Children's Hospital

Rum Thomas MB BS DNB (Paediatrics) FRCPCH, Consultant in Paediatric Critical Care, Sheffield Children's NHS Foundation Trust; Clinical Lead, Paediatric Critical Care Operational Delivery Network Yorkshire and Humber South

Hanna Tilly BSc BMedSci BMBS, Specialist Registrar in Paediatrics, North Central and East London

Mark Worrall MB ChB FRCA MRCPCH FFICM, Consultant in Paediatric Intensive Care and Paediatric Anaesthesia, Royal Hospital for Children, Glasgow; Consultant in Paediatric Critical Care Transport, ScotSTAR, Scottish Ambulance Service

RCEM Intercollegiate group

Anne Frampton MPhil BSc MB ChB MRCP DipIMC DCH FRCEM, Consultant in Emergency Medicine (Paediatrics), Bristol Royal Hospital for Children, UHBW NHS FT

Michelle Jacobs BSc MB BCh FRCEM ARSM, Consultant in Paediatric Emergency Medicine, ED Clinical Lead for Paediatric Emergency Department, London North West University Healthcare NHS Trust (Northwick Park Hospital)

Damian Roland B(Med)Sci BMBS FRCPCH PhD, Honorary Professor and Consultant in Emergency Medicine, Head of Service, Children's Emergency Department, Leicester Hospitals and University

Rob Stafford MBBS MRCA PGCertMedEd FHEA FRCEM, Consultant in Adult and Paediatric Emergency Medicine; Chair, RCEM Paediatric Emergency Medicine Professional Advisory Group

We would like to thank, in advance, those of you who will attend the Advanced Paediatric Life Support course and others using this text for your continued constructive comments regarding the future development of both the course and the manual.

Contact details and further information

ALSG: www.alsg.org

For details on ALSG courses visit the website or contact:
Advanced Life Support Group
ALSG Centre for Training and Development
29–31 Ellesmere Street
Swinton, Manchester
M27 0LA
Tel: +44 (0) 161 794 1999
Email: enquiries@alsg.org

Updates

The material contained within this book is updated on approximately a 4-yearly cycle. However, practice may change in the interim period. We will post any changes on the ALSG website, so we advise you to visit the website regularly to check for updates (www.alsg.org).

References

To access references, visit the ALSG website www.alsg.org – references are on the course pages as well as at the end of this book.

On-line feedback

It is important to ALSG that the contact with our providers continues after a course is completed. We now contact everyone 6 months after their course has taken place asking for on-line feedback on the course. This information is then used whenever the course is updated to ensure that the course provides optimum training to its participants.

PART 1

Introduction

CHAPTER 1

Introduction and structured approach to paediatric emergencies

---

Learning outcomes

After reading this chapter, you will be able to:

- Appreciate the focus and principles of the APLS course
- Describe the structured approach to identifying and managing paediatric emergencies
- Identify the important differences in children and the impact these have on the management of emergencies
- Appreciate that the absolute size and relative body proportions change with the age of the child
- Identify the approach to triage of a child

1.1 Introduction

The Advanced Paediatric Life Support (APLS) course equips those caring for children with the necessary skills and structured approach to identify and safely manage ill or injured children whenever or wherever they encounter them.

Children continue to die from preventable causes throughout the world. The reasons for their deaths differ between countries, however the structure and principles for managing the underlying causes are universal.

Child mortality is the lowest it has ever been and has halved in the last three decades, which is a huge achievement (12.5 million deaths of under 5-year-olds worldwide in 1990 compared with 5 million in 2020).

Worldwide data from the World Health Organization (WHO) show the leading cause of death in this age group is pneumonia, followed by preterm birth and then diarrhoeal illnesses. This compares with recent data from the USA showing the leading cause in children to be gun-related injuries. In the UK, Office for National Statistics (ONS) data show that cancer is the leading cause of death in all children followed by accidents and then congenital abnormalities.

The COVID-19 pandemic has not directly had a significant impact on child mortality. However, there are ongoing concerns about the indirect impact due to strained and under-resourced health systems; a reduction in care-seeking behaviours; a reduced uptake of preventative measures such as vaccination and nutritional supplements; and socioeconomic challenges.

1.2 The APLS approach

In the structured approach it is essential to remember that:

- The child's family will need support from a qualified member of the team
- Absolute size and body proportions change with age
- Observations and therapy in children must be related to their age and weight
- The psychological needs of children must be considered
- It is key to support each other as the clinical team

Physiological differences

Children, especially young ones, have significantly lower physiological reserves than adults. As a consequence, they may deteriorate rapidly when severely ill or injured and respond differently from adults to various interventions. It is essential to manage and support their respiratory and cardiovascular systems in a timely and structured manner to prevent further deterioration or even cardiovascular arrest. (See normal ranges table, inside front cover.)

Relationship between disease progression and outcomes

The further a disease process is allowed to progress, the worse the outcome is likely to be. The outcomes for children who have a cardiac arrest out of hospital are generally poor. This may be because cardiac arrest in children is less commonly related to cardiac arrhythmia, but is more commonly a result of hypoxaemia and/or shock with associated organ damage and dysfunction. By the time that cardiac arrest occurs, there has already been substantial damage to various organs. This is in contrast to situations (more common in adults) where the cardiac arrest is the consequence of cardiac arrhythmia – with preceding normal perfusion and oxygenation. Thus the focus of the course is on early recognition and effective management of potentially life-threatening problems before there is progression to respiratory and/or cardiac arrest (Figure 1.1).

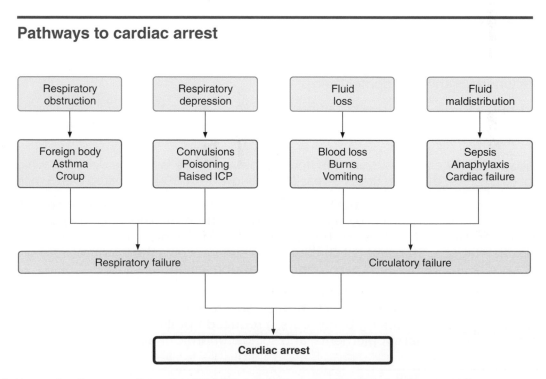

Figure 1.1 Pathways leading to cardiac arrest in childhood (with examples of underlying causes)
ICP, intracranial pressure

Standardised structure for assessment and stabilisation

A standardised approach for resuscitation enables the provision of a standard working environment and access to the necessary equipment to manage ill or injured children. The use of the standardised structure enables the whole team to know what is expected of them and in which sequence.

Once basic stabilisation has been achieved, it is appropriate to investigate the underlying diagnoses and provide definitive therapy.

> Definitive therapy (such as surgical intervention) may be a component of the resuscitation

Resource management

Provision of effective emergency treatment depends on the development of teams of healthcare providers working together in a coordinated, well-led manner (Figure 1.2). It is important that all training in paediatric life support focuses on how to best use the equipment and human resources available and emphasises the key nature of effective communication.

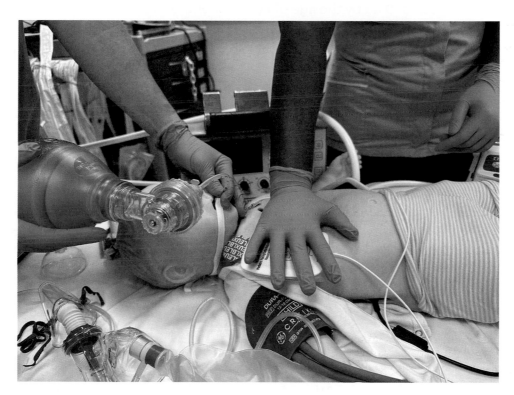

Figure 1.2 Advanced paediatric life support (APLS) in action

Early referral to appropriate teams for definitive management

Emergency departments are unlikely to be able to provide definitive management for all paediatric emergencies, and a component of stabilisation of critically ill or injured children is the capacity to call for help as soon as possible, and where necessary transfer the child to the appropriate site safely.

Ongoing care until admission to appropriate care

In most parts of the world it is impossible to transfer critically ill children into intensive care units or other specialised units within a short time of their arrival in the emergency area. Therefore, it is important to provide training in the ongoing therapy that is required for a range of relatively common conditions once initial stabilisation has been completed.

1.3   Important differences in children

Children are a diverse group, varying enormously in weight, size, shape, intellectual ability and emotional responses. At birth a child is, on average, a 3.5 kg, 50 cm long individual with small respiratory and cardiovascular reserves and an immature immune system. They are capable of limited movement, have immature emotional responses though still perceive pain and are dependent upon adults for all their needs. At the other end of childhood, the adolescent may be more than 60 kg, 160 cm tall and look physically like an adult, often exhibiting a high degree of independent behaviour but who may still require support in ways that are different from adults.

Competent management of a seriously ill or injured child who may fall anywhere between these two extremes requires a knowledge of these anatomical, physiological and emotional differences and a strategy of how to deal with them.

Weight

The most rapid changes in weight occur during the first year of life. An average birth weight of 3.5 kg will have increased to 10 kg by the age of 1 year. After that time weight increases more slowly until the pubertal growth spurt. This is illustrated in the weight charts shown in Figure 1.3.

As most drugs and fluids are given as the dose per kilogram of body weight, it is important to determine a child's weight as soon as possible. The most accurate method for achieving this is to weigh the child on scales; however, in an emergency this may be impracticable. Very often, especially with infants, the child's parents or carer will be aware of a recent weight. If this is not possible, various formulae or measuring tapes are available. The Broselow or Sandell tapes use the height (or length) of the child to estimate weight. The tape is laid alongside the child and the estimated weight read from the calibrations on the tape. This is a quick, easy and relatively accurate method. Various formulae may also be used although they should be validated to the population in which they are being used.

> If a child's age is known, the normal ranges table will provide you with an approximate weight (inside front cover) and allow you to prepare the appropriate equipment and drugs for the child's arrival in hospital. Whatever the method, it is essential that the carer is sufficiently familiar with the tools to use them quickly and accurately under pressure. When the child arrives, you should quickly review their size to check if it is much larger or smaller than predicted. If you have a child who looks particularly large or small for their age, you can go up or down one age group.

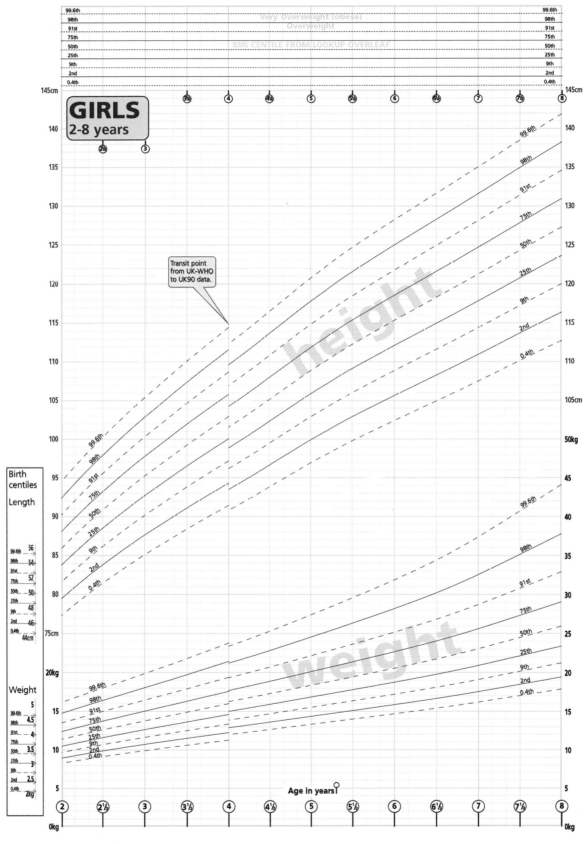

Figure 1.3 Example of centile chart for weight in girls (2–18 years)

©Reproduced with kind permission of RCPCH and Harlow Printing Limited

(*Continued*)

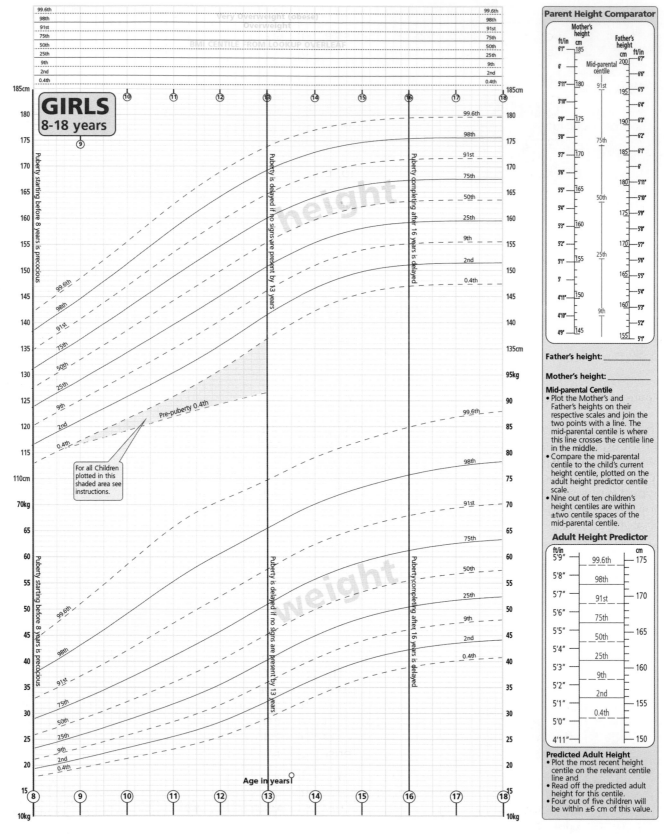

Figure 1.3 (*Continued*)

Anatomical

As the child's weight increases with age the size, shape and proportions of various organs also change. Particular anatomical changes are relevant to emergency care.

Airway

The airway is influenced by anatomical changes in the tissues of the mouth and neck. In a young child the occiput is relatively large and the neck short, potentially resulting in neck flexion and airway narrowing when the child is laid flat in the supine position. The face and mandible are small, and teeth or orthodontic appliances may be loose. The tongue is relatively large and not only tends to obstruct the airway in an unconscious child, but may also impede the view at laryngoscopy. Finally, the floor of the mouth is easily compressible, requiring care in the positioning of fingers when holding the jaw for airway positioning. These features are summarised in Figure 1.4.

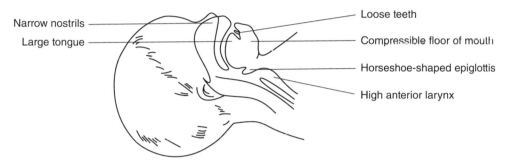

Narrow nostrils

Large tongue

Loose teeth

Compressible floor of mouth

Horseshoe-shaped epiglottis

High anterior larynx

Figure 1.4 Summary of significant upper airway anatomy

The anatomy of the airway itself changes with age, and consequently different problems affect different age groups. Infants less than 6 months old are primarily nasal breathers. As the narrow nasal passages are easily obstructed by mucous secretions, and as upper respiratory tract infections are common in this age group, these children are at particular risk of airway compromise. Adenotonsillar hypertrophy may be a problem at all ages, but is more usually found between 3 and 8 years. This not only tends to cause obstruction, but also may cause difficulty when the nasal route is used to pass pharyngeal, gastric or tracheal tubes.

The trachea is short and soft. Overextension of the neck as well as flexion may therefore cause tracheal compression. The short trachea and the symmetry of the carinal angles (the angle between the right and left main bronchi) mean that not only is tube displacement more likely, but a tube or a foreign body is also just as likely to be displaced into the left as the right main-stem bronchus.

Breathing

The lungs are relatively immature at birth. The air–tissue interface has a relatively small total surface area in the infant (less than 3 m^2). In addition, there is a 10-fold increase in the number of small airways from birth to adulthood. Both the upper and lower airways are relatively small and are consequently more easily obstructed. As resistance to flow is inversely proportional to the fourth power of the airway radius (halving the radius increases the resistance 16-fold), seemingly small obstructions can have significant effects on air entry in children. This may partially explain why so much respiratory disease in children is characterised by airway obstruction.

Infants rely mainly on diaphragmatic breathing. Their muscles are more likely to fatigue as they have fewer type I (slow-twitch, highly oxidative, fatigue-resistant) fibres compared with adults. Preterm infants' muscles have even fewer type I fibres. These children are consequently more prone to respiratory failure.

The ribs lie more horizontally in infants, and therefore contribute less to chest expansion. In the injured child, the compliant chest wall may allow serious parenchymal injuries to occur without necessarily incurring rib fractures. For multiple rib fractures to occur the force must be very large; the parenchymal injury that results is consequently very severe and flail chest is tolerated badly.

Circulation

At birth the two cardiac ventricles are of similar weight; by 2 months of age the RV : LV weight ratio is 0.5. These changes are reflected in the infant's electrocardiogram (ECG). During the first months of life the right ventricle (RV) dominance is apparent, but by 4–6 months of age the left ventricle (LV) is dominant. As the heart develops during childhood, the sizes of the P wave and QRS complex increase, and the P-R interval and QRS duration become longer.

The child's circulating blood volume per kilogram of body weight (70–80 ml/kg) is higher than that of an adult, but the actual volume is small. This means that in infants and small children, relatively small absolute amounts of blood loss can be critically important.

Body surface area

The body surface area (BSA) to weight ratio decreases with increasing age (Figure 1.5). Small children, with a high ratio, lose heat more rapidly and consequently are relatively more prone to hypothermia. At birth, the head accounts for 19% of BSA; this falls to 9% by the age of 15 years.

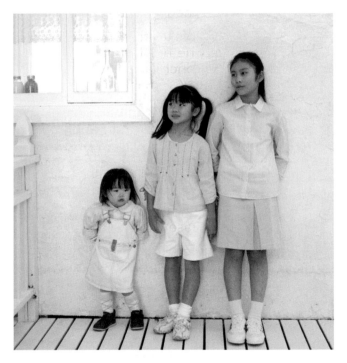

Figure 1.5 Differences in children
TAGSTOCK2/Adobe Stock

Physiological

Respiratory

The infant has a relatively greater metabolic rate and oxygen consumption. This is one reason for an increased respiratory rate. However, the tidal volume remains relatively constant in relation to body weight (5–7 ml/kg) through to adulthood. The work of breathing is also relatively unchanged at about 1% of the metabolic rate, although it is increased in the preterm infant.

In the adult, the lung and chest wall contribute equally to the total compliance. In the newborn, most of the impedance to expansion is due to the lung, and is critically dependent on the presence of surfactant. The lung compliance increases over the first week of life as fluid is removed from the lung. The infant's compliant chest wall leads to prominent sternal recession when the airways are obstructed or lung compliance decreases. It also allows the intrathoracic pressure to be less 'negative'. This reduces small airway patency. As a result, the lung volume at the end of expiration is similar to the closing volume (the volume at which small-airway closure starts to take place).

The combination of high metabolic rate and oxygen consumption with low lung volumes and limited respiratory reserve means that infants in particular will desaturate much more rapidly than adults. This is an important consideration during procedures such as endotracheal intubation.

At birth, the oxygen dissociation curve is shifted to the left and P_{50} (PO_2 at 50% oxygen saturation) is greatly reduced. This is due to the fact that 70% of the haemoglobin (Hb) is in the form of fetal haemoglobin (HbF); this gradually declines to negligible amounts by the age of 6 months.

The immature infant lung is also more vulnerable to insult. Following prolonged respiratory support of a preterm infant, chronic lung disease of the newborn may cause prolonged oxygen dependence. Many infants who have suffered from bronchiolitis remain 'chesty' for a year or more.

Cardiovascular

The infant has a relatively small stroke volume (1.5 ml/kg at birth) but has the highest cardiac index seen at any stage of life (300 ml/min/kg). Cardiac index decreases with age and is 100 ml/min/kg in adolescence and 70–80 ml/min/kg in the adult. At the same time the stroke volume increases, the heart gets bigger and muscle mass relative to connective tissue increases. As cardiac output is the product of stroke volume and heart rate, these changes underlie the heart rate changes seen during childhood. In addition, the average infant is only able to increase their heart rate by approximately 30% versus the adult who may be able to increase heart rate under stress by up to 300%.

As the stroke volume is small and relatively fixed in infants, cardiac output is principally related to heart rate. The practical importance of this is that the response to volume therapy is blunted when normovolaemic because stroke volume cannot increase greatly to improve cardiac output. By the age of 2 years, myocardial function and response to fluid are similar to those of an adult.

Systemic vascular resistance rises after birth and continues to do so until adulthood is reached. This is reflected in the changes seen in blood pressure.

Immune function

At birth the immune system is immature and, consequently, babies are more susceptible than older children to many infections such as bronchiolitis, septicaemia, meningitis and urinary tract infections. Maternal antibodies acquired across the placenta provide some early protection but these progressively decline during the first 6 months. These are replaced slowly by the infant's antibodies as they grow older. Infants may be particularly susceptible to infectious diseases in the period between the waning of maternal antibodies and development of their own antibodies (sometimes in response to immunisation). Breastfeeding provides increased protection against respiratory and gastrointestinal infections.

Psychological

Fear

Children vary enormously in their intellectual ability and their emotional response. A knowledge of child development assists in understanding a child's behaviour and formulating an appropriate management strategy. Particular challenges exist in communicating with children. Many situations that adults would not classify as fearful, engender fear in children. This causes additional distress to the child and adds to parental anxiety. Physiological parameters, such as pulse rate and respiratory rate, are often raised because of it, and this in turn makes clinical assessment of pathological processes such as shock more difficult.

Fear is a particular problem in the pre-school child who often has a 'magical' concept of illness and injury. This means that the child may think that the problem has been caused by some bad wish or thought that they have had. School-age children and adolescents may have fearsome concepts of what might happen to them in hospital because of ideas they have picked up from adult conversation, films and television.

> Knowledge allays fear and it is important to explain things as clearly as possible to the child in language they understand

Play can be used to help with explanations (e.g. applying a bandage to a teddy first), and also helps to maintain some semblance of normality in a strange and stressful situation. Parents must be allowed to stay with the child at all times (including during resuscitation if at all possible); importantly, they too must be supported and fully informed at all times.

Communication

Infants and young children either have no language ability or are still developing their speech. This causes difficulty when symptoms such as pain need to be described. Even children who are usually fluent may remain silent in healthcare settings when unwell or injured. Information has to be gleaned from the limited verbal communication and from the many non-verbal cues (such as facial expression and posture) that are available. Older children are more likely to understand aspects of their illness and treatment and so be reassured by adequate age-appropriate communication.

> Children with developmental differences due to pre-existing conditions such as autism, chromosome abnormalities or cerebral palsy may require different means of communication

1.4   Structured approach to paediatric emergencies

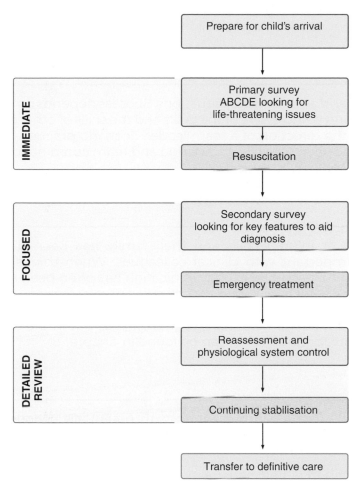

Structured approach to paediatric emergencies

Figure 1.6 **Structured approach to paediatric emergencies**

A structured approach to paediatric emergencies will enable a clinician to manage emergencies in a logical and effective fashion and assist in ensuring that vital steps are not forgotten even in unfamiliar or infrequent emergency situations (Figure 1.6). This allows:

- Identification of life-threatening situations: closed or obstructed airway, absent or ineffective breathing, or absent pulse or shock requiring immediate interventions which comprise resuscitation
- Following resuscitation, looking for key features which signpost likely working diagnosis
- Initiation of emergency treatment
- Stabilisation and transfer for definitive care

Remember to utilise newer techniques such as point of care ultrasound (POCUS) if practitioners have the skill set to do so (see Appendix I).

Throughout this book, in the virtual learning environment (VLE) and on APLS courses, the same structure will be used so that the clinician will become familiar with the approach and be able to apply it to any clinical emergency situation.

1.5 Preparation

If warning has been received of the child's arrival then preparations can be made:

- Ensure that appropriate help is available: critical illness and injury need a team approach
- Work out the likely drug, fluid and equipment needs

For unexpected emergencies, ensure that all areas where children may be treated are stocked with the drugs, fluid and equipment needed for any childhood emergencies.

1.6 Teamwork

A well-functioning team is vital in all emergency situations. Success depends on each team member carrying out their own tasks and being aware of the tasks and the skills of other team members. The whole team must be under the direction of a team leader. Scenario practice by teams who work together is an excellent way to keep up skills, knowledge and team coordination in preparation for the 'real thing'. See Chapter 2 on non-technical skills.

1.7 Communication

Communication with the ill or injured child and their family has been discussed previously. Communication is no less important with clinical colleagues. When things have gone wrong, investigations have identified that an issue in communication has often been involved. Structured communication tools may be useful in ensuring that all relevant information is conveyed to all the teams involved in the child's care. Contemporaneous recording of clinical findings, of the child's history and of test results and management plans seems obvious but in the emergency situation may be overlooked. A template for note taking can be found in Chapter 8.

1.8 Triage

Triage is the process whereby each child presenting with potentially serious illness or injury is assigned a clinical priority. It is an essential clinical risk management step, and also a tool for optimisation of resource allocation in any emergency.

In the UK, Canada and Australia, five-part national triage scales have been agreed. Such a scale is shown in Table 1.1. While the names of the triage categories and the target times assigned to each name vary from country to country, the underlying concept does not.

Table 1.1	Triage scale		
Number	**Colour**	**Name**	**Maximum time to clinician**
1	Red	Immediate	0 min
2	Orange	Very urgent	10 min
3	Yellow	Urgent	60 min
4	Green	Standard	240 min
5	Blue	Non-urgent	N/A

Triage is used to identify children who require urgent intervention.

Accuracy of triage and assigning a priority is an important basis for any triage system. However, there are instances when even for lower acuity patients the management may be deemed urgent, for example in an epidemic it may be important to get potentially uninfected children away from possible infection as soon as possible but the assessed triage priority will not change, just the action post triage. Never forget the need for repeated triage/reassessment – children can deteriorate rapidly and if there is no reassessment process, this may be missed.

Remember also that being triaged green does not mean that a child does not have a serious problem that requires specialist attention. It simply means the risk has been assessed and it would be acceptable for that child to wait for definitive management.

It is important to make sure that the family understands the nature of the triage process (and why they will see other children receiving treatment who arrived after their child).

Triage decision making

There are many models of decision making, each including: identification of a problem, determination of the alternatives and selection of the most appropriate alternative.

Discriminators are factors normally expressed as a word or short statement that allow patients to be allocated to one of five clinical priorities as in the algorithm in Figure 1.7. They can be general or specific. The former apply to all patients irrespective of their presentation and include life threat, pain, haemorrhage, conscious level and temperature and appear across the priorities (e.g. very hot, hot and warm). Specific discriminators tend to relate to key features of particular conditions, for example an asthmatic child 'unable to talk in sentences'. Thus severe pain is a general discriminator, but cardiac pain and pleuritic pain are specific discriminators.

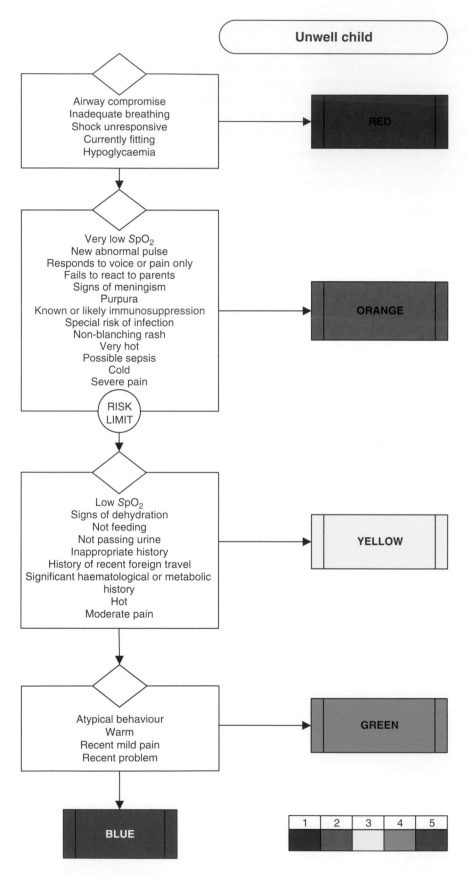

Figure 1.7 Paediatric triage for an unwell child

Secondary triage

It may not be possible to carry out all the assessments necessary at the initial triage encounter – this is particularly so if the workload of the department is high. In such circumstances, the necessary assessments should still be carried out, but as secondary procedures by the receiving healthcare professional. The actual initial clinical priority cannot be set until the process is finished. More time-consuming assessments (e.g. blood glucose estimation and peak flow measurement) are often left to the secondary stage.

1.9   Summary

This chapter has given an overview of management of paediatric emergencies, outlining the structured approach which is central to APLS. Subsequent chapters will focus in depth on the elements of the ABCDE approach in both the ill and the injured child.

CHAPTER 2

Getting it right: non-technical factors and communication

Learning outcomes

After reading this chapter, you will be able to:

- Describe how clinical human factors affect the performance of individuals and teams in the healthcare environment

---

2.1   Introduction

This chapter provides a brief introduction to some of the non-technical skills that can affect the performance of individuals and teams in the healthcare environment. Non-technical skills, also referred to as human factors or ergonomics, is an established scientific discipline and clinical human factors have been described as:

Enhancing clinical performance through an understanding of the effects of teamwork, tasks, equipment, workspace, culture and organisation on human behaviour and abilities and application of that knowledge in clinical settings. (Kohn et al., 2010)

2.2   Extent of healthcare error

In 2000 an influential report entitled *To Err is Human: Building a Safer Health System* suggested that across the USA somewhere between 44 000 and 98 000 deaths each year could be attributed to medical error. A pilot study in the UK demonstrated that approximately one in 10 patients admitted to healthcare experienced an adverse event.

Healthcare has been able to learn from a number of other high-risk industries including the nuclear, petrochemical, space exploration, military and aviation industries about how team issues have been managed. These lessons have been gradually adopted and translated to healthcare.

Specialist working groups and national bodies have been instrumental in promoting awareness of the importance of human factors in healthcare. One such example of this in the UK is the Human Factors Clinical Working Group.

2.3 Causes of healthcare error

Consider this example of an adverse event:

A child needs to receive an infusion of a particular drug. An error occurs and the child receives an incorrect drug. There are a number of potential causes of this situation. A few of these are given below.

Prescription error	Wrong drug prescribed
Prescription error	Incorrect amount prescribed
Preparation error	Correct drug prescribed but misread
Preparation error	Contents mislabelled during manufacture
Drawing up error	Incorrect drug selected
Administration error	Patient ID mix-up, drug given to wrong patient

However many checks and procedures are put in place, mistakes will still occur and may cause harm to patients. It is vital therefore that we look to work in a way that, wherever possible, reduces the occurrence of mistakes and ensures that when they do occur the chance of the error resulting in harm to children in our care is minimised. Reason's taxonomy of errors (Figure 2.1) provides further insight by illustrating how errors can be sharp or blunt or a combination of the two.

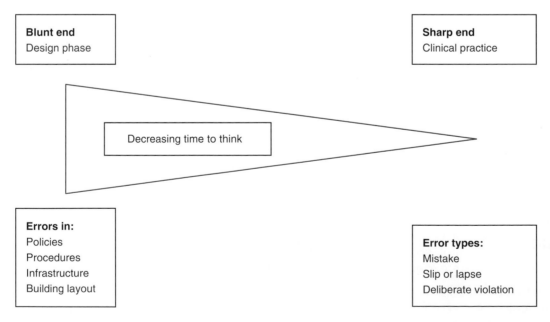

Figure 2.1 Reason's taxonomy of errors

Because errors are multifactorial, it is typically found that the organisational or blunt issues often coexist with the clinical or sharp errors; in fact it is rare for an isolated error to occur – often there is a chain of events that results in the adverse event. Apparently random, unconnected events and organisational decisions can all make errors more likely. Conversely, a standardised system with good defences can often capture these errors and prevent adverse events and subsequent impact on the patient.

In the example of drug error just given, the first potential error is the doctor writing the prescription, the second is the organisation's drug policy, the third is the nurse who draws up the drug and the fourth is the nurse who second checks the drug.

Now consider the following:

- What if the doctor is very junior and not familiar with that area or drugs used?
- What if the doctor is very senior and makes untested assumptions about drugs available?
- What if the organisation has failed to develop a robust drug policy that is fit for purpose?
- What if the nurse is a bank nurse who does not normally work on this ward and is not familiar with commonly used drugs?
- What if this area is always short of staff so that other staff do not routinely attempt to get the drug second checked?

The end result is that multiple defences have been weakened or removed and error is not only more likely to occur, but, if it does, there is a greater chance that it will cause harm.

2.4   Improving team and individual performance

Raising awareness of clinical human factors and being able to practise these skills and behaviours within multiprofessional teams allows the development of effective teams in all situations. Simulation activity allows a team to explore these new ideas, practise them and develop them. To do this we need feedback on our performance within a safe environment where no patient is at risk and egos and personal interests can be set aside. Consider how you developed a clinical skill. It was something that needed to be practised again and again until eventually it started to become automatic and routine. The same applies for our non-technical behaviours. In addition, recognising our inherent human limitations and the situations when errors are more likely to occur, will encourage us to aim to be hypervigilant when required. It is important to remember that paying attention alone does not guarantee improved awareness of a situation as attentional control is subconscious and therefore beyond volitional control.

2.5   Communication

Poor communication is a leading cause of adverse events. This is not surprising; to have an effective team there needs to be good communication. The leader needs to communicate with the followers, and followers need to communicate with leaders and other followers. Communication is not just saying something – it is ensuring that information is accurately passed on and received. There are multiple components to effective communication (Table 2.1).

Table 2.1 Elements of communication				
Sender	**Sender**	**Transmitted**	**Receiver**	**Receiver**
Thinks of what to say	Says message	Through air, over phone, via email	Hears it	Thinks about it and acts

When communicating face-to-face, in an emergency setting, a message is often announced to a room where nobody acknowledges it. Targeting our communications towards specified individuals in what is sometimes referred to as 'directed communication' is now seen to be an essential element in improving communication. Many emergency settings, where staff change frequently, have people's names prominently displayed to encourage this.

Information is also transmitted non-verbally and processed in different ways by different people dependent on cultural, linguistic, neurodivergent and contextual variables. Communication can be more difficult when talking across professional, cultural, specialty or hierarchal barriers as we do not always talk the same technical language, have the same levels of understanding, or even have a full awareness of the other person's role.

There are a variety of tools to aid communication, such as SBAR (situation, background, assessment and recommendation) which facilitates planning and organising a message, making it succinct and focused. A good SBAR provides a handover in a logical and expected order. It is also an empowerment tool allowing the sender (who may be more junior) to request an action from a more senior individual.

Effective communication with a feedback loop

Consider a busy clinical situation and the team leader shouts '*We need an ECG connecting*' while looking at the blood pressure – what happens? The majority of times nothing – nobody goes to connect the electrocardiogram (ECG) because responsibility for the task has been diffused. The larger the group, the more likely it is that no-one will take responsibility for this vaguely phrased request. So how can this be improved? Most obviously an individual can be identified to perform the task, by name: '*Michael can you please connect the ECG?*' If Michael says '*Yes*', effective communication might be assumed, but not always. What has Michael heard and what will he do? At the moment we do not really know what message has been received. Michael might dash over with the defibrillator as this is what he thought he heard. This may seem a slightly strange thing to happen, but how often in a clinical emergency have you asked for something and been presented with something else? People are less likely to ask questions in emergencies as everyone is busy. This could be the catalyst for an error or precipitate a missed task. So how do we find out what message Michael received? The easiest way is to include a feedback loop in which we request that the other person let us know when they've completed the task.

Now the conversation goes:

Team leader	'Michael, can you please connect the ECG, and let me know when you've done it?'
Michael	'Okay'
Michael (later)	'I have connected the ECG'

We now know that the message has been transmitted and received correctly. For this process to work both parties (the sender and receiver) need to understand and expect it – again demonstrating the need for us to practise and train together.

2.6   Team working, leadership and followership

At a basic level a team is a group of individuals with a common cause. Historically we have tended to train individually or in professional silos; the risk here is that we are making a 'team of experts' rather than an 'expert team'. Often within healthcare, our teams form at short notice and arrive at different times. Emphasis tends to be placed on the significance of the role of the leader, but a leader cannot be a team on their own. As much emphasis should be given to developing the other team members, the active followers. A good leader will be able to swap from the role of leader to follower as more senior staff arrive and agree to take over.

The leader

The leader's role is multifaceted and includes directing the team, assigning tasks and assessing performance, motivating and encouraging the team to work together, and planning and organising. Additionally, a leader needs to maintain standards, support others and see where needs arise. All leadership skills and behaviours need to be developed and practised. Constructive feedback on efficacy of communication should both be given and sought in order to facilitate continuously improving performance.

It is important to clearly identify who is leading. The leader may change as more people arrive in an emergency situation. If there is a scribe recording events, they should record and update who is leading at any time.

As soon as the leader becomes hands on, and task focused, they are primarily concentrating on the task at hand. This becomes the focus of their thoughts and they lose situation awareness, their objective overview of the situation. The leader should be standing in an optimal position where they can gather all the information and ideally view the patient, the team members and the monitoring and diagnostic equipment. This enables them to recognise when a member is struggling with a task or procedure and support them appropriately.

Team roles

Ideally, the team should meet before the event and have the opportunity to introduce themselves to each other and clarify roles and actions in emergencies. Sometimes this can be facilitated at the beginning of a shift but at other times it is impossible to predict or arrange. It is important, therefore, that individuals identify themselves to the leader as they arrive and roles are agreed, allocated and understood. Much of the time their role may be determined purely in relation to the specific bleep the individual carries, but it is important that team members are flexible, for example if three airway providers are first on the scene we would expect other tasks to also be allocated and undertaken.

Followership

Followers are expected to work within their scope of practice and take the initiative. They should be attentive to the needs of the rest of the team and know where they fit within the bigger picture. It is important to think about the level of communication required between the leader and followers. If it is obvious that a team member is doing a task, this does not need to be communicated, but there are times when it is important that followers signal if they have a problem or request the leader's attention.

Hierarchy

Within the team there needs to be a hierarchy. This is the power gradient; the leader is at the top of this as the person coordinating, directing and making the decisions. However, this should not be absolute. If the power gradient is too steep the leader's decisions cannot be questioned and the followers blindly follow the orders. This is not safe because leaders are humans too and also make errors – their team is their safety net. Safe practice is achieved where the followers feel they can raise concerns or question instructions. This must always be understood by the leaders as much as by the followers. One way to reduce the hierarchy is for the leader to invite the team's thoughts and concerns, particularly around patient safety issues. It is also important for the follower to learn how to raise concerns appropriately.

One method that is sometimes used to raise concerns appropriately is PACE (probing, alerting, challenging or declaring an emergency).

Stage	Level of concern
P Probe	*I think you need to know what is happening*
A Alert	*I think something bad might happen*
C Challenge	*I know something bad will happen*
E Emergency	*I will not let it happen*

These stages are described with examples below:

- **Probe** – this is used where a person notices something they think might be a problem. They verbalise the issue, often as a question. 'Have you noticed that this child is cyanosed?'
- **Alert** – the observer strengthens and directs their statement and suggests a course of action. 'Dr Brown, I am concerned, the child is deeply cyanosed, should we start bag–valve–mask ventilation?'
- **Challenge** – the situation requires urgent attention. One of the key protagonists needs to be directly engaged. If possible, the speaker places themself into the eye line of the person with whom they wish to communicate. 'Dr Brown, you must listen to me now, this child needs help with their ventilation'
- **Emergency** – this is used where all else has failed and/or the observer perceives a critical event is about to occur. Where possible, a physical signal or physical barrier should be employed together with clear verbalisation. 'Dr Brown, you are overlooking this child's respiratory state, please move out of the way as I am going to ventilate them'

The PACE structure can be commenced at any appropriate level and escalated until a satisfactory response is gained. If an adverse event is imminent then it may be relevant to start at the declaring 'emergency' stage, whereas a much lower level of concern may well start at a 'probing' question.

An alternative approach that many healthcare settings are using is CUSS. It helps if standard phrases are used because these can act as collective triggers.

C	Concerned	*I am concerned*
U	Uncomfortable	*I am uncomfortable*
S	Safety issue	*This is unsafe*
S	Stop	*You need to stop*

At each of these levels, which increase in assertiveness, the reasoning needs to be re-stated in a clear, unambiguous way.

2.7 Situation awareness

A key element of good team working and leadership is to be conscious of what is happening; this is termed situation awareness. It not only involves seeing what is happening, but also captures how this is interpreted and understood, how decisions are made and, ultimately, planning ahead. We can distinguish between individual situation awareness, shared situation awareness and team situation awareness.

Consider Figure 2.2 which illustrates just how easy it is to misinterpret data:

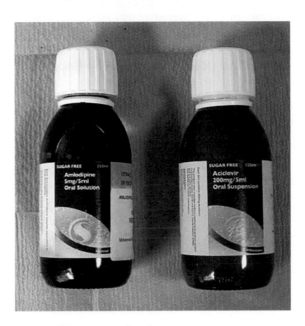

Figure 2.2 Similar package design of two different medications

We see what we expect to see, and misperceiving is particularly likely to happen when we are over-loaded, distracted or the mental demands on us are too high.

Distractions

Within healthcare, distractions become the norm to such an extent individuals are often not even aware of them. The risk is that mistakes are made and information is missed. It is important to try to challenge interruptions when doing critical tasks, and when they do occur restart the task from the beginning, rather than from where it is considered the interruption occurred. Some organisations have specific quiet areas for critical tasks such as prescribing. Whatever the local set up, the key is to develop and maintain everyone's awareness of how distraction greatly increases the chance of error.

Decision making

To make a good decision a person needs to assess all aspects of a problem and ensure they have the key information. Good situation awareness is a basic prerequisite for this process. The whole team should be on the alert for ambiguities or conflicting information. Any inconsistent facts should be treated as a potential marker for faulty situation awareness. They should never be brushed off as unimportant anomalies in the absence of evidence to support such a decision.

Where there are no time pressures, the decision-making process should not be concluded until the team is satisfied they have all the information and have considered all the options. Where time is a pressure, a certain amount of pragmatism must be employed. There is plenty of evidence to confirm that practise and experience can mitigate some of the negative effects of abbreviating a decision-making process. Those making decisions under such circumstances need to remain aware of the shortcuts they have taken. They should be ready to receive feedback from their team, particularly if any member of the team has significant concerns about the proposed course of action.

Mental models

Our mental models are affected by our previous experiences but also by the information/briefing that we received before the experience. A good pre-brief, where possible, will positively influence how the team frame the situation and which mental models they draw on. Where a briefing is accurate it is extremely helpful, where it is inaccurate, because it influences how we interpret information, it can lead to error. We are more likely to fit what we see to what we expect to see and therefore make inaccurate conclusions. Practising good briefings and handovers is time well spent. There can be a number of reasons why we might fail to have accurate situation awareness.

- Lack of or poor mental model
- A tendency to seek confirming evidence and ignore disconfirming evidence
- Overload on our working memory leading to forgetting vital information

> We see what we expect to see

Team situation awareness

We gather information from the world around us using our five senses. Because there is too much information constantly assaulting us, we selectively attend to only some of it based on our previous experiences and on what jumps out at us at the time. Different people attend to different aspects of a complex event, so individuals in a team will have a differing awareness of the situation.

> The team's situation awareness will often be greater than any one individual's, therefore the leader should actively encourage this sharing of perspectives

2.8 Improving team and individual performance

In addition to effective communication, team working, situation awareness, leadership and followership skills, there are a number of other ways that team and individual performance can be further developed and improved.

Awareness of situations when errors are more likely

If we are aware that errors are more likely we can be more proactive in detecting them. Two common situations that make errors more likely are stress and fatigue. Stress is not only a source of error when we are overworked and overstimulated, but also, at the other end of the spectrum, when we are understimulated we become inattentive.

The acronym HALT has been used to describe situations when error is more likely:

H	Hungry
A	Angry
L	Late
T	Tired

IMSAFE has been used as a checklist in the aviation industry, asking whether the individual may be affected by:

I	Illness
M	Medication
S	Stress
A	Alcohol
F	Fatigue
E	Emotion

Ideally, individuals who are potentially compromised need to be supported appropriately, allowed time to recover and the team made aware. How this can be achieved in the middle of a night shift can be problematic.

Awareness of error traps

A common trap that people fall into is only seeing or registering the information that fits in with their current mental model. This is known as a *confirmation bias*. When this occurs people favour information that confirms their preconceptions or hypotheses regardless of whether the information is true. This may be observed within the healthcare setting during the process of a referral or handover. An example of this might be a clinician receiving a phone call requesting them to attend the ward to review an acutely deteriorating child. The clinician is advised that the patient is a known asthmatic. On their way to the ward the clinician builds up a series of preconceived expectations around what they will find upon their arrival. They may even formulate a management plan whilst travelling to the scene, based upon their expectations. Once this mindset is established it can be difficult to shift.

On arrival, the clinician examines the systems affected by the presumed diagnosis. They seek to confirm their expectation by focusing on an auscultation of the chest at the expense of a thorough assessment. Upon hearing bilateral wheeze their preconceived ideas are confirmed and the remainder of the assessment is completed without due attention and more as a rehearsed exercise than an open-minded exploration. They fail to notice that the patient also has a soft stridor and is hypotensive. In this case the eventual diagnosis of anaphylaxis becomes at best a very late consideration, or at worst a situation that requires an objective newcomer to the team to point out the obvious.

Cognitive aids: checklists, guidelines and protocols

Well-constructed cognitive aids such as guidelines and algorithms are important because the human memory is not infallible. They also confer team understanding through the use of a standardised response. This reduces stress. This is especially true where an uncommon emergency event occurs. The team may be unfamiliar with one another and each member will be trying to remember what to do, what treatments are required and in what order. A good team leader will use the available cognitive aids as a prompt and the team members can use them as a resource so that they can plan ahead. Safe practice is promoted through the use of these tools in an emergency rather than relying on memory.

Calling for help early

Trainee staff are often reluctant to call for senior help, partly due to not recognising the severity of the situation and partly due to concerns about wasting the time of seniors. With all emergency events, and in particular with paediatric emergencies, escalation and appropriate help should be summoned as soon as possible. Remember, help will not arrive instantly, but it is helpful to state when help is needed and to be clear about what that help should be.

Debriefing

Wherever possible a debriefing should be facilitated following clinical events, even if brief, as this encourages us to normalise talking about difficult situations. A debrief immediately after an event is described as a 'hot' debrief and it has the aim of ensuring psychological safety. There is a place for this at the end of a shift or difficult emergency to ensure that staff are ok as they go home. The 'hot' debrief is not about learning points or establishing what happened. That can wait for the 'cold' debrief, days or even weeks after the event. This is usually facilitated by a trained individual with the intention of learning from the event and providing pointers moving forwards.

2.9 Summary

In this chapter we have given a brief introduction to the clinical human factors that can lead to poor team working, patient harm and adverse events. It is important for you to use every opportunity to reflect and develop your own performance and influence the development of others and the team.

PART 2
The seriously ill child

CHAPTER 3

Structured approach to the seriously ill child

Learning outcomes

After reading this chapter, you will be able to:

- Describe how to recognise the seriously ill child
- Describe a structured approach to the assessment of the seriously ill child
- Describe a structured approach to resuscitation and treatment of the seriously ill child focusing on the early management

---

3.1 Introduction

Paediatric cardiac arrests are uncommon and generally have a very poor outcome in comparison to adults with their primary cardiac causes. Therefore, earlier recognition and management of **potential** respiratory, circulatory or central neurological failure will reduce mortality and secondary morbidity. Rapid, effective assessment and initiation of correct treatment are key and this needs to be done in a calm, structured way with clear communication to both other team members (if present) but also to the family and/or child if appropriate.

The structured approach is outlined on the next page (Figures 3.1 and 3.2).

This can either be done by an individual or ideally with a team working together.

The primary survey and resuscitation involve assessment and management of the vital ABCDE functions. This primary assessment and any necessary resuscitation must be initiated before the more detailed secondary assessment is performed. Once the child's vital functions are supported, the secondary survey and emergency treatment begins. Illness-specific pathophysiology is sought and emergency treatments are instituted.

Advanced Paediatric Life Support: A Practical Approach to Emergencies, Seventh Edition. Edited by Stephanie Smith.
© 2023 John Wiley & Sons Ltd. Published 2023 by John Wiley & Sons Ltd.

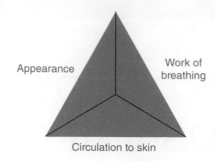

Appearance	Work of breathing	Circulation to skin
Abnormal tone	Abnormal sounds	Pallor
Decreased interaction	Abnormal position	Mottling
Decreased consolability	Retractions	Cyanosis
Abnormal look/gaze	Flaring	
Abnormal speech/cry	Apnoea/gasping	

Figure 3.1 Paediatric assessment triangle

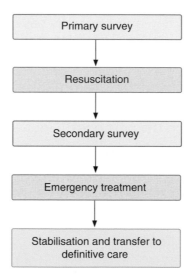

Figure 3.2 Structured approach to paediatric emergencies

During the secondary survey, vital signs should be checked frequently to detect any change in the child's condition. If there is deterioration, then return to the primary survey.

3.2 Primary survey and resuscitation of the airway

Assess patency of the airway by:

- Looking for chest and/or abdominal movements
- Listening for breath sounds
- Feeling for expired air

Vocalisations, such as crying or talking, indicate ventilation and some degree of airway patency.

- If there is obvious spontaneous ventilation, note other signs that may suggest upper airway obstruction such as the presence of stridor or evidence of recession
- If there is no evidence of air movement, then head tilt/chin lift or jaw thrust manoeuvres must be carried out. Reassess the airway after any airway-opening manoeuvres
- If there continues to be no evidence of air movement then airway patency can be assessed by performing an airway-opening manoeuvre while giving rescue breaths (see Chapter 16)

Resuscitation

If the airway is not patent, then this can be secured by:

- Head tilt/chin lift or jaw thrust
- Use of an airway adjunct
- Tracheal intubation

3.3   Primary survey and resuscitation of breathing

A patent airway does not ensure adequate ventilation. The latter requires an intact respiratory centre and adequate pulmonary function augmented by coordinated movement of the diaphragm and chest wall.

The **effort**, **efficacy** and **effect** of breathing need to be assessed bearing in mind the effects of respiratory inadequacy on other organs in the child's body.

Effort of breathing

The degree of effort of breathing is an indication of the severity of respiratory disease. It is important to assess the following:

1. **Respiratory rate**. Normal resting respiratory rates at differing ages are shown in the normal ranges table (inside front cover). Normal rates are higher in infancy and fall with increasing age. Care should be taken in interpreting single measurements: infants can show wide variation in respiratory rates depending on their state of activity. The World Health Organization (WHO) uses a cut-off of 60 breaths per minute for pneumonia in infants and young children. Most useful are trends in the measurement as an indicator of improvement or deterioration. At rest, tachypnoea indicates that increased ventilation is needed because of either lung or airway disease, or metabolic acidosis. A slow respiratory rate indicates fatigue, cerebral depression or a pre-terminal state.
2. **Recession**. Intercostal, subcostal, sternal or suprasternal (tracheal tug) recession shows increased effort of breathing. This sign is more apparent in younger infants as they have a compliant chest wall. If present in older children (i.e. over 6 years) this sign suggests severe respiratory compromise. The degree of recession gives an indication of the severity of respiratory difficulty, however in the child who has become exhausted through increased effort of breathing, recession decreases as respiratory failure develops.
3. **Inspiratory or expiratory noises**. An inspiratory noise while breathing (*stridor*) is a sign of laryngeal or tracheal obstruction. In severe obstruction stridor may also occur in expiration, but the inspiratory component is usually more pronounced. *Wheezing* indicates lower airway narrowing and is more pronounced in expiration. A prolonged expiratory phase also indicates lower airway narrowing. The volume of the noise is not an indicator of severity, as it may disappear in the pre-terminal state.
4. **Grunting**. This is produced by exhalation against a partially closed glottis. It is an attempt to generate a positive end-expiratory pressure and prevent airway collapse at the end of expiration in children with 'stiff' lungs. This is a sign of severe respiratory distress and is characteristically seen in infants with pneumonia or pulmonary oedema. It may also be seen with raised intracranial pressure, abdominal distension or peritonism.

5. **Accessory muscle use**. As in adult life, the sternomastoid muscle may be used as an accessory respiratory muscle when the effort of breathing is increased. In infants, this is ineffectual and just causes the head to bob up and down with each breath.
6. **Flaring of the nostrils**. This is seen especially in infants with respiratory distress.
7. **Gasping**. Gasping is a sign of severe hypoxia and may be pre-terminal.

Exceptions

There may be minimal or no increased effort of breathing if the child with respiratory failure has:
1. Fatigue due to prolonged respiratory effort; exhaustion is a pre-terminal sign
2. Cerebral depression from raised intracranial pressure, poisoning or encephalopathy. These children will have respiratory inadequacy without increased effort of breathing. The respiratory inadequacy in this case is caused by decreased respiratory drive
3. Neuromuscular disease (e.g. spinal muscular atrophy or muscular dystrophy) who may present in respiratory failure without increased effort of breathing

The diagnosis of respiratory failure in these children is made by observing the efficacy of breathing and looking for other signs of respiratory inadequacy, as described

---

Efficacy of breathing

Observations of the degree of chest expansion (or, in infants, abdominal excursion) provide an indication of the amount of air being inspired and expired. Similarly, important information is given by auscultation of the chest. Listen for reduced, asymmetrical or bronchial breath sounds. **A silent chest is an extremely worrying sign.**

Pulse oximetry can be used to measure the arterial oxygen saturation (SpO_2). A good plethysmographic (pulse) waveform is important to help confirm the accuracy of measurements. In severe shock and hypothermia, there may be poor or absent pulse detection. Measurements are also not as accurate when the SpO_2 is less than 80%, with motion artefact or high levels of ambient light and in the presence of carboxy- or methaemoglobin. Oximetry in air gives a good indication of the efficacy of breathing, although to assess the adequacy of ventilation, some measure of carbon dioxide should be obtained. Any supplemental oxygen will mask problems with oxygenation due to ineffective breathing unless the hypoxia is severe. Normal SpO_2 in an infant or child in air at sea level is 97–100%, however the aim for oxygen treatment would be 94–98%.

Effects of respiratory inadequacy on other organs

1. **Heart rate**. Hypoxia produces tachycardia in the older infant and child. Anxiety and fever will also contribute to tachycardia, making this a non-specific sign. **Severe or prolonged hypoxia leads to bradycardia. This is a pre-terminal sign.**
2. **Skin colour**. Hypoxia produces vasoconstriction and skin pallor (via catecholamine release). **Cyanosis is a late and pre-terminal sign of hypoxia** as it usually becomes apparent when SpO_2 falls to less than 80%, and only in the absence of anaemia. By the time central cyanosis is visible in acute respiratory disease, the child is close to respiratory arrest. In the anaemic child, cyanosis may never be visible despite profound hypoxia. A few children will be cyanosed because of cyanotic heart disease, but may have adequate oxygen uptake within the lungs, and their cyanosis will be largely unchanged by oxygen therapy.
3. **Mental status**. The hypoxic or hypercapnic child will be agitated and/or drowsy. Gradually drowsiness increases and eventually consciousness is lost. These extremely useful and important signs are often more difficult to detect in small infants. The parents may say that the infant is just 'not himself'. The healthcare practitioner must assess the child's state of alertness by gaining eye contact and noting the response to voice and, if necessary, to painful stimuli. A generalised muscular hypotonia also accompanies hypoxic cerebral depression.

Resuscitation

All children with breathing difficulties should receive oxygen as soon as the airway is opened to attain SpO_2 94–98%. This can be achieved by using a flow up to 10-15 l/min via a non-rebreathing mask with reservoir bag, or by using high-flow nasal cannula (HFNC) oxygen therapy. With decreasing oxygen need, low-flow nasal cannula or prongs can be used.

In the child with inadequate respiratory effort, breathing should be supported either with bag–mask ventilation (two-person technique ideally) or intubation and ventilation with capnography. Cuffed tubes are now recommended in most instances.

3.4   Primary survey and resuscitation of the circulation

The cardiovascular status needs to be assessed bearing in mind the effects of circulatory inadequacy on other organs.

Factors to assess

1. ***Heart rate***. Normal rates are shown in the normal ranges table (inside front cover). The heart rate initially increases in shock due to catecholamine release and as compensation for decreased stroke volume. Fit adolescents can have a heart rate below 60 beats/min without circulatory problems.

> **An abnormally slow pulse rate, or bradycardia, is defined as less than 60 beats/min or a rapidly falling heart rate associated with poor systemic perfusion. This is a pre-terminal sign**

2. ***Pulse volume***. Although blood pressure (BP) in children is maintained until shock is severe, an indication of perfusion can be gained by comparative palpation of both peripheral and central pulses. Absent peripheral pulses and weak central pulses are serious signs of advanced shock and indicate that hypotension is already present. Bounding pulses may be caused by an increased cardiac output (e.g. septicaemia), arteriovenous systemic shunt (e.g. patent arterial duct) or hypercapnia.
3. ***Capillary refill time***. Following cutaneous pressure on the centre of the sternum for 5 seconds, capillary refill should occur within 2 seconds. A slower refill time than this can indicate poor skin perfusion, a sign which may be helpful in early septic shock, when the child may otherwise appear well, with warm peripheries. The presence of fever does not affect the sensitivity of delayed capillary refill in children with hypovolaemia but a low ambient temperature reduces its specificity. Poor capillary refill and differential pulse volumes are neither sensitive nor specific indicators of shock in infants and children but are useful clinical signs when used in conjunction with the other signs described. They should not be used as the only indicators of shock nor as quantitative measures of the response to treatment. In children with pigmented skin, the sign is more difficult to assess. In these cases, the nail beds are used and additionally the soles of the feet in young babies.
4. ***Blood pressure***. Normal systolic pressures are shown in the normal ranges table (inside front cover). In septic shock, aim for these normal values and respond to trends along with the other indicators of shock. Use of the correct cuff size is crucial if an accurate blood pressure measurement is to be obtained. This caveat applies to both auscultatory and oscillometric devices. The width of the cuff should be more than 40% of the length of the upper arm and the bladder more than 80% of the arm's circumference (Figure 3.3). It is important to recognise that BP can be raised due to pain, movement and being upset, and that it is vital to address these and reassess to obtain a true BP. A manual device, which is generally tolerated much better, may need to be used. **A fall in BP is a late and pre-terminal sign of shock.**

(a)

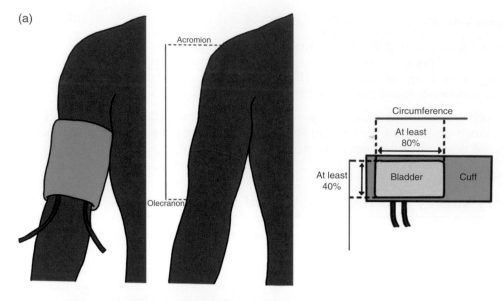

(b)

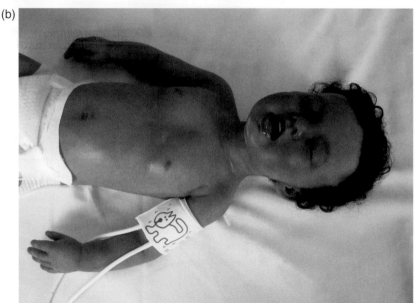

Figure 3.3 (a, b) Size and position of cuff
(b) Children's Health Queensland/CC BY 4.0

Effects of circulatory inadequacy on other organs

1. *Respiratory system.* A rapid respiration rate with an increased tidal volume but without recession, may be compensatory for the metabolic acidosis resulting from circulatory failure.

Cardiac failure

The following features suggest a cardiac cause of respiratory inadequacy:
- Cyanosis, not correcting with oxygen therapy
- Tachycardia out of proportion to respiratory difficulty
- Raised jugular venous pressure (older child/teenager)
- Gallop rhythm/murmur
- Enlarged liver
- Absent femoral pulses

2. *Skin*. Mottled, cold, pale skin peripherally indicates poor perfusion. A line of coldness may be felt to move centrally as circulatory failure progresses.
3. *Mental status*. Agitation and then drowsiness leading to unconsciousness are characteristic of circulatory failure. These signs are caused by poor cerebral perfusion. In an infant, parents may say that their child is 'not himself'.
4. *Urinary output*. A urine output of less than 1 ml/kg/h in children and less than 2 ml/kg/h in infants may indicate inadequate renal perfusion during shock. A history of reduced wet nappies or urine production should be sought.

Resuscitation

In every child with an inadequate circulation (shock):

- Give high-flow oxygen via a non-rebreathing mask with reservoir bag, or by using HFNC oxygen therapy, or via an endotracheal tube if intubation has been necessary for airway control or inadequate breathing
- Venous or intraosseous (IO) access should be gained without delay and an immediate infusion of balanced crystalloid (10 ml/kg) given. Urgent blood samples, especially blood glucose and preferably also a blood gas, may be taken at this point.

3.5 Primary assessment and resuscitation of disability (neurological evaluation)

Neurological assessment should only be performed after airway (A), breathing (B) and circulation (C) have been assessed and treated. **There are no neurological problems that take priority over ABC.** Both hypoxia and shock can cause a decrease in conscious level. Any problem with ABC must be addressed before assuming that a decrease in conscious level is due to a primary neurological problem.

Both respiratory and circulatory failure will have central neurological effects. Conversely, some conditions with direct central neurological effects (e.g. meningitis, raised intracranial pressure from trauma, and status epilepticus) may also have respiratory and circulatory consequences. These must be addressed to improve the neurological status. In addition, any patient with a decreased conscious level or convulsions must have an initial glucose stick test performed.

Primary assessment of neurological function

1. *Conscious level*. A rapid assessment of conscious level can be made by assigning the patient to one of the categories shown in the box below.

A	**A**lert
V	Responds to **V**oice
P	Responds only to **P**ain
U	**U**nresponsive to all stimuli

If the child does not respond to voice, it is important that response to pain is then assessed. A painful central stimulus can be delivered by sternal pressure, by massaging the mastoid process or by supraorbital ridge pressure. Commonly, a child who is unresponsive or who only responds to pain has a significant degree of coma, equivalent to 8 or less on the Glasgow Coma Scale (GCS) and their airway must be supported. Carry out formal GCS assessment to monitor their response to treatment.

2. *Posture*. Many children who are suffering from a serious illness in any system are hypotonic. Stiff posturing such as that shown by decorticate (flexed arms, extended legs) or decerebrate (extended arms, extended legs) children is a sign of serious brain dysfunction (Figure 3.4). These

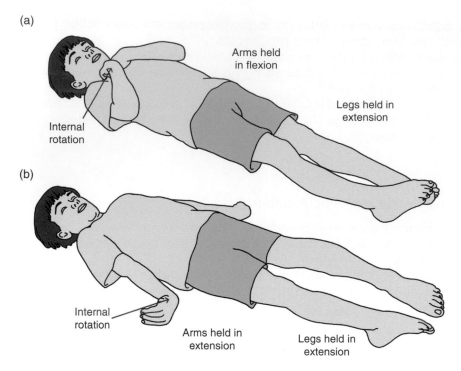

(a)

Arms held in flexion

Legs held in extension

Internal rotation

(b)

Internal rotation

Arms held in extension

Legs held in extension

Figure 3.4 (a) Decorticate posturing, and (b) decerebrate posturing

postures can be mistaken for the tonic phase of a convulsion. Alternatively, a painful stimulus may be necessary to elicit these postures. Severe extension of the neck due to upper airway obstruction can mimic the opisthotonos that occurs with meningeal irritation. A stiff neck and full fontanelle in infants are signs that suggest meningitis.

3. *Pupils.* Many drugs and cerebral lesions have effects on pupil size and reactions. However, the most important pupillary signs to seek are dilatation, unequal sizes and lack of reactivity, which indicate possible serious brain disorders if new. See Chapter 6 for a more detailed explanation.

Effects of neurological inadequacy on other organs

1. *Respiratory effects of central neurological failure.* There are several recognisable breathing pattern abnormalities with raised intracranial pressure. However, they are often changeable and may vary from hyperventilation to Cheyne–Stokes breathing to apnoea. The presence of any abnormal respiratory pattern in a child with coma suggests mid- or hindbrain dysfunction. This is different from Kussmaul breathing, due to the profound acidosis of diabetic ketoacidosis.

2. *Circulatory effects of central neurological failure.* Systemic hypertension with sinus bradycardia (Cushing response) indicates compression of the medulla oblongata caused by herniation of the cerebellar tonsils through the foramen magnum. **This is a late and pre-terminal sign.**

Resuscitation

- Consider intubation to stabilise the airway in any child with a conscious level recorded as P or U (only responding to painful stimuli or unresponsive)
- If hypoglycaemia has been found, treat hypoglycaemia (less than 2.8 mmol/l or 50 mg/dl) with a bolus of glucose (3 ml/kg of 10% glucose) followed by an IV infusion of glucose, after taking blood for glucose measurement in the laboratory and a sample for further studies
- For prolonged or recurrent seizures, treat reversible causes such as hypoglycaemia or hyponatraemia, then follow the status epilepticus algorithm found in Chapter 6
- Manage raised intracranial pressure if present (see Chapter 6 for further details)

3.6   Primary survey and resuscitation of issues found during exposure

The examination of the seriously ill child involves examination for markers of illness that will help provide specific emergency treatment. There are a few key indicators:

- *Temperature.* A fever suggests an infection as the cause of the illness but may also be the result of prolonged convulsions or shivering. In young infants, infection may present with a low body temperature
- *Rash and bruising.* Examination is carried out for rashes, such as urticaria in allergic reactions, purpura, petechiae and bruising in septicaemia or trauma (accidental or inflicted), or maculopapular and erythematous rashes in allergic reactions and some forms of sepsis
- *Resuscitation.* Depends on what factor is identified. Urticarial rash with airway/circulatory compromise requires IM adrenaline (0.01 ml/kg of 1:1000) immediately. Purpuric rash synonymous with meningococcal sepsis requires early IV/IO access with administration of IV antibiotics and resuscitation fluids if indicated. Unexplained bruising requires measurement of coagulation factors and a thorough examination with a very detailed history with the appreciation that there may be significant trauma such as head injuries or subtle abdominal trauma, which will require appropriate treatment.

Summary: rapid clinical assessment of an infant or child

Airway and Breathing
- Effort of breathing
- Respiratory rate/rhythm
- Stridor/wheeze
- Auscultation
- Skin colour
- Oximetry

Circulation
- Heart rate
- Pulse volume
- Capillary refill
- Skin temperature

Disability
- Mental status/conscious level
- Posture
- Pupils

Exposure
- Fever
- Rashes and bruising

The whole assessment should take less than a minute

Remember to obtain information from pre-hospital staff about the initial condition of the child and any treatment given

Once airway (A), breathing (B) and circulation (C) are clearly recognised as being stable or have been stabilised, then definitive management of the underlying condition should be started

---

Reassessment

Single observations on respiratory and heart rates, degree of recession, blood pressure, conscious level, pupils, etc. are useful but much more information can be gained by frequent, repeated observations to detect a trend in the child's condition. These are commonly now combined into a scoring system to provide an early warning of deterioration, such as the paediatric early warning system (PEWS). There is no single validated tool yet, with different systems being used in different institutions.

3.7   Secondary survey and emergency treatment

The secondary survey takes place once vital functions have been assessed and the treatment of life-threatening conditions has been instituted. It includes:

- A focused medical history from parents/carers or child
- A review of notes if available and attention to information obtained from pre-hospital staff
- A clinical examination and specific investigations

It differs from a standard medical history and examination in that it is designed to establish which further immediate measures are required to stabilise the child. Time is limited and a focused approach is essential. At the end of the secondary survey, the practitioner should have a better understanding of the illness affecting the child and may have formulated a differential diagnosis. Emergency treatments will be appropriate at this stage – either to treat specific conditions (e.g. asthma) or processes (e.g. raised intracranial pressure). The establishment of a definite diagnosis is part of definitive care.

Some children will present with an acute exacerbation of a known condition such as asthma or epilepsy. Such information is helpful in focusing attention on the appropriate system, but the practitioner should be wary of dismissing new pathologies in such children. The structured approach prevents this problem. Unlike trauma (which is dealt with later), illness affects systems rather than anatomical areas.

After the presenting system has been dealt with, all other systems should be assessed, and any additional treatments commenced as appropriate.

The secondary survey is not intended to complete the diagnostic process, but rather is intended to identify any problems that require further emergency treatment.

The following gives an outline of a structured approach of emergency care. It is not exhaustive but addresses the majority of emergency conditions that are amenable to specific emergency treatments in this time period. The symptoms, signs and treatments relevant to each emergency condition are elaborated in the relevant chapters that follow.

Respiratory

Secondary survey

Box 3.1 gives common symptoms and signs that should be sought in the respiratory system. Emergency investigations are suggested.

Box 3.1 Common symptoms and signs that should be sought in the respiratory system

Symptoms
- Breathlessness
- Coryza
- Cough
- Noisy breathing – grunting, stridor, wheeze
- Drooling and inability to drink
- Abdominal pain
- Chest pain
- Apnoea
- Feeding difficulties
- Hoarseness

Signs
- Cyanosis
- Tachypnoea
- Recession
- Grunting
- Stridor
- Wheeze
- Chest wall crepitus
- Tracheal shift
- Abnormal percussion note
- Crepitations on auscultation
- Acidotic breathing

Investigations
- Oxygen saturation
- Peak flow if asthma is suspected
- End-tidal/transcutaneous carbon dioxide if hypoventilation is suspected
- Blood culture if infection is suspected
- Chest X-ray/ultrasound (selective)
- Blood gases (selective)
- Viral polymerase chain reaction (PCR)/swab

Emergency treatment

- If 'bubbly' noises are heard, the airway is full of secretions, which may require clearance by suction
- If there is a harsh stridor associated with a barking cough and severe respiratory distress, upper airway obstruction due to severe croup should be suspected and the child given nebulised budesonide or adrenaline
- If there is a quiet stridor, drooling and a short history in a sick-looking child, consider epiglottitis or tracheitis. Intubation is likely to be urgently required, preferably by a senior anaesthetist. Do not jeopardise the airway by any unpleasant or frightening interventions. Give IV cefotaxime or ceftriaxone once the airway is secure
- With a sudden onset and significant history of inhalation, consider a foreign body within the airway. If the 'choking child' procedure has been unsuccessful, the child may require laryngoscopy. Do not jeopardise the airway by unpleasant or frightening interventions but contact a senior anaesthetist/ENT surgeon urgently. However, in extreme cases of life threat, immediate direct laryngoscopy to remove a visible foreign body with a Magill forceps may be necessary
- Stridor following ingestion/injection of a known allergen suggests anaphylaxis. Children in whom this is likely should receive IM adrenaline
- Children with a history of asthma or with wheeze and significant respiratory distress, decreased peak flow and/or hypoxia should receive oxygen therapy and inhaled β_2-agonists. Infants with wheeze and respiratory distress are likely to have bronchiolitis and require only oxygen if hypoxic
- In acidotic breathing, take a blood sample for acid–base balance and blood sugar. Treat diabetic ketoacidosis with IV fluid and insulin

Cardiovascular (circulation)

Secondary survey

Box 3.2 gives common symptoms and signs that should be sought in the cardiovascular system. Emergency investigations are suggested.

Box 3.2 Common symptoms and signs that should be sought in the cardiovascular system

Symptoms
- Breathlessness
- Fever
- Palpitations
- Feeding difficulties
- Sweating with feeds in infants
- Drowsiness
- Pallor
- Shock
- Poor urine output

Signs
- Tachy- or bradycardia
- Hypo- or hypertension
- Abnormal pulse volume or rhythm
- Abnormal skin perfusion or colour
- Cyanosis/pallor
- Hepatomegaly
- Crepitations on auscultation
- Cardiac murmur
- Peripheral oedema
- Absent femoral pulses
- Raised jugular venous pressure
- Hypotonia
- Purpuric rash

Investigations
- Urea and electrolytes
- Liver function tests
- Full blood count
- Blood gas, lactate
- Coagulation studies
- Blood culture
- Electrocardiogram
- Chest X-ray (selective)

Emergency treatment

- Further boluses of fluid should be given to shocked children who have not had a sustained improvement to the first bolus given at resuscitation
- Consider inotropes, intubation and invasive arterial blood pressure monitoring particularly if more than 40 ml/kg of fluid is needed with signs of ongoing shock
- Consider IV third generation cephalosporin in shocked children with no obvious fluid loss as sepsis is likely
- If a child has a cardiac arrhythmia the appropriate protocol should be followed
- If anaphylaxis is suspected, give IM adrenaline in addition to fluid boluses
- Give an IV infusion of dinoprostone (prostaglandin or PGE2) or alprostadil (PGE1) urgently if duct-dependent congenital heart disease is suspected, for instance in neonates with unresponsive hypoxia or shock
- Surgical advice and intervention may be needed for gastrointestinal emergencies. The following symptoms and signs may suggest this:
  - Symptoms – bilious vomiting, blood per rectum, abdominal pain
  - Signs – abdominal tenderness, abdominal mass, abdominal distension

Neurological (disability)

Secondary survey

Box 3.3 gives common symptoms and signs that should be sought in the nervous system. Emergency investigations are suggested.

Box 3.3 Common symptoms and signs that should be sought in the nervous system

Symptoms
- Headache
- Convulsions
- Change in behavior
- Change in conscious level
- Weakness
- Visual disturbance
- Fever

Signs
- Altered conscious level
- Altered pupil size and reactivity
- Abnormal posture
- Abnormal oculocephalic reflexes
- Meningism
- Papilloedema or retinal haemorrhage
- Altered deep tendon reflexes
- Hypertension
- Slow pulse
- Full and tense anterior fontanelle

Investigations
- Urea and electrolytes
- Blood sugar
- Liver function tests
- Ammonia
- Blood culture
- Blood gas
- Coagulation studies
- Blood and urine toxicology including carboxyhaemoglobin level
- Computed tomography brain scan
- Metabolic screen

Emergency treatment

- For convulsions follow the status epilepticus protocol (see Chapter 6)
- If there is evidence of raised intracranial pressure (decreasing conscious level, asymmetrical pupils, abnormal posturing and/or abnormal ocular motor reflexes) then the child should undergo:
  - **Ventilation to maintain end-tidal CO_2 ($ETCO_2$) 3.5–4.0 kPa (26–30 mmHg) (this is equivalent to arterial $PaCO_2$ 4.0–4.5 kPa (30–34 mmHg)**
  - Nursing with head in-line and 20° head-up position (to help cerebral venous drainage)
  - **Infusion of IV 3% sodium chloride (3 ml/kg) or mannitol 0.25–0.5 g/kg (i.e. 1.25–2.5 ml/kg of 20% solution IV over 15 minutes)**
- Consider dexamethasone (only for oedema surrounding a space-occupying lesion) 0.5 mg/kg 6-hourly
- In a child with a depressed conscious level or convulsions, consider meningitis/encephalitis. Give third generation cephalosporins and aciclovir with or without ampicillin and with or without corticosteroids
- In drowsiness with sighing respirations, check blood sugar, acid–base balance and salicylate level. Treat diabetic ketoacidosis with IV fluids and insulin
- In unconscious children with pinpoint pupils, consider opiate poisoning. A trial of naloxone could be considered

External

Secondary survey

Box 3.4 gives common symptoms and signs that should be sought externally.

Box 3.4 Common symptoms and signs that should be sought externally

Symptoms	*Signs*
• Rash	• Purpura
• Swelling of lips/tongue	• Urticaria
• Fever	• Angioedema

Emergency treatment

- In a child with circulatory or neurological symptoms and signs, a purpuric rash suggests septicaemia/meningitis. The child should receive cefotaxime or ceftriaxone as soon as possible
- In a child with respiratory or circulatory difficulty, the presence of an urticarial rash or angioedema suggests anaphylaxis. Give IM adrenaline immediately

Further history

Developmental and social history

Knowledge of the child's developmental progress and immunisation status may be useful, particularly in a small child or infant.

Drugs and allergies

Any medication that the child is currently on or has been on should be recorded. If poisoning is a possibility, it is important to document any medication in the home that the child might have had access to, as even relatively benign over-the-counter medications for adults may cause serious toxicity in small children. A history of allergies should be sought.

3.8 Summary

This chapter has described the structured approach to the seriously ill child which enables the practitioner to focus on diagnosis and emergency treatment.

The primary survey and resuscitation are concerned with the maintenance of vital functions, while the secondary survey and emergency treatment allow more specific urgent therapies to be started.

CHAPTER 4

Airway and Breathing

Learning outcomes

After reading this chapter, you will be able to:

- Describe why infants and young children are susceptible to respiratory failure
- Assess and treat children with breathing difficulties
- Resuscitate a child with life-threatening breathing difficulties

---

4.1   Introduction

Respiratory diseases have the highest prevalence in childhood, accounting for up to 30–40% of acute hospital admissions of children. Acute respiratory illnesses, such as pneumonia, account for 1.8 million deaths per year in children under 5 years of age, more than any other illness, in every region of the world. Disorders outside the respiratory system may also cause breathing difficulties, including cardiac disease, metabolic and neurological disorders and poisoning (Table 4.1).

Most respiratory illnesses are self-limiting minor infections, but some present as potentially life-threatening emergencies, especially in children with underlying co-morbidity. Accurate diagnosis and prompt initiation of appropriate treatment are essential if unnecessary morbidity and mortality are to be avoided in such cases.

Table 4.1   Causes of breathing difficulty in children, according to mechanism

Mechanism	Cause
Upper airway obstruction	Croup/epiglottitis, foreign body inhalation
Lower airway obstruction	Tracheitis, bronchiolitis, asthma, foreign body inhalation
Disorders affecting the lungs	Pneumonia, lung oedema (e.g. in cardiac disease)
Disorders around the lungs	Pneumothorax, pleural effusion or empyema, rib fractures
Disorders of the respiratory muscles	Neuromuscular disorders
Disorders below the diaphragm	Peritonitis, abdominal distension
Increased respiratory drive	Diabetic ketoacidosis, shock, anxiety attack and hyperventilation
Decreased respiratory drive	Coma, convulsions, raised intracranial pressure, poisoning

Advanced Paediatric Life Support: A Practical Approach to Emergencies, Seventh Edition. Edited by Stephanie Smith.
© 2023 John Wiley & Sons Ltd. Published 2023 by John Wiley & Sons Ltd.

4.2   Susceptibility to respiratory failure

Severe respiratory illness may result in the development of respiratory failure, defined as an inability of physiological compensatory mechanisms to ensure adequate oxygenation and ventilation (carbon dioxide (CO_2) elimination), resulting in hypoxia with or without hypercapnia. Young children and infants develop respiratory failure more readily than older children and adults, reflecting important differences in their immune status and the structure and function of the respiratory system.

- Children, and particularly infants, are susceptible to infection with many viruses and bacteria to which adults have acquired immunity
- The airways in children are smaller and more easily obstructed by mucosal swelling, secretions or a foreign body. Airway resistance is inversely proportional to the fourth power of the radius of the airway: a reduction in the radius by a half causes a 16-fold increase in airway resistance. Thus, 1 mm of mucosal oedema in an infant's trachea of 5 mm diameter results in a much greater increase in resistance than the same degree of oedema in a trachea of 10 mm diameter
- The thoracic cage of young children is much more compliant than that of adults. When there is airway obstruction and increased effort, this leads to marked recession and a reduction in the efficiency of breathing. The compliant thorax also provides less support in maintaining lung volume
- In infants, lung volume at end expiration is similar to closing volume, increasing the tendency to small airway closure and hypoxia
- Children have fewer alveoli, which makes them more susceptible to ventilation–perfusion mismatch
- The respiratory muscles of young children are relatively inefficient. In infancy, the diaphragm is the principal respiratory muscle while intercostal and accessory muscles make relatively little contribution. Fatigue can develop rapidly, resulting in respiratory failure or apnoea
- The pulmonary vascular bed is relatively muscular in infancy, increasing the tendency with which pulmonary vasoconstriction can occur in, for example, hypoxia. In turn, this can lead to right-to-left shunting, ductal opening (in the early neonatal period), ventilation–perfusion mismatch and further hypoxia
- In the first 1–2 months of life there may be a paradoxical inhibition of respiratory drive. This may result in infections presenting with apnoea or hypoventilation rather than the usual increased effort

4.3   Clinical presentations of the child with breathing difficulties

Respiratory conditions can present with respiratory symptoms but also with symptoms within other systems:

Respiratory	Breathlessness, tachypnoea, sub-/intercostal recessions, head bobbing (only in infants), nasal flaring
	Cough
	Noisy breathing (stridor, wheeze, grunting)
	Chest pain
Non-respiratory	Poor feeding (infant)
	Abdominal pain
	Hypotonia, change in conscious level
	Tachycardia, change in colour

Noisy breathing may be normal for the child or suggest pathology. Parents and carers commonly understand different meanings from those understood by doctors and nurses for the terms used to describe breathing noises or may have their own terms. Useful historical features include relieving or aggravating factors (e.g. sleep, crying, feeding, position, exercise) and whether the voice or vocalisations are normal.

Stridor is a high-pitched sound usually on inspiration from obstruction of the upper airway and should be distinguished from *stertor* or *snoring*, which are lower pitched inspiratory noises suggestive of poor airway positioning or pharyngeal obstruction. *Bubbly noises* suggest pharyngeal secretions, often seen in the child with neurodisability who may have long-standing poor airway control and inability to spontaneously clear secretions. *Wheeze* is predominantly expiratory from lower airway obstruction. *Grunting* is a physiological response (partial closure of the glottis during expiration) to prevent end-expiratory alveolar collapse in pneumonia or pulmonary oedema.

Chest pain is an unusual symptom in children. It does not usually reflect cardiac disease as it so often does in adults but can suggest pneumonia or pleuritis. Similarly, pneumonia may present as abdominal pain.

While parents are usually alerted to breathing difficulties in toddlers and older children, abnormal respiration may be more difficult for them to detect in infants. Infants with breathing difficulties may present with acute feeding problems. Feeding for an infant is one of the most strenuous activities, and its ease is often taken by parents as a gauge of their infant's well-being.

Some features suggest a cardiac cause of respiratory inadequacy. These are:

- Cyanosis, not correcting with oxygen therapy
- Tachycardia out of proportion to respiratory difficulty
- Raised jugular venous pressure (difficult to see in young children)
- Gallop rhythm/murmur
- Enlarged liver
- Absent femoral pulses

4.4   Primary survey and resuscitation

This is dealt with in Chapter 2. In general, the following ABCDE principles apply to all children with breathing difficulties.

Airway

- A patent airway is the first requisite. If the airway is not patent, an airway-opening manoeuvre should be used and, if needed, secured with a pharyngeal airway device or by intubation with experienced senior help

Breathing

- All children with breathing difficulties should receive oxygen as soon as the airway is opened to attain SpO_2 94–98%. This can be achieved by using a flow of 10–15 l/min via a non-rebreathing mask with reservoir bag, or by using high-flow nasal cannula (HFNC) oxygen therapy. With decreasing oxygen need, a low-flow nasal cannula or prongs can be used

- Warning: a child requiring more than 50% oxygen through a mask of HFNC to achieve SpO_2 94–98% is significantly hypoxaemic and may be at risk of sudden deterioration and cardiac arrest. Get senior help and urgent review from the critical care team

- If the child is hypoventilating with a slow rate or weak effort, respiration should be supported with oxygen via a bag–valve–mask device and experienced senior help summoned

Circulation

Fluid intake may have been reduced, particularly in infants with feeding difficulties. Consider a fluid bolus (10 ml/kg of balanced fluids) if there are signs of circulatory failure.

4.5 Secondary survey and looking for key features

While the primary survey and resuscitation are being carried out, a focused history of the child's health and activity over the previous days and any significant previous illness should be gained. All children with breathing difficulties will have varying degrees of respiratory distress and cough, so these are not useful diagnostic discriminators. Certain key features can point the clinician to the likeliest working diagnosis for emergency treatment.

- Inspiratory stridor points to upper airway obstruction
- Expiratory wheeze points to lower airway obstruction
- Fever without upper airway symptoms suggests pneumonia
- Signs of heart failure point to congenital/acquired heart disease
- Acute history, allergen exposure and urticarial rash point to anaphylaxis
- Suspicion of ingestion and no clear cardiorespiratory pathology point to poisoning

4.6 General approach to the child with upper airway obstruction

Obstruction of the upper airway is potentially life threatening. Its small cross-sectional area renders the young child particularly vulnerable to obstruction by oedema, secretions or an inhaled foreign body. Table 4.2 shows the different aetiologies of upper airway obstruction in children.

Table 4.2 Causes of upper airway obstruction		
Incidence (UK)	**Diagnosis**	**Clinical features**
Very common	Croup, viral laryngotracheobronchitis	Coryzal, barking cough, mild fever, hoarse voice
Uncommon	Foreign body aspiration	Sudden onset, history of choking
Rare	Epiglottitis	Drooling, muffled voice, septic appearance, absent cough
	Bacterial tracheitis	Harsh cough, chest pain, septic appearance
	Trauma	Neck swelling, crepitus, bruising
	Retropharyngeal or peritonsillar abscess	Drooling, septic appearance
	Inhalation of hot gases	Facial burns, perioral soot
	Infectious mononucleosis	Sore throat, tonsillar enlargement
	Angioneurotic oedema	Itching, facial swelling, urticarial rash
	Diphtheria	Travel to endemic area, unimmunised

In the child with a compromised but functioning airway, an important principle in all cases is to avoid worsening the situation by upsetting the child. Crying and struggling may quickly convert a partially obstructed airway into a completely obstructed one. Parents should be encouraged to help soothe and settle the child.

Airway

Is the airway partially obstructed or narrowed and what is the likely cause? Note the presence of inspiratory noises.

- 'Bubbly' noises suggest pharyngeal secretions requiring clearance. This might suggest that the child is fatigued or has a depressed conscious level and is unable to clear secretions with their own cough

- Stertorous (snoring) noises suggest partial airway obstruction due to a depressed conscious level
- A harsh stridor and barking cough are suggestive of croup; a quiet stridor in a sick-looking child without cough point at epiglottitis or tracheitis
- A stridor of sudden onset with no prodromal symptoms or a history suggestive of inhalation, could mean foreign body aspiration

Breathing

- What degree of effort is needed for breathing and what is its efficacy and effect? The answer to this question will inform the clinician as to the severity of the upper airway obstruction. A pulse oximeter should be put in place and the oxygen saturation noted both on breathing air and high-flow oxygen

4.7   Specific approach to the child with upper airway obstruction

Most cases of upper airway obstruction in children are the result of infection, but inhalation of a foreign body or hot gases (house fires), anaphylaxis and trauma can all result in obstruction. The airway may also become obstructed in the unconscious, supine child.

Partial obstruction from secretions or a depressed conscious level

- Use suction to clear secretions as long as there is no stridor
- Support the airway with the chin lift or jaw thrust manoeuvre in a child with stertorous breathing due to a depressed conscious level or extreme fatigue and seek senior airway support
- Further maintenance of the airway can be accomplished with an oro- or nasopharyngeal airway, but the child may require intubation
- Whilst help is summoned, continuous positive airway pressure (CPAP) can be given to children with a reduced conscious level using a face mask, oxygen flow and breathing circuit (e.g. an anaesthetic breathing circuit (Ayre's T-piece)), if familiar with using such circuits

Croup

Background

Croup (acute laryngotracheobronchitis) is defined as an acute clinical syndrome with inspiratory stridor, a barking cough, hoarseness and variable degrees of respiratory distress. Parainfluenza viruses are the commonest pathogens, but others include respiratory syncytial virus, influenzavirus and adenovirus. The peak incidence of croup is in the second year of life and most hospital admissions are in children aged between 6 months and 5 years. Between 1% and 5% of children with croup are admitted.

The typical features (Figure 4.1) of a barking cough, harsh stridor and hoarseness are often preceded by fever and coryza for 1–3 days. The symptoms usually start, and are worse, at night. Many children have stridor and a mild fever (less than 38.5°C) with little or no respiratory difficulty. If tracheal narrowing is minor, stridor will be present only when the child hyperventilates or is upset. As the narrowing progresses, the stridor becomes both inspiratory and expiratory, and is present even when the child is at rest. Some children, and particularly those below the age of 3 years, develop the features of increasing obstruction with marked sternal and subcostal recession, tachycardia, tachypnoea and hypoxia leading to agitation. If the infection extends distally to the bronchi, wheeze may also be audible. Some children have repeated episodes of croup.

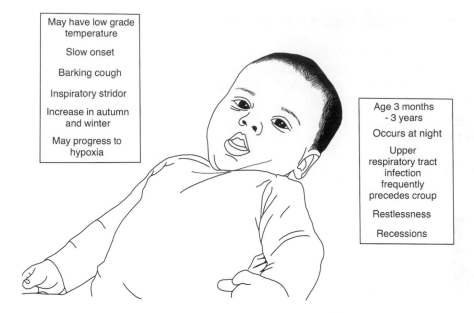

May have low grade temperature

Slow onset

Barking cough

Inspiratory stridor

Increase in autumn and winter

May progress to hypoxia

Age 3 months - 3 years

Occurs at night

Upper respiratory tract infection frequently precedes croup

Restlessness

Recessions

Figure 4.1 Croup

Treatment

Steroids modify the natural history of croup – they give rise to clinical improvement within 30 minutes, and decrease the need for hospitalisation, the duration of hospitalisation and the need for intubation. Oral steroids (*dexamethasone 0.15–0.6 mg/kg* or *prednisolone 1–2 mg/kg*) are the treatment of choice, but if the child will not take oral medication or is vomiting, then *nebulised budesonide 2 mg* can be used. Dexamethasone can be repeated after 24 hours if clinically indicated; budesonide aerosol can be given more regularly (every 30–60 minutes) based on clinical response.

A small proportion of children will need admission to hospital. Based on clinical severity aerosol with budesonide or adrenaline will be needed. In both cases they should also receive steroids, such as dexamethasone.

- Give *nebulised adrenaline 5 ml of 1:1000* with oxygen through a face mask to children with severe respiratory distress, provided it does not unduly upset the child. This will produce a transient improvement beginning within 10–30 minutes and lasting for up to 2 hours, giving time for the corticosteroids to take effect. It may need to be repeated, and if so, additional measures should be taken to ensure the airway is managed by senior staff. Children should be observed closely with continuous monitoring (three-lead electrocardiogram (ECG) and SpO_2), as they may still deteriorate and require intubation. Adrenaline may contribute to a tachycardia, but other side effects are uncommon. This treatment is best used to 'buy time' in which to assemble an experienced team to treat a child with severe croup. Failure to respond to nebulised adrenaline should question the diagnosis of croup – consider bacterial tracheitis, epiglottitis or foreign body
- Give *humidified oxygen* and monitor SpO_2. Hypoxia is a late sign of croup reflecting alveolar hypoventilation secondary to airway obstruction and ventilation–perfusion mismatch. The respiratory rate and the degree of recession are more valuable clinical indicators of severity and response to treatment
- A very small proportion of these children require intubation. The decision to intubate is a clinical one based on increasing tachycardia, tachypnoea and chest retraction, or the appearance of cyanosis, exhaustion or confusion. Ideally, the procedure should be performed under gas induction anaesthesia by an experienced (paediatric) anaesthetist, unless there is respiratory arrest. A tube of smaller gauge than usual is often required. If there is doubt about the diagnosis or difficulty in intubation is anticipated, an ENT surgeon capable of performing a tracheotomy should be present (see Figure 19.8)

Epiglottitis

Background

Acute epiglottitis shares some clinical features with croup, but it is a quite distinct entity. Although much less common than croup, its importance is that unless the diagnosis is made rapidly and appropriate treatment commenced, total obstruction and death may ensue. Epiglottitis is due to infection with *Haemophilus influenza* b (Hib), which causes intense swelling of the epiglottis and the surrounding tissues and obstruction of the larynx (Figure 4.2). It is thus less commonly seen in countries where Hib immunisation is routine but may still occur in cases of vaccine failure or unimmunised children.

(a) (b)

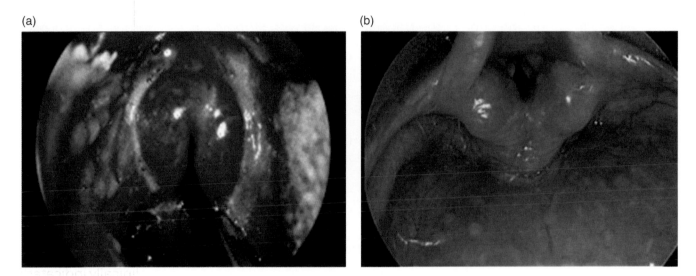

Figure 4.2 (a) Larynx in epiglottitis, and (b) normal larynx

Epiglottitis is most common in children aged 2–6 years, but it can occur in any age group. The onset of the illness is usually acute with high fever, lethargy, a soft inspiratory stridor and rapidly increasing respiratory difficulty over 3–6 hours. In contrast to croup, cough is minimal or absent. Typically, the child sits immobile, with the chin slightly raised and the mouth open, drooling saliva. The child appears very toxic and pale and has poor peripheral circulation (most are septicaemic). There is usually a high fever (over 39°C). Because the throat is so painful, the child is reluctant to speak and unable to swallow drinks or saliva.

Treatment

> Disturbance of the child, and particularly attempts to lie the child down, to examine the throat with a tongue depressor or insertion of an intravenous cannula should only be considered in the presence of appropriate senior support

- Intubation is likely to be required. Contact a senior anaesthetist and an ENT surgeon capable of performing a tracheotomy urgently. When deeply anaesthetised, the child can be laid on their back to allow laryngoscopy and intubation. Tracheal intubation may be difficult because of the intense swelling of the epiglottis ('cherry red epiglottis') (Figure 4.2a). A smaller tube than the one usually required for the child's size will be necessary

- After securing the airway, blood should be sent for culture and treatment with intravenous cefotaxime or ceftriaxone commenced. With appropriate treatment most children can be extubated after 24–36 hours and they recover fully within 3–5 days. Complications such as hypoxic cerebral damage, pulmonary oedema or accompanying *H. influenza* meningitis are rare. In countries where the Hib vaccine is in use, there should be an investigation into vaccine failure

Bacterial tracheitis

Background

Bacterial tracheitis or pseudomembranous croup is an uncommon but life-threatening form of upper airway infection. Infection of the tracheal mucosa with *Staphylococcus aureus*, streptococci or Hib results in copious, purulent secretions and mucosal necrosis. The child appears toxic, with a high fever and signs of progressive upper airway obstruction. The croupy cough, absence of drooling and a longer history help distinguish this condition from epiglottitis.

Treatment

Over 80% of children with this illness need intubation and ventilatory support to maintain an adequate airway, as well as intravenous antibiotics (cefotaxime or ceftriaxone plus flucloxacillin).

Foreign body aspiration

Background

Foreign body aspiration (FBA) must be suspected for any witnessed choking episode. It is commonest in children less than 3 years of age – a history of a witnessed choking event is very suggestive as the child is often too young to give a history. Children have a smaller airway than adults and their larynx is in a relatively high position with the epiglottis close to the root of the tongue, increasing the risk of aspiration. Incisors bite through food while molars are necessary to masticate food in preparation for swallowing. Molars erupt approximately 6 months after incisors thus infants are unable to pulp their food and the bite-sized food they generate is the ideal shape to obstruct an airway if aspirated. Children often run around and talk while chewing, may put non-organic foreign bodies in their mouth while playing and may be inattentive and easily distractible. Foodstuffs (nuts, grapes, sweets and meat) are the commonest foreign bodies. In contrast to croup there is usually no history of prodromal viral upper respiratory tract infection or pyrexia.

Most suspected FBA should have a chest radiograph. Flat objects such as coins tend to align in the sagittal plane in the trachea whereas objects in the oesophagus tend to align in the coronal plane. The majority of foreign bodies are radiolucent and therefore not visible on radiographs, but there may be secondary evidence of localised gas trapping, atelectasis or mediastinal shift. In approximately 20% of FBA cases, the chest radiograph is normal. Although a history of inhalation may be elicited from the parent, FBA cannot be excluded on either normal physical examination or chest radiograph.

Treatment

Removal through a bronchoscope under general anaesthetic should be performed as soon as possible because there is a risk that coughing will move the object into the trachea and cause life-threatening obstruction.

- Do not jeopardise the airway by unpleasant or frightening interventions but contact a senior anaesthetist/ENT surgeon capable of performing a tracheotomy urgently. In the case of a stridulous child with a relatively stable airway and a strong suspicion of foreign body inhalation, careful gaseous induction of anaesthesia should be used so the foreign body can then be removed under controlled conditions

- In extreme cases of life threat, immediate direct laryngoscopy with Magill's forceps to remove a visible foreign body (Figure 4.3) may be necessary

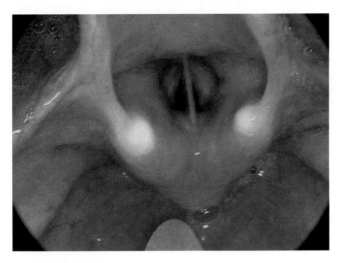

Figure 4.3 Larynx with foreign body obstruction

Anaphylaxis

Background

Anaphylaxis is a potentially life-threatening, immunologically mediated reaction with respiratory or circulatory effects that develop over minutes, often associated with skin or mucosal changes. Laryngeal oedema causing upper airway obstruction is one manifestation. Food, especially nuts, drugs (including contrast media and anaesthetic drugs) and venom are the commonest causes of this. Prodromal symptoms of flushing, itching, facial swelling and urticaria usually precede stridor. Abdominal pain, diarrhoea, wheeze and shock may be additional or alternative manifestations of anaphylaxis. A severe episode of anaphylaxis can be predicted in children with a previous severe episode or a history of increasingly severe reaction, a history of asthma or treatment with β-blockers.

See Chapter 5 for further details and emergency treatment of anaphylaxis.

Other causes of upper airways obstruction

Although croup accounts for the large majority of cases of acute upper airway obstruction, several other uncommon conditions need to be considered.

Diphtheria is seen only in children who have not been immunised against the disease. Always ask about immunisations in any child with fever and signs of upper airway obstruction, particularly if they have been to endemic areas recently. Specific treatment of diphtheric croup includes penicillin, steroids and antitoxin.

Attempts at endotracheal intubation may push a laryngeal membrane into the trachea causing total airway obstruction; a tracheostomy may be required for children with laryngeal diphtheria.

Marked tonsillar swelling in *infectious mononucleosis* or *severe acute tonsillitis* can occasionally compromise the upper airway. The passage of a nasopharyngeal tube may give instant relief. If there is impending airway obstruction, corticosteroids often work fast.

Retropharyngeal or peritonsillar abscesses are uncommon, but both can present with fever and upper airway obstruction together with feeding difficulties. Treatment is by surgical drainage and intravenous antibiotics.

4.8   Approach to the child with wheeze

The two common causes of lower respiratory obstruction are:

- Acute severe asthma
- Bronchiolitis

Bronchiolitis is mostly confined to the under 1-year-olds and asthma is much more commonly diagnosed in the over 1-year-olds.

Acute severe asthma

Background

Acute exacerbation of asthma is the commonest reason for a child to be admitted to hospital in the UK. One in 11 children is currently receiving treatment for asthma. In 2018, asthma caused 20 deaths in under 14-year-olds in England and Wales; reviews of such cases often identify preventable factors in both the recognition and management of the condition. The classic features of acute asthma are *cough*, *wheeze* and *breathlessness*.

In young children there may be no triggers other than viral infections and no interval symptoms. Such cases are often termed viral-induced wheeze or episodic viral wheeze but should be treated as acute asthma. An increase in symptoms and decreasing response to bronchodilators, along with difficulty in walking, talking or sleeping, all indicate worsening asthma.

Common exacerbation triggers include:

- Poor adherence to therapy, specifically inhaled corticosteroids
- Viral upper respiratory tract infections (URTIs) (most common in the pre-school child)
- Aero-allergen exposure (e.g. house dust mite, pollens, moulds): it is difficult to attribute a cause and effect relationship because of their ubiquitous nature and the delay in the allergic response
- Air quality: cold air, exposure to a smoky or polluted atmosphere, or chemical irritants such as paints and domestic aerosols
- Exercise-induced symptoms
- Emotional upset or excitement

Disease severity

Before progressing to specific treatment for acute asthma in any setting, it is essential to assess accurately the *severity* of the child's condition.

Historical features associated with severe or life-threatening asthma flares include:

- A long duration of symptoms and/or regular nocturnal awakening
- Poor response to treatment already given in this episode
- A severe course of previous attacks, including the use of intravenous therapy and admission to a paediatric critical care unit (PCCU)

Assessing severity can be difficult since clinical signs correlate poorly with the severity of airway obstruction. Some children with acute severe asthma do not appear distressed, and young children with severe asthma are especially difficult to assess. The following clinical signs should be recorded regularly, for example every 30–60 minutes, or before and after each dose of bronchodilator:

- Pulse rate
- Respiratory rate, degree of recession, use of accessory muscles of respiration
- Degree of agitation and conscious level

- SpO_2 (for assessing severity, monitoring progress and predicting outcome in acute asthma. More intensive inpatient treatment is likely to be needed if the SpO_2 is less than 90% in air after initial bronchodilator treatment)
- Peak flow (can be valuable, but under-6-year-olds and those who are very dyspnoeic are usually unable to produce reliable readings)

Examination features that are poor signs of severity include the degree of wheeze, respiratory rate and pulsus paradoxus.

A chest radiograph is indicated only if there is severe dyspnoea, uncertainty about the diagnosis, asymmetry of chest signs or signs of severe infection.

Two degrees of severity are described to indicate the appearance of asthmatic children at the most severe end of the spectrum: severe and life-threatening asthma (Table 4.3 and Figure 4.4).

Table 4.3 Levels of severity of acute asthma attacks in children

Moderate acute asthma	Able to talk in sentences	
	$SpO_2 \geq 92\%$	
	PEF ≥50% best or predicted	
	Heart rate:	≤140/min in children aged 1–5 years
		≤125/min in children >5 years
	Respiratory rate:	≤40/min in children aged 1–5 years
		≤30/min in children >5 years
Acute severe asthma	Can not complete sentences in one breath or too breathless to talk or feed	
	$SpO_2 <92\%$	
	PEF 33–50% best or predicted	
	Heart rate:	>140/min in children aged 1–5 years
		>125/min in children >5 years
	Respiratory rate:	>40/min in children aged 1–5 years
		>30/min in children >5 years
Life-threatening asthma	Any one of the following in a child with severe asthma:	
	Clinical signs	**Measurements**
	Exhaustion	PEF <33% best or predicted
	Hypotension	$SpO_2 <92\%$
	Cyanosis	
	Silent chest	
	Poor respiratory effort	
	Confusion	

Reproduced from SIGN158: https://www.sign.ac.uk/media/1773/sign158-updated.pdf (last accessed March 2023)
PEF, peak expiratory flow.

Treatment of asthma

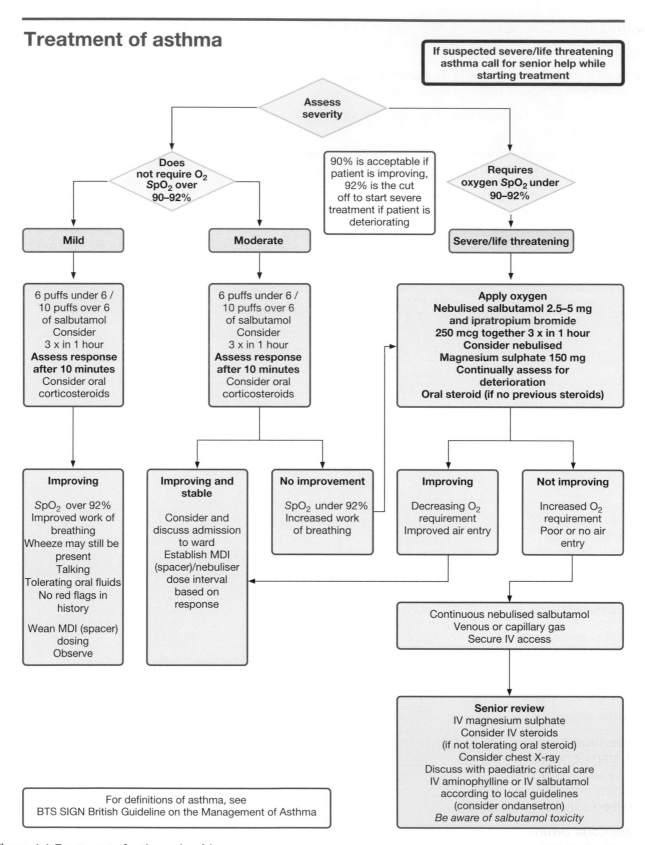

Figure 4.4 Treatment of asthma algorithm
MDI, metered dose inhaler

Treatment

Drugs

The cornerstone in the treatment of a severe asthma attack is the repetitive administration of β_2-*bronchodilator* (to relieve bronchoconstriction), the early introduction of systemic *corticosteroids* (to relieve inflammation and bronchial thickening) and controlled or titrated flow oxygen supplementation.

Short acting β_2-agonist (SABA), such as salbutamol:

- In those with moderate asthma maintaining SpO_2 greater than 92% in air, give *600 micrograms (6 puffs)* to children aged under 6 years, and *1000 micrograms (10 puffs)* for those over 6 years old (practice may differ, follow local guidelines). Use a valved holding chamber (spacer) with/without a face mask. Children aged 4 years or under are likely to require a face mask connected to the mouthpiece of a spacer for successful drug delivery. Inhalers should be sprayed into the spacer in individual puffs and inhaled immediately by tidal breathing. Spacers help the medication get straight to where it is needed in the lungs, with less medication ending up in the child's mouth or throat
- In those with severe or life-threatening asthma with oxygen need, use nebulised salbutamol *2.5 mg (under 6 years)* or *5 mg (over 6 years)* with oxygen at a flow of 6–8 l/min in order to provide small enough particle sizes. Higher flows may be used, but more of the nebulised drug may be lost from the face mask. This can be repeated every 10–20 minutes. If the child is on high-flow oxygen therapy ultrasonic devices can be used to enhance and fasten drug delivery

Although inhaled drugs should be given first as they are accessible and more acceptable to the child, intravenous salbutamol has a place in life-threatening episodes that do not respond promptly to inhaled therapy. A *loading dose (15 micrograms/kg in children over 2 years, 5 micrograms/kg under 2 years)* can be given, but if frequent doses of nebulised salbutamol were used this can be omitted and *continuous infusion (1–5 micrograms/kg/min)* can be started immediately. Important side effects include sinus tachycardia and hypokalaemia: serum potassium levels should be checked regularly, and supplementation may be needed. If high doses are used, salbutamol-induced lactic acidosis can occur in the absence of poor circulation. β_2-adrenergic agents increase glycolysis and pyruvate production, which is then converted to lactate. The diagnosis of salbutamol-induced lactic acidosis must be made by elimination, and could lead to increased tachypnea despite regression of bronchospasm. It is, however, transient and normalises after stopping or decreasing salbutamol.

Corticosteroids expedite recovery from acute asthma. Give an initial dose equivalent to *prednisolone 1–2 mg/kg (max. 40 mg)* on the first day, followed by a further 1 mg/kg/day for 2 days. Unless the child is vomiting, there is no advantage in giving steroids parenterally.

Nebulised ipratropium bromide should be added only in severe or life-threatening asthma (250 micrograms in nebulised solution in children over 2 years, 125 micrograms in nebulised solution under 2 years) three times during the first hour. If used as an adjunctive therapy, lung function is improved and hospitalisation rates are decreased.

Intravenous magnesium sulphate is a safe treatment for acute asthma if the child fails to respond to inhaled or nebulised SABA. A dose of 40 mg/kg (max. dose 2 g) by slow infusion (over 20 minutes) may be used. Studies of efficacy for severe childhood asthma unresponsive to more conventional therapies have shown evidence of benefit. *Nebulised magnesium sulphate* (150 mg added to nebulised solution) may be useful in severe asthma.

Intravenous aminophylline can have a role as a third line bronchodilator in the child who fails to respond adequately, after considering other add-on treatment options. In view of its poor efficacy and safety profile and the greater effectiveness and relative safety of SABA, its use is no longer routinely recommended. However, if needed in severe or life-threatening asthma unresponsive to other treatment, a 5 mg/kg loading dose for 20 minutes followed by a continuous infusion at 1 mg/kg/h can be considered. Monitoring of serum levels is necessary and if the child is vomiting then stopping the infusion should be considered.

There is no evidence to support the routine use of inhaled steroids given in addition to systemic corticosteroids for the treatment of acute asthma in childhood. There is limited support for inhaled heliox therapy, which may be considered in children who do not respond to standard therapy. If the child is still unresponsive, cannot inhale bronchodilators, or is considered to be peri-arrest, consider IV adrenaline 10 micrograms/kg.

Emergency treatment

- Assess ABCDE and give controlled or titrated low oxygen via a face mask with a reservoir bag or via a HFNC. Aim to keep SpO_2 at 94–98%
- Give salbutamol 600–1000 micrograms via a spacer in moderate or severe asthma, or nebulised salbutamol 2.5–5 mg with ipratropium bromide in life-threatening asthma. This can be repeated every 10–20 minutes or even continuously as breaks between doses can lead to a rebound of symptoms
- Give oral corticosteroids or, if too dyspnoeic to swallow or vomiting, give intravenously
- If an infant or child is clearly in respiratory failure with poor respiratory effort, a depressed conscious level and poor saturation despite maximum oxygen therapy, attempt to support ventilation with a bag–valve–mask and arrange for urgent intubation. Give an IV bronchodilator such as salbutamol
- Reassess ABCDE and monitor the response to treatment carefully. Assessment is based on physical signs and continuous monitoring of oxygen saturation measurements

If not responding or condition deteriorating

- For severe or life-threatening asthma, intravenous bronchodilators are effective: consider IV magnesium sulphate or salbutamol
- Contact the PCCU or the retrieval service and senior anaesthetic support
- The evidence regarding non-invasive ventilation in children during acute asthma exacerbations is limited. Invasive mechanical ventilation is rarely required. There are no absolute criteria, as the decision to intubate is usually based on the clinical condition of the child. If respiratory effort is poor or deteriorating, or conscious level is depressed, or SpO_2 is low and falling despite maximum oxygen therapy, attempt to support ventilation with a bag–valve–mask device, or with bag–mask ventilation or T-piece and bag with high-flow oxygen, whilst arranging for urgent intubation. Intubation is usually preceded by either rapid sequence induction with IV ketamine or inhalational anaesthesia; both may help bronchodilatation

In cases of acute severe asthma that responds to treatment, there is usually little value to be gained from routine blood gas measurement. However, in those responding poorly, a blood gas with raised CO_2 should expedite the decision to intubate. Children with acute asthma who require mechanical ventilation need to be transferred to the PCCU. The prognosis is good, but complications such as air leak and lobar collapse are common. All intubated children must have continuous end-tidal CO_2 monitoring.

If responding and improving

- If there has been improvement (SpO_2 92% or more in air, minimal recession, peak expiratory flow 50% or more of normal value), it may be possible to consider discontinuing intravenous treatment
- When oxygen is no longer needed, change from a nebulised bronchodilator to the use of sprays of a β_2-agonist inhaler
- Reduce the frequency of inhaled therapy gradually from every 30 minutes to 4-hourly, further reducing frequency as improvement occurs

Inhaler technique should be checked, and an asthma action plan provided. The child's maintenance treatment should be reviewed and altered if inadequate. Ensure that the child has appropriate medical follow-up.

Other measures

- Reassure the child and avoid upset
- Monitor the heart rhythm and SpO_2
- Ensure that there is avoidance of any identifiable trigger
- Intravenous fluids: restrict to two-thirds of the normal requirements
- Antibiotics are usually not indicated as most asthma attacks are triggered by viral infections

Bronchiolitis

Background

Bronchiolitis is the most common serious respiratory infection of childhood: 10% of infants are affected and 2–3% are admitted to hospital with the disease in their first year of life. Ninety per cent of patients are aged 1–9 months; it is unusual after 1 year of age. There is usually an annual winter epidemic. Respiratory syncytial virus (RSV) is the pathogen in 60–70% of cases, the remainder being caused by other respiratory viruses such as influenza or parainfluenza, human metapneumovirus (hMPV) and adenoviruses. Secondary bacterial involvement is uncommon.

Fever and a clear nasal discharge precede a dry, sharp cough and increasing breathlessness. Wheezing or fine end-expiratory crackles may be audible on auscultation. There is tachypnoea and subcostal and intercostal recession, often with head bobbing in the infant. Feeding difficulties associated with increasing dyspnoea are often the reason for admission to hospital. Apnoea is a serious and potentially fatal complication and is seen particularly in infants born prematurely. Infants with co-morbidities including premature birth, immunodeficiency, congenital heart disease or chronic lung diseases are more **prone to develop severe disease**, as are very young infants (less than 6 weeks old). The natural history of bronchiolitis is of a self-limiting disease that usually lasts 7–10 days.

Infants with bronchiolitis rarely need a chest radiograph. If performed it usually shows hyperinflation and often evidence of collapse or consolidation, particularly in the upper right lobe (Figure 4.5).

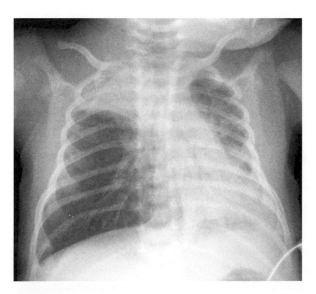

Figure 4.5 Chest radiograph demonstrating lung hyperinflation with a flattened diaphragm and bilateral atelectasis in the right apical and left basal regions in a 16-day-old infant
Matteo Di Nardo / Wikimedia Commons / CC BY 2.0

RSV and other viruses can be identified on nasopharyngeal secretions. Blood gas analysis, which is required in only the most severe cases, shows lowered oxygen and raised CO_2 levels.

Bronchiolitis may trigger heart failure in an infant with a previously undiagnosed cardiac lesion. On the other hand, bronchiolitis and cardiac decompensation can have a similar clinical picture in an infant. Table 4.4 lists features to help in distinguishing between these conditions.

Table 4.4 Features that help distinguish heart failure from bronchiolitis

Heart failure	Bronchiolitis
Feeding difficulty with growth failure	Feeding difficulty
	Coryzal and harsh cough
Tachycardia and tachypnoea	Tachycardia, tachypnoea, dyspnoea
Pallor, sweating and cool peripheries	Restlessness, sweating
Large heart with displaced apex beat	Normal or apparently small heart
Large liver	Liver lower than normal due to hyperinflation
Gallop rhythm	
Murmur	No murmur
Pulmonary congestion and large heart on chest X-ray	Hyperinflation on chest X-ray

Treatment

Management is *primarily supportive* – fluid replacement, gentle suctioning of nasal secretions, prone position (if in hospital), oxygen therapy and respiratory support if necessary.

- Assess ABCDE
- Ensure that the *airway* is patent: use of a suction catheter can clear the nose and nasopharynx, which can have a significant impact on an infant's respiratory distress. Installation of sodium chloride nasal drops may help to 'thin' and clear nasal secretions
- Give a high concentration of oxygen via a nasal cannula (max. 2 l/min). Aim at SpO_2 94–98%. Consider using humidity, prone positioning and HFNC humidified systems (flows of 2 l/kg/min for the first 10 kg, then 0.5 l/kg/min)
- Maintain hydration and nutrition. In infants with significant respiratory distress, maintain hydration by feeding via a nasogastric tube; intravenous fluid (at two-thirds the usual maintenance) is seldomly needed. Breastfeeding may be too stressful, in which case breast milk should be expressed and given via a nasogastric tube
- Monitor for apnoea/hypoventilation (especially in those less than 2 months old), SpO_2, respiratory frequency and PCO_2 (transcutaneous, capillary or end-tidal)
- HFNC therapy and non-invasive continuous positive airway pressure (nCPAP) are both believed to improve the work of breathing by preventing dynamic airway collapse during expiration, thereby reducing air trapping and improving gas exchange. Their place is as rescue therapies when low-flow oxygen has failed
- Mechanical ventilation is required in 2% of infants admitted to hospital. Indications to intubate include recurrent apnoea, impending exhaustion or severe respiratory distress. After intubation SpO_2 and end-tidal or transcutaneous PCO_2 should be continuously monitored
- Both nebulised 3% sodium chloride and nebulised adrenaline with oral corticosteroids have been subjected to trials, but without showing substantial benefit. Bronchodilators, steroids and physiotherapy are not useful. Antibiotics should only be considered if concomitant bacterial infection is strongly suspected

4.9 Approach to the child with fever and breathing difficulties

Although many causes of breathing difficulties are associated with infection, a high fever is usually associated only with *pneumonia, epiglottitis* and *bacterial tracheitis*. Many cases of asthma are precipitated by an URTI, but the asthmatic child is rarely febrile, and a low-grade fever is characteristic of bronchiolitis. Therefore, in the absence of stridor and wheeze, breathing difficulties in association with a significant fever are likely to be due to pneumonia.

Pneumonia

Background

Pneumonia in childhood was responsible globally for 14% of deaths of children aged under 5 years in 2019 (WHO data). Infants, and children with congenital abnormalities or chronic illnesses, are at particular risk. A wide spectrum of pathogens causes pneumonia in childhood, and different organisms are important in different age groups. The incidence of viral infections decreases with increasing age, while the incidence of bacterial infections remains stable across all ages. Viral infections typically peak during the autumn and winter season, whereas bacterial pneumonia exhibits less marked seasonal fluctuation.

Pathogens at different ages	
Newborn	*Escherichia coli*, other Gram-negative bacilli Group B β-haemolytic *Streptococcus* *Chlamydia trachomatis*
Infancy	Viruses: respiratory syncytial virus (RSV), influenza, parainfluenza, bocavirus, human metapneumovirus Adeno- and rhinoviruses *Streptococcus pneumoniae* *Haemophilus influenza* *Staphylococcus aureus* *Bordetella pertussis*
School age	*Streptococcus pneumoniae* *Mycoplasma pneumoniae* *Chlamydia pneumoniae* Respiratory viruses (see above)

Fever, cough, breathlessness and *chest recession* in the younger child and lethargy are the usual presenting symptoms of pneumonia. The cough is often dry initially but then becomes loose. Older children may produce purulent sputum but in those below the age of 5 years it is usually swallowed. *Pleuritic chest pain, neck stiffness* and *abdominal pain* may be present if there is pleural inflammation. Classic signs of consolidation such as decreased percussion, decreased breath sounds and bronchial breathing are often absent, particularly in infants, and a *chest radiograph* or *ultrasound* is needed. This may show lobar consolidation, widespread bronchopneumonia or, rarely, cavitation of the lung. Pleural effusions may occur, particularly in bacterial pneumonia and this may organise to empyema. An *ultrasound* of the chest will delineate the size and nature of pleural collection and if needed will guide placing of a chest drain. Blood cultures, swabs for viral isolation and a full blood count can be performed.

Treatment

- Assess ABCDE
- Provide a high concentration of oxygen via a face mask with reservoir bag or HFNC or low-flow oxygen via a nasal cannula. Attach a pulse oximeter and aim at SpO_2 greater than or equal to 92%. Airway and breathing support may be especially needed in children with neurodisability or

neuromuscular weakness, who may have poor airway control and weak respiratory muscles even when well. These children could also benefit from secretion management techniques which are usually not needed in previously healthy children with community-acquired pneumonia

---

Techniques for secretion management

Airway positioning and suctioning
Nebulised sodium chloride or ipratroprium
Increased humidification: high-flow nasal cannula
Antisialagogues*: hyoscine, glycopyrronium, atropine
Mucolytics: nebulised acetylcysteine, erdosteine, DNAse
Physiotherapeutic adjuvants: use of positive pressure, airway vibration or oscillation

* Use with caution in children with a poor cough (often seen in children with neurodisability) as they may be prone to mucous plugging and lower airway obstruction

---

- Maintain hydration: extra fluid may be needed to compensate for loss from fever and tachypnoea, or restriction (70%) may be needed because of an increase in antidiuretic hormone secretion leading to SIADH (syndrome of inappropriate antidiuretic hormone). Fluid overload can contribute to worsening breathlessness
- It is not possible to differentiate reliably between bacterial and viral infection on clinical, haematological or radiological grounds, so children diagnosed as having significant pneumonia should receive *antibiotics*. Oral antibiotics are sufficient in most cases, unless there is vomiting or severe respiratory distress: that is, infants and children who look toxic, have definite dyspnoea, an SpO_2 below 92%, grunting or signs of dehydration. The initial choice of antibiotics depends on the age of the child and local policy. Newborns and young infants should receive broad-spectrum intravenous antibiotics. For older infants and preschool children, oral amoxicillin is suitable. Check for any antibiotic allergy. Antibiotics should be given for 3–10 days (or as per local policy) although complicated pneumonias (e.g. with empyema) may require several weeks' duration. Other options include the use of:
  - Flucloxacillin – if *Staphylococcus aureus* is suspected
  - Macrolides – if atypical pneumonia (school-aged children) or pertussis is suspected
- Clinical examination and the chest radiograph may reveal a pleural effusion (Figure 4.6). This should be confirmed with ultrasound and, if large, it should be *drained* to relieve breathlessness, aid diagnosis and allow the instillation of intrapleural fibrinolytic agents. Ultrasound may guide the positioning of a chest drain. Details of the procedure can be found in Chapter 21

(a)　　　　　　　　　　　(b)

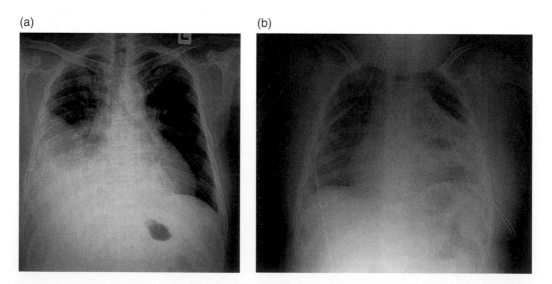

Figure 4.6 (a, b) Chest X-rays of pneumonia with a chest drain in place (b)
(a) Tewan Banditrakkanka/Shutterstock.com

Mechanical ventilation is rarely required unless there is a serious underlying condition. Transfer to the PCCU should be considered with the following: an FiO_2 of more than 0.6 to keep SpO_2 more than 94%, shock, impending exhaustion, rising PCO_2, apnoea or irregular breathing. If a child has recurrent or persistent pneumonia, they should be referred to a respiratory specialist so further investigation may be undertaken.

4.10   Other conditions that may present as breathing difficulties

Heart failure

Infants and children with serious cardiac pathology may present with breathlessness, cyanosis or cardiogenic shock. The immediate management of shock is described in Chapter 5.

Causes of heart failure that may present as breathing difficulties

Left ventricular volume overload or excessive pulmonary blood flow

Ventricular septal defect (VSD)	Atrioventricular septal defect (AVSD)
Common arterial trunk	Patent ductus arteriosus (PDA)

Left heart obstruction

Hypertrophic cardiomyopathy	Critical aortic stenosis
Aortic coarctation	Hypoplastic left heart syndrome

Primary 'pump' failure

Myocarditis	Cardiomyopathy

Dysrhythmia

Supraventricular tachycardia	Complete heart block

Background

In infancy, heart failure is usually secondary to *structural heart disease*, and medical management is directed at improving the clinical condition prior to definitive surgery. There are some complex congenital heart defects in which the presence of a patent ductus arteriosus (PDA) is essential to maintain pulmonary or systemic flow. The normal ductus arteriosus closes functionally in the first 24 hours of life. Infants with duct-dependent right or left heart lesions present in the first few days of life as the ductus arteriosus starts closing in response to transition from fetal to postnatal life. With modern obstetric management, many infants with congenital heart disease are now diagnosed antenatally so that they may be delivered within cardiac units. Newborns also more commonly undergo newborn oximetry screening, which also allows earlier detection of cases. This has resulted in fewer infants with serious congenital heart disease, including those with duct-dependent disease, presenting to paediatric or emergency departments.

In the older child, *myocarditis and cardiomyopathy* are the usual causes of the acute onset of heart failure. Although there are many causes for myocarditis, in most children it is triggered by an infection, usually viral. Presenting features include fatigue, effort intolerance, anorexia, abdominal pain and cough. The presence of chest pain and arrhythmia should also be included as clues towards a diagnosis of myocarditis. On examination, a marked sinus tachycardia, hepatomegaly and raised jugular venous pressure are found with inspiratory crackles on auscultation. ECG and cardiac enzymes may be helpful in diagnosis.

Emergency treatment of heart failure

- Assess ABCDE
- If needed, give *high-flow oxygen* by face mask with a reservoir or HFNC
- If there are signs of shock – poor pulse volume or low blood pressure with extreme pallor and depressed conscious level – treat the child for *cardiogenic shock* (see Chapter 5)

- If circulation is adequate and SpO_2 is normal or improves significantly with oxygen but there are signs of heart failure, then breathing difficulties are due to pulmonary congestion secondary to a large left-to-right shunt. The shunt may be through an atrioventricular septal defect (AVSD), ventricular septal defect (VSD), PDA or, more rarely, an aortopulmonary window or truncus arteriosus. In many cases a heart murmur will be heard. A chest X-ray usually provides supportive evidence in the form of cardiomegaly and increased pulmonary vascular markings. *Diuretics* should be commenced, for example a combination of loop diuretics (furosemide) with a potassium-sparing diuretic (amiloride or spironolactone) in twice or thrice daily doses. Electrolytes should be checked prior to commencing diuretics
- Babies in the first few days of life who present with breathlessness and increasing cyanosis largely unresponsive to oxygen supplementation are likely to have duct-dependent congenital heart disease such as tricuspid or pulmonary atresia. Start *prostaglandin* to maintain the patency of the ductus arteriosus (see Chapter 3 for further details)
- Children of all ages who present with breathlessness from heart failure may have myocarditis. This is characterised by a marked sinus tachycardia and the absence of signs of structural abnormality. The patients should be treated with *oxygen* and *diuretics*, but often are transferred to the PCCU in need of inotropes or vasopressors

A full blood count and measurements of serum urea and electrolytes, calcium, glucose, heart enzymes, inflammatory parameters and (arterial) blood gases with lactate should be performed on all children in heart failure. A routine infection screen including blood cultures is recommended, especially in infants. A full 12-lead ECG and a chest radiograph are essential. All patients suspected of having heart disease should be discussed with a paediatric cardiologist, as transfer to a tertiary centre will usually be required. Echocardiography will establish the diagnosis in most cases.

Diabetic ketoacidosis

As hyperventilation is a feature of the severe acidosis produced by diabetes, occasionally a child may present with a primary breathing difficulty. The correct diagnosis is usually easy to establish, and management is described in Appendix B.

Intoxication

There may be apparent breathing difficulties following the ingestion of a number of poisons. The respiratory rate may be increased by poisoning with:

- Salicylates
- Ethylene glycol (antifreeze)
- Methanol
- Cyanide

However, usually only poisoning with salicylates causes any diagnostic dilemma. Poisoning with drugs that cause a depression of ventilation will present as a diminished conscious level. The management of the poisoned child is dealt with in Appendix F.

4.11 Summary

This chapter has discussed the range of mechanisms and possible causes that make children and infants particularly susceptible to respiratory failure. The clinician should take a structured approach to assessing, managing and treating the child with breathing difficulties.

CHAPTER 5

Circulation

Learning outcomes

After reading this chapter, you will be able to:

- Describe the pathophysiology of shock
- Identify the causes of circulatory failure in infants and children
- Describe how to assess children with cardiovascular failure
- Describe how to resuscitate the child with life-threatening shock
- Describe the emergency treatment of the different causes of circulatory failure including arrhythmias
- Identify the properties of different resuscitation fluids

5.1   Introduction

The role of the cardiovascular system is to ensure that adequate oxygen is delivered to the end organs and tissues, and to facilitate the removal of waste products away from tissues. Failure of the cardiovascular system to carry out this role can lead to critical illness and shock. Before considering the pathophysiology of shock, it is important to understand some basic normal physiology.

5.2   Normal physiology of oxygen delivery

Oxygen delivery (DO_2) to tissues is dependent on two factors: (i) the cardiac output; and (ii) the content of oxygen in arterial blood. Both are needed to ensure tissues are well perfused with adequate amounts of oxygen.

Cardiac output is the volume of blood ejected from the heart per minute and is calculated as a product of heart rate multiplied by stroke volume (volume of blood ejected from the heart per beat). Children have a limited capacity to acutely increase stroke volume, meaning that to increase the cardiac output in times of illness the main physiological mechanism is to increase the heart rate.

> This is important as an isolated tachycardia in a child can be the first warning sign that the cardiac output is compromised

Advanced Paediatric Life Support: A Practical Approach to Emergencies, Seventh Edition. Edited by Stephanie Smith.
© 2023 John Wiley & Sons Ltd. Published 2023 by John Wiley & Sons Ltd.

The stroke volume is reliant on three components, all of which can be compromised in critical illness:

1. *Preload:*
   - The circulating volume that returns to the heart (filling of the heart or end diastolic volume)
   - This can be reduced in situations such as major haemorrhage, fluid loss (e.g. gastroenteritis) or fluid redistribution (e.g. capillary leak in sepsis)
2. *Contractility:*
   - The strength of the cardiac muscle contraction to generate the pressure to allow blood to eject
   - This can be reduced in situations such as cardiomyopathy or myocarditis
3. *Afterload:*
   - The resistance the heart must eject against
   - This is increased when the circulation is vasoconstricted or when there is a fixed obstruction such as aortic stenosis, and decreased when the circulation is vasodilated (e.g. some presentations of sepsis). Positive pressure ventilation also reduces left ventricular afterload

Content of oxygen in arterial blood

The arterial oxygen content of blood is mostly dependent on the amount of haemoglobin and the percentage of haemoglobin carrying oxygen (oxygen saturation usually measured by peripheral pulse oximetry). There is also a very small amount of oxygen dissolved in plasma.

Oxygen delivery (DO_2) can therefore be calculated by applying an equation to the these concepts (Figure 5.1). This means when dealing with inadequate oxygen delivery in critical illness (shock), patient management needs to be orientated to optimising the various aspects of this equation.

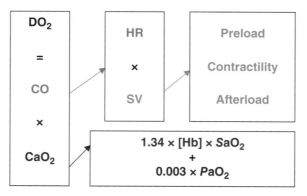

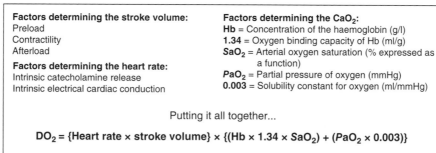

Factors determining the stroke volume:
Preload
Contractility
Afterload

Factors determining the heart rate:
Intrinsic catecholamine release
Intrinsic electrical cardiac conduction

Factors determining the CaO_2:
Hb = Concentration of the haemoglobin (g/l)
1.34 = Oxygen binding capacity of Hb (ml/g)
SaO_2 = Arterial oxygen saturation (% expressed as a function)
PaO_2 = Partial pressure of oxygen (mmHg)
0.003 = Solubility constant for oxygen (ml/mmHg)

Putting it all together...

$$DO_2 = \{Heart\ rate \times stroke\ volume\} \times \{(Hb \times 1.34 \times SaO_2) + (PaO_2 \times 0.003)\}$$

Figure 5.1 Oxygen delivery equation
Hb, haemolglobin; HR, heart rate; SV, stroke volume

5.3 Pathophysiology of shock

Shock describes a clinical situation of circulatory failure, with inadequate oxygen delivery to tissues to meet their metabolic demands. This leads to cellular hypoxia and if not recognised and treated quickly leads to worsening cellular hypoxia, acidosis and loss of normal organ function and subsequently death.

Whilst the causes of the shock can vary, the fundamental physiology remains the same: oxygen delivery to tissues is inadequate (e.g. cardiomyopathy), oxygen consumption (VO_2) is higher than normal (e.g. in sepsis), oxygen carriage is abnormal (e.g. haemoglobinopathies) or a combination of these reasons.

Without intervention shock will progress, and whilst becoming more clinically obvious will also carry higher morbidity and mortality with delaying intervention. It is important to have early recognition of shock to try and fully reverse it before end-organ injury occurs.

Homeostasis describes the physiological responses that maintain normal body function, and in this case, normal oxygen delivery. In young people homeostasis is often very effective, making it difficult to spot changes in oxygen delivery in the early stages of illness so the clinician must have a low threshold for considering early shock.

In early shock (sometimes referred to as compensated shock), the body activates a variety of physiological processes to redirect oxygenated blood to the key organs (i.e. heart and brain). Sympathetic nervous activity leads to a tachycardia (to increase oxygen delivery by increasing the cardiac output) and causes vasoconstriction of peripheral vasculature to increase preload and redivert blood away from non-essential tissues. There may be a mild tachypnoea to increase oxygen intake and carbon dioxide (CO_2) removal to compensate for the developing metabolic acidosis due to activation of anaerobic metabolism as a source of energy production. Children can compensate for early shock very well. Often an isolated tachycardia or tachypnoea are the only clues.

As shock progresses, the body's homeostasis starts to fail (often referred to as uncompensated shock). At this point cellular hypoxia has worsened and multiorgan failure starts to develop.

If shock is still not managed appropriately then the cellular damage cannot be reversed despite full management, and cardiac arrest and death will occur. This is often known as irreversible shock.

It is vital that the features of shock are identified before it becomes irreversible, remembering that not all features will be present as shock is a spectrum. A low threshold for considering shock should be present when there are only one or two of these features:

General clinical features

- Tachycardia
- Tachypnoea
- Failure to detect pulse oximeter probe tracing
- Cool or very warm, flushed peripheries
- Weak or bounding pulses
- Prolonged capillary refill time OR very rapid (flash) refill time
- Grey/mottled/pale skin appearances or very flushed
- Blood pressure may be normal or low. Sometimes only the diastolic is low with a wide pulse pressure
- Blood pressure can also be high due to peripheral vasoconstriction, sometimes with a narrow pulse pressure
- Changes in activity level: agitation, not responding to usual social cues, drowsiness or unconsciousness
- Reduced urine output

Blood gas results

- Raised lactate
- Metabolic acidosis
- Low $PaCO_2$ (due to hyperventilation to compensate for metabolic acidosis)

Laboratory results

- Disseminated intravascular coagulation (raised international normalised ratio (INR) and activated partial thromboplastin time ratio (aPTTr) and low fibrinogen and low platelets)
- Acute kidney injury (raised urea and creatinine)
- Acute liver injury (raised alanine transaminase/aspartate aminotransferase, bilirubin)
- Bone marrow suppression (low platelets, low haemoglobin)

5.4 Classification of causes of shock

Shock is classically divided into five categories based on aetiology: hypovolaemic, distributive, cardiogenic, obstructive or dissociative. Several mechanisms often coexist.

Some of the potential classifications and causes of shock are listed in Table 5.1. The most common cause in paediatric patients is hypovolaemia from several different conditions. It must be stated again that the cause of shock can be multifactorial. For example, in septic shock, hypovolaemia, cardiogenic and distributive shock frequently occur simultaneously.

Table 5.1   Categories and example causes of shock

Categories	Aetiology	Cause
Hypovolaemic	Loss of fluid	Haemorrhage Gastroenteritis Surgical abdomen *(e.g. intussusception, volvulus, perforation)* Burns Diabetic ketoacidosis Third space fluid loss *(e.g. sepsis, pancreatitis)*
Distributive	Alterations in vascular tone	Sepsis Anaphylaxis Vasodilating drugs *(e.g. anaesthesia)* Spinal cord injury
Cardiogenic	Pump failure	Arrhythmias Cardiomyopathy/myocarditis Congenital heart diseases *(e.g. coarctation of the aorta)* Valvular disease Myocardial contusion
Obstructive	Flow restriction	Congenital heart disease *(e.g. coarctation of the aorta, hypoplastic left heart, aortic stenosis)* Pneumothorax Pleural effusions/haemothorax Cardiac tamponade Pulmonary embolism
Dissociative	Oxygen-carrying ability problem	Profound anaemia Carbon monoxide poisoning Methaemoglobinaemia Cyanide poisoning

5.5 Approach to the child in circulatory failure

Early recognition and treatment of cardiovascular failure leading to shock is crucial and requires a high index of suspicion. The initial ABCDE approach is generic and used whatever the underlying cause, However, it is helpful to have a working knowledge of the conditions that predispose children of different ages and co-morbidities to shock. For example, it is important to know if there is a history of congenital heart disease, immunodeficiency, trauma, surgery, toxin ingestion or allergies. Other than certain obvious causes of shock like external haemorrhage, signs and symptoms of early compensated shock can be easily missed.

The child may present with fever, rash, pallor, poor feeding or drowsiness. A high level of vigilance should be maintained during the entire assessment of any patient. It may be difficult to recognise shock in children with neurodisability as their baseline physiology may include cool peripheries, and they may be unresponsive to voice and painful stimuli. A high index of suspicion is needed to diagnose circulatory shock in these children.

Parents or carers can be valuable in knowing what is normal for these children. Evaluation of cardiac output is a challenge for any clinician, so multiple parameters should be actively assessed. One 'good' value can be often misleading, for example capillary refill time can be normal in toxic shock syndrome despite shock being present.

5.6   Primary survey and resuscitation

Children with circulatory failure have a high likelihood of collapse and even cardiac arrest. There should be a low threshold for using a medical emergency call to gather a team with advanced skills in paediatric resuscitation.

Although our approach is based on the sequential ABCDE method, a well-trained team can do multiple assessments and tasks simultaneously. When using this team-based approach an understanding of human factors is essential and situational awareness is required of the team leader as well as different team members (see Chapter 2).

[A] Airway

- Ensure the airway is open: consider airway-opening manoeuvres, airway adjuncts or urgent induction of anaesthesia and intubation to secure the airway

[B] Breathing

- There is often tachypnoea to compensate for metabolic acidosis
- Children can have a combined respiratory and circulatory problem
- Point of care ultrasound (POCUS) may be used for rapid assessment (see Appendix I)

Emergency treatment

- If the child is obviously shocked give high-flow oxygen through a face mask with a reservoir or start HFNC
- Use pulse oximetry and aim for SpO_2 greater than or equal to 94–98%
- If hypoventilating support with oxygen via a bag–valve–mask device or breathing circuit such as the Ayres T-piece and seek experienced help for early intubation and mechanical ventilation

[C] Circulation

- Monitor the heart rate/rhythm with a continuous three- or five-lead electrocardiogram (ECG). Measure non-invasive blood pressure and use a short cycle time (1–5 minutes) if possible. Note capillary refill time and central and peripheral pulsations
- If the heart rate is above 200 beats/min in an infant, above 150 beats/min in a child or very slow, consider arrhythmia and do a 12-lead ECG
- POCUS may be used for rapid assessment of cardiac function (see Appendix I)

Emergency treatment

- Gain intravenous (IV) or intraosseous (IO) access:
  - Insert one, or ideally two, IV cannulae if possible; immediately proceed to IO access if peripheral venous access is difficult
  - Central access (femoral, jugular or subclavian) can be used when peripheral or IO access is impossible and experienced help is available (see Chapter 20)
- Take blood for blood gas (normally includes lactate, glucose, haemoglobin, sodium, potassium and ionised calcium). A raised lactate is a key discriminator of critical illness in the presence of

clinical signs of shock and resuscitation should begin immediately. If the lactate is above 4 mmol/l, referral to paediatric critical care should be made without delay. Other laboratory tests are not a priority and depend on the potential underlying cause (e.g. full blood count (FBC), electrolytes, renal and liver function tests, C-reactive protein (CRP) or procalcitonin, blood culture, bacterial polymerase chain reaction (PCR), crossmatch and coagulation studies)

- Primary treatment of potential *hypovolaemic shock* is fluid resuscitation. Give 10 ml/kg of isotonic crystalloid over 5–10 minutes and reassess after each bolus. Titrate fluid resuscitation at the bedside to reverse shock (tachycardia, hypotension, capillary refill time, peripheral pulses, lactate and level of consciousness). If there is no improvement after 20–40 ml/kg of fluid, prepare vasoactive drugs (e.g. adrenaline infusion). Rarely, the total volume of fluid resuscitation can be as high as 60–80 ml/kg in special circumstances. In settings without easy access to intensive care facilities which have inotropes and mechanical ventilation, more caution is warranted. If fluid boluses worsen signs of shock, pulmonary oedema or hepatomegaly then stop giving fluid
- Expert advice regarding intubation and ventilation should be sought in children with shock who have not responded to fluid resuscitation. Mechanical ventilation decreases the energy requirements of the heart and respiratory muscles and helps reduce the risk of development of pulmonary oedema
- Be cautious in those with primary *cardiogenic shock* or in those with signs of *raised intracranial pressure* (ICP): the first group may still benefit from a judicious fluid bolus (5 ml/kg) to optimise preload but seek the urgent advice of a paediatric cardiologist or paediatric intensivist for further treatment. In children with signs suggestive of raised ICP (i.e. relative bradycardia and hypertension, posturing or seizures), hypotension is detrimental for cerebral perfusion, but excessive fluids carry the theoretical risk of worsening cerebral oedema; hence fluids should be given cautiously
- Also be cautious with fluids in children with *diabetic ketoacidosis*; follow local guidelines, which usually start with a 10 ml/kg fluid bolus
- Catheterise the child and measure hourly urine output
- In non-hypotensive children with *severe haemolytic anaemia* (severe malaria or sickle cell crises), blood transfusion is superior to crystalloid boluses
- In children with suspected severe *dengue* as the cause of the shock, refer to dengue-specific resuscitation guidelines (WHO, 2022)
- Give a broad-spectrum antibiotic such as ceftriaxone or cefotaxime for those with an obvious or suspected diagnosis of septicaemia, or in those where the aetiology is unknown. Blood cultures should be obtained before administering antibiotics when possible, but this should not delay their administration
- In children with trauma, haemorrhage must be looked for and controlled for effective management of shock (see Chapter 8)
- If a tachy-/bradyarrhythmia is identified as the cause of shock, special algorithms should be used (see Section 5.14)
- If anaphylaxis is likely (e.g. in urticarial rash or possible recent allergen exposure) then give IM adrenaline (see Figure 5.3)

[D] Disability

- Conscious level (AVPU): agitation at first, evolving to obtundation and coma
- Posture: children in shock are usually hypotonic
- If there is coexistent evidence of raised ICP, manage as in Chapter 6

[E] Exposure

- Rash can help identify the cause of shock, but can also be absent. Haemorrhagic purpura, although characteristic of meningococcal sepsis, may be seen in sepsis of other aetiologies particularly pneumococcal sepsis. Generalised erythema, conjunctivitis and mucositis may indicate toxic shock syndrome
- Bruising may suggest occult trauma due to inflicted injury
- Fever suggests an infective cause

'Don't ever forget glucose' (DEFG)

Hypoglycaemia may give a similar clinical picture to that of compensated shock. This must always be excluded by an urgent glucose bedside test and blood glucose estimation. Shock and hypoglycaemia may coexist due to limited glycogen reserves and the fact that ill children may not have had adequate nutritional intake.

Treat hypoglycaemia (blood glucose less than 2.8 mmol/l or 50 mg/dl) with a bolus of 3 ml/kg 10% glucose.

5.7   Key features of the child in shock

While the primary survey and resuscitation are being carried out, a focused history of the child's health and activity over the previous 24 hours and any significant previous illness should be gained. Certain key features that will be identified from this – and the initial blood test results – can point the clinician to the likeliest working diagnosis for emergency treatment.

- A history of vomiting and/or diarrhoea points to fluid loss either externally (e.g. gastroenteritis) or into the abdomen (e.g. volvulus, intussusception or ruptured appendix)
- The presence of fever and/or rash points to septicaemia
- The presence of urticaria, angioneurotic oedema or a history of allergen exposure points to anaphylaxis
- The presence of cyanosis unresponsive to oxygen or a grey colour/pallor with signs of heart failure in a baby within the first 4 weeks of life points to duct-dependent congenital heart disease
- The presence of heart failure in an older infant or child points to cardiomyopathy or myocarditis
- A history of sickle cell disease, a history of glucose-6-phosphate dehydrogenase (G6PD) deficiency or a recent diarrhoeal disease are suggestive of haemolytic uraemic syndrome, and a very low haemoglobin points to acute haemolysis. A history of sickle cell disease, abdominal pain and enlarged spleen points to acute splenic sequestration
- An immediate history of trauma points to blood loss or, more rarely, tension pneumothorax, haemothorax, cardiac tamponade or spinal cord transection. Inflicted injury may present with no history or an inconsistent history of trauma but with clinical signs of injury such as bruising
- The presence of severe tachy-/bradycardia or an abnormal rhythm on the ECG points to a cardiac cause for shock
- A history of polyuria, the presence of acidotic breathing and a very high blood glucose points to diabetic ketoacidosis
- A history of drug ingestion points to poisoning

5.8   Approach to the child with gastrointestinal fluid loss

Infants are more likely than older children to present with shock due to sudden and rapid fluid losses due to gastroenteritis or with concealed fluid loss secondary to a 'surgical abdomen' such as a volvulus.

In infants, gastroenteritis may occasionally present as circulatory collapse with little or no significant history of vomiting or diarrhoea. This is due to sudden massive loss of fluid from the bowel wall into the gut lumen, causing a depletion of intravascular volume. The infecting organism can be any of the usual diarrhoeal pathogens, of which viruses are the most common.

Emergency treatment

Having completed the primary survey and resuscitation and identified by means of the key features that fluid loss is the most likely diagnosis, the child is reassessed to identify the response to the start of fluid resuscitation.

Reassess ABCDE

- Repeat 10 ml/kg boluses of isotonic crystalloid if the shock is responding to fluid but is not fully resolved. In gastroenteritis, 10–40 ml/kg boluses usually restore circulating volume. Once signs of shock are reversed, rehydration should continue but transitioning to the enteral route (oral or nasogastric) (see Appendix B) should be started with normal feeding within 4–6 hours
- Do not persist with fluid resuscitation if shock is not improving. Consider vasoactive support, intubation and ventilation, in discussion with the paediatric critical care team, when shock is refractory to fluid resuscitation
- Recheck acid–base status and electrolytes:
  - Acidosis will usually be corrected by treatment of shock; bicarbonate losses need to be corrected only in children who have proven large bicarbonate losses (e.g. in stool). There is very little role for bicarbonate replacement in paediatric resuscitation
  - Severe hyponatraemia may occur, and this may cause convulsions. If convulsions are present, give a dose of 3% sodium chloride 3 ml/kg (range 3–5 ml/kg) over 15 minutes, aiming for a serum sodium of 125 mmol/l or seizure termination. This dose of sodium chloride may be repeated once if there is no response to the first dose. Once the seizure has stopped, or if there is asymptomatic hyponatraemia, slowly correct serum sodium (maximum 8–12 mmol/l/day)
- Consider the diagnostic possibilities:
  - Abdominal X-ray or ultrasound to detect distended bowel or intra-abdominal air or fluid
  - Consider urgent surgical referral especially if bile-stained vomiting or abdominal guarding is present
  - Consider sepsis, which maybe secondary to a surgical abdominal problem, and give appropriate intravenous antibiotics. It is worth noting that sepsis can present with generalised abdominal pain without specific abdominal pathology
- The bladder should be catheterised to accurately assess urinary output
- Treatment with an appropriate antiemetic may be helpful

5.9   Approach to the child with septic shock

The Third International Consensus in 2016 (Sepsis-3) defined sepsis in adults as 'life-threatening organ dysfunction caused by a dysregulated host response to infection' and septic shock as 'a subset of sepsis in which particularly profound circulatory, cellular and metabolic abnormalities are associated with a greater risk of mortality than with sepsis alone'. Although formal revisions to paediatric-specific definitions are outstanding, the clinical manifestations of septic shock are essentially comparable throughout a person's life:

- Hypotension (late sign in children who compensate well)
- Reliance on vasoactive agents to maintain a normal blood pressure
- Signs of inadequate tissue perfusion (in particular lactate greater than 2 mmol/l, but also other signs such as increased capillary refill time and oliguria) in the absence of hypovolaemia (after initial fluid resuscitation)

Shock associated with sepsis can be *hypovolaemic* (negative fluid balance because of fever, diarrhoea, vomiting and anorexia and/or capillary leak syndrome causing loss of fluid from the intravascular compartment), *cardiogenic* (both the host inflammatory response and infecting organisms can cause myocardial suppression) or *distributive* (caused by widespread vasodilatation resulting in a low systemic vascular resistance). Children with sepsis can also develop impaired cellular oxygen utilisation at the mitochondrial level (distributive).

The burden of sepsis in children is considerable and is the cause of 8% of admissions to paediatric critical care units in high-income countries. The mortality is 4–50% depending on illness severity, risk factors and geographical location. In 2020, the First International Consensus guidelines for the care of children with septic shock and other sepsis-associated organ dysfunction were published by the Surviving Sepsis Campaign (SSC). These guidelines form the basis for the most recent tools for the recognition and management of sepsis in children, published by the Academy of Medical Royal Colleges in May 2022, which are shown in Figure 5.2. The guidelines use the UK national paediatric early warning system (PEWS) score.

SEPSIS SCREENING TOOL ACUTE ASSESSMENT – CHILD | AGE <16

PATIENT DETAILS:

DATE:

NAME:

DESIGNATION:

SIGNATURE:

TIME:

01 START IF THE CHILD IS LIKELY TO HAVE AN INFECTION, AND EITHER YOU'RE WORRIED CLINICALLY OR PEWS HAS TRIGGERED

ADDITIONAL FACTORS PROMPTING SCREENING FOR SEPSIS INCLUDE:

- ☐ Parent or carer concern
- ☐ Known (or risk of) immunosuppression
- ☐ Age less than one year
- ☐ Recent surgery/ trauma or indwelling lines

YES

CALCULATE PEWS SCORE USING LATEST VITAL SIGNS & MEASURE LACTATE USING VBG/CAP IF AVAILABLE

02 IS PEWS 9 OR ABOVE?

OR IS PEWS BETWEEN 5 AND 8 AND LACTATE → 4 MMOL/L

OR DOES THE CHILD LOOK EXTREMELY UNWELL TO A HEALTH PROFESSIONAL?

NO ### 03 IS PEWS BETWEEN 5 AND 8?

OR IS THERE PERSISTING SIGNIFICANT PARENTAL CONCERN?

IF LACTATE → 4 MMOL/L ESCALATE TO RED FLAG SEPSIS

YES

RED FLAG SEPSIS

START PAEDIATRIC SEPSIS SIX

YES

SEND FULL SET OF BLOODS

ENSURE SENIOR CLINICAL REVIEW (ST4+) WITHIN 30 MINUTES

IF ANTIMICROBIALS ARE NEEDED, THESE SHOULD BE GIVEN AND A PLAN MADE FOR ESCALATION & SOURCE CONTROL WITHIN 3 HOURS

I have prescribed antimicrobials ☐

This patient does not require antimicrobials as:

- I don't think this child has an infection ☐
- This child is already on appropriate antimicrobials ☐
- Other _____

NAME: GRADE:
DATE: TIME: ☐☐ : ☐☐☐

SIGNATURE:

NO AMBER CRITERIA = ROUTINE CARE / CONSIDER OTHER DIAGNOSIS

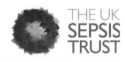

THE UK SEPSIS TRUST

UKST CHILD INPATIENT 2022 1.2 PAGE 1 OF 2

Figure 5.2 Sepsis Screening Tool
Courtesy of Nutbeam T and Daniels R on behalf of the UK Sepsis Trust, https://sepsistrust.org/professional-resources/clinical/ (last accessed March 2023)

(*Continued*)

SEPSIS SCREENING TOOL - THE SEPSIS SIX | AGE <16

PATIENT DETAILS:

DATE: **TIME:**
NAME:
DESIGNATION:
SIGNATURE:

COMPLETE ALL ACTIONS WITHIN ONE HOUR

01 ENSURE SENIOR CLINICIAN ATTENDS

NOT ALL PATIENTS WITH RED FLAGS WILL NEED THE 'SEPSIS 6' URGENTLY. A SENIOR DECISION MAKER MAY SEEK ALTERNATIVE DIAGNOSES/ DE-ESCALATE CARE. RECORD DECISIONS BELOW

TIME

02 OXYGEN IF REQUIRED

START IF O2 SATURATIONS LESS THAN 92% OR THERE IS EVIDENCE OF SHOCK

TIME

03 OBTAIN IV/IO ACCESS, TAKE BLOODS

BLOOD CULTURES (FULLY FILL AEROBIC BOTTLE FIRST!), BLOOD GLUCOSE, LACTATE, FBC, U&E'S, CRP AND CLOTTING LUMBAR PUNCTURE IF INDICATED

TIME

04 GIVE IV ANTIBIOTICS, THINK SOURCE CONTROL

MAXIMUM DOSE BROAD SPECTRUM THERAPY
CONSIDER: LOCAL POLICY / ALLERGY STATUS / ANTIVIRALS
EVALUATE NEED FOR IMAGING/ SPECIALIST REVIEW
IF SOURCE AMENABLE TO DRAINAGE ENSURE ACHIEVED AS SOON AS POSSIBLE BUT ALWAYS WITHIN 12H

TIME

05 GIVE IV FLUIDS

IF LACTATE 2-4 mmol/L GIVE FLUID BOLUS 10 ml/kg WITHOUT DELAY IF LACTATE →4 mmol/L CALL PICU. (REPEAT FLUID BOLUS IF REQUIRED)

TIME

06 CONSIDER INOTROPIC SUPPORT

CONSIDER INOTROPIC SUPPORT IF NORMAL PHYSIOLOGY IS NOT RESTORED AFTER ≥20 ml/kg FLUID (10 ml/kg IN NEONATES), AND CALL PICU OR A REGIONAL CENTRE URGENTLY

TIME

RED FLAGS AFTER ONE HOUR – ESCALATE TO CONSULTANT NOW

RECORD ADDITIONAL NOTES HERE:

e.g. allergy status, arrival of specialist teams, de-escalation of care, delayed antimicrobial decision making, variance from Sepsis Six

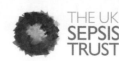

THE UK
SEPSIS
TRUST

UKST CHILD INPATIENT 2023 2.0 PAGE 2 OF 2

Figure 5.2 *(Continued)*

Emergency treatment using the Sepsis Six

Steps 01, 02 and 03

Sepsis is a life-threatening emergency and children should be attended to by senior clinicians without delay. Oxygen is indicated if the SpO_2 is less than 92% or in the presence of shock. Intravenous access can be difficult and can be an obstacle to time-critical escalation of investigation and resuscitation of critically unwell children. Attempts should be limited in number and time, and intraosseous access used as an alternative when indicated. A sample should be taken straight away for blood gas analysis, including lactate, which is a key discriminator of critical illness. Glucose should be checked and hypoglycaemia corrected. Blood should also be taken for culture, FBC, urea and electrolytes, liver function tests, CRP, pro-calcitonin (if available), calcium, phosphate, magnesium and a coagulation screen but this is of secondary importance and should not delay administration of antimicrobials or escalation of ABCDE support. Lumbar puncture should be deferred in children with signs of critical illness.

Step 04

GIVE IV ANTIBIOTICS, THINK SOURCE CONTROL.

Ensure intravenous antibiotics are given as soon as possible at the maximum dose and according to local guidance. A third-generation cephalosporin, such as cefotaxime or ceftriaxone, is usual but there are some specific considerations:

- Aciclovir should be given when sepsis is suspected in the neonatal period to cover herpes simplex virus
- Clindamycin is usually added in suspected toxic shock syndrome aimed at halting bacterial exotoxin production
- Amoxicillin is often added in under 3-month old infants to cover *Listeria*
- Cefotaxime is sometimes preferred to ceftriaxone in premature or jaundiced infants, if there is hypoalbuminaemia or if a calcium-containing infusion is being used
- Piperacillin/tazobactam ± an aminoglycoside is often used if there is a high risk of Gram-negative sepsis (e.g. in immunocompromise, urosepsis or known colonisation with a resistant Gram-negative organism)
- If there are previous cultures of a resistant organism, give the appropriate antibiotic (e.g. methicillin-resistant *Staphylococcus aureus* (MRSA): add vancomycin; extended-spectrum β-lactamases (ESBL): add meropenem)
- If central venous catheters have been in place for more than 48 hours consider adding vancomycin

Source control should be considered part of resuscitation for sepsis. Urgently look for sources of infection and address. For example, surgical problems such as appendicitis or necrotising fasciitis, or an infected line which must be removed.

Steps 05 and 06

GIVE IV FLUIDS AND CONSIDER INOTROPIC SUPPORT.

Healthcare systems with access to intensive care

If the lactate is more than 2 mmol/l and there are no signs of fluid overload, give 10 ml/kg of isotonic crystalloid (based on ideal body weight). Assess the haemodynamic response at the bedside and repeat if there is evidence of improvement but still signs of shock. If there are signs of fluid overload do not give further boluses of fluid. POCUS or echocardiography can be used to assess myocardial function. If myocardial function is impaired, consider starting an adrenaline infusion (0.1–1 micrograms/kg/min).

If normal physiology has not been restored after ≥20 ml/kg of fluid boluses (≥10 ml/kg in neonates) or earlier if there are signs of fluid overload, then vasoactive drugs should be considered. These are usually adrenaline and/or noradrenaline infusions (0.1–1 micrograms/kg/min) and should be done in discussion with the paediatric critical care service. If the lactate is greater than 4 mmol/l, referral to paediatric critical care should be made without delay.

Healthcare settings without access to intensive care

The FEAST (Fluid Expansion As Supportive Therapy) study was published in 2011 and showed that in a resource-limited setting in Africa, without access to intensive care, children with severe febrile illnesses and evidence of impaired perfusion who were treated with fluid boluses had a significantly increased mortality compared with controls. In systems without access to intensive care, the SSC guidelines only recommend fluid boluses if there is evidence of both impaired perfusion and hypotension. In the absence of hypotension, maintenance fluid with vasoactive support (if available) is recommended. In this context, hypotension is defined as a systolic blood pressure less than 50 mmHg in children aged less than 1 year, less than 60 mmHg for age 1–5 years and less than 70 mmHg for over 5 years.

Intubation and ventilation

There are no clear recommendations for the timing of intubation and ventilation in septic shock. Some children present in extremis and intubation is required as part of the initial ABCDE resuscitation. In other children, respiratory failure may be a presenting feature or may develop as a result of fluid boluses. Intubation and ventilation should also be strongly considered in children with fluid refractory shock, even without evidence of respiratory failure. Mechanical ventilation reduces oxygen consumption and positive intrathoracic pressure reduces left ventricular afterload, therefore improving oxygen supply and reducing demand. Septic shock can be associated with an impaired level of consciousness and agitation is a common barrier to delivering the care that is required, which is another indication for intubation. Meningitis causes raised ICP and there should be a low threshold for induction of anaesthesia and intubation as part of the medical management of raised ICP (see Chapter 6). When vasoactive infusions are required to support the circulation, a central line, arterial line, urinary catheter and continuous saturation and ECG monitoring are required. The reality in many children is that this can only realistically be delivered after intubation and there should be a low threshold for doing this. Induction of anaesthesia should be with ketamine (1 or 2 mg/kg) and a rapid acting muscle relaxant (e.g. rocuronium 1–2 mg/kg). Adrenaline should be prepared to support the circulation (see Chapter 19).

Refractory shock

Hydrocortisone (2–4 mg/kg 6 hourly, maximum 100 mg) can be given if shock remains refractory to fluid and vasoactive drugs. Veno-arterial or veno-venous extracorporeal life support (ECLS) for refractory shock or oxygenation/ventilation failure (after addressing other causes of shock and respiratory failure) could be considered in discussion with the regional paediatric critical care service.

Causative organisms

The most common causes of community-acquired sepsis in children include *Streptococcus pneumoniae*, *Neisseria meningitidis*, *Streptococcus pyogenes* (group A *Streptococcus*) and *Staphylococcus aureus*, with epidemiology varying depending on geographical region and vaccination access/coverage. *Streptococcus agalactiae* (group B *Streptococcus*) and Gram-negative sepsis are more prevalent in the neonatal age range. Herpes simplex virus should also not be forgotten as a possible cause of neonatal sepsis and early empirical IV aciclovir should be considered.

The cardinal sign of meningococcal septicaemia is a purpuric rash in an ill child. At the onset, however, the rash may be absent or mistaken for viral exanthems and a careful search should be made for purpura in any unwell child. In about 15% of children with meningococcal septicaemia, a blanching erythematous rash replaces or precedes a purpuric one, and in 7% of cases no rash occurs.

In toxic shock syndrome the initial clinical picture includes a high fever, diffuse erythema, headache, confusion, conjunctival and mucosal hyperaemia (strawberry tongue), scarlatiniform rash (can look like sunburn), subcutaneous oedema, vomiting and watery diarrhoea. Findings may include a trivial injury such as an infected wound, cut, scratch, minor burn or scald, surgical wound infection or coexistent deep-seated infection such as pneumonia or bone/joint infection. Early administration of intravenous antibiotics (e.g. ceftriaxone and clindamycin), concurrent with initial resuscitation, is vital. Intravenous immunoglobulin should be considered in discussion with infectious disease specialists, along with urgent drainage of any localised abscess.

Source control and further investigations

It is important to seek expert advice from the microbiology/infectious diseases team after initial empirical management, especially if there has been a slow response to treatment. Further investigations might include specific PCRs (*N. meningitidis, Streptococcus pneumoniae, S. pyogenes, S. agalactiae Staphylococcus aureus,* Enterobacterales) or broad-range PCR (16S) depending on the most likely pathogens.

5.10   Approach to the child with anaphylaxis

Anaphylaxis is a serious systemic hypersensitivity reaction that is usually rapid in onset and may cause death. Severe anaphylaxis is life threatening and may present with either shock and/or severe respiratory distress. Life-threatening features include breathing difficulties (due to upper airway swelling and/or bronchospasm) and/or shock (due to acute vasodilatation, fluid loss from the intravascular space caused by increased capillary permeability and cardiac involvement). Any of these may lead to respiratory or cardiac arrest.

Symptoms of anaphylactic shock include dizziness, collapse, pallor and floppiness; peripheral perfusion may be compromised (cold extremities) or warm due to systemic vasodilatation. Respiratory symptoms of anaphylaxis include swelling of the throat, stridor or wheeze and may or may not be associated with shock. Other allergic symptoms/signs include skin flushing, itchy rash (urticaria), facial swelling, abdominal pain and vomiting; these may or may not precede shock. Skin symptoms/signs are absent in 10–20% of cases.

Individuals allergic to food allergens will often have a history of previous allergic reactions; some may have a 'medic-alert' bracelet or carry their own adrenaline autoinjector device. Possible risk factors for more severe reactions include:

- Previous poor response to IM adrenaline
- Poorly controlled asthma
- Treatment with β-blockers

Symptoms and signs vary according to the body's response to the allergen. These are shown in Table 5.2.

Table 5.2 Symptoms and signs in allergic reaction		
	Symptoms	**Signs**
Allergic reactions	Itchy mouth/lips/throat, throat clearing, feeling of warmth, nausea, vomiting, abdominal pain, loose bowel motions, sweating	Urticarial rash, angioedema, conjunctivitis, erythema/flushing
Anaphylaxis	Difficulty breathing, noisy breathing, persistent cough, cyanosis, agitation, collapse	Wheeze, stridor, tachycardia, hypotension, poor pulse volume and pallor, respiratory or cardiac arrest

IM adrenaline 1:1000 dosages
- Under 6 months: 100 micrograms or 0.1 ml
- 6 months to 6 years: 150 micrograms or 0.15 ml
- 6 to 12 years: 300 micrograms or 0.3 ml
- Over 12 years: 500 micrograms or 0.5 ml

Many hospitals use adrenaline auto-injectors (e.g. Epipen®) for a first dose of adrenaline, in which case a dose of 300 or 500 micrograms is appropriate. Importantly, if further doses are needed, these should be given by ampoule/needle/syringe

Emergency treatment of anaphylaxis

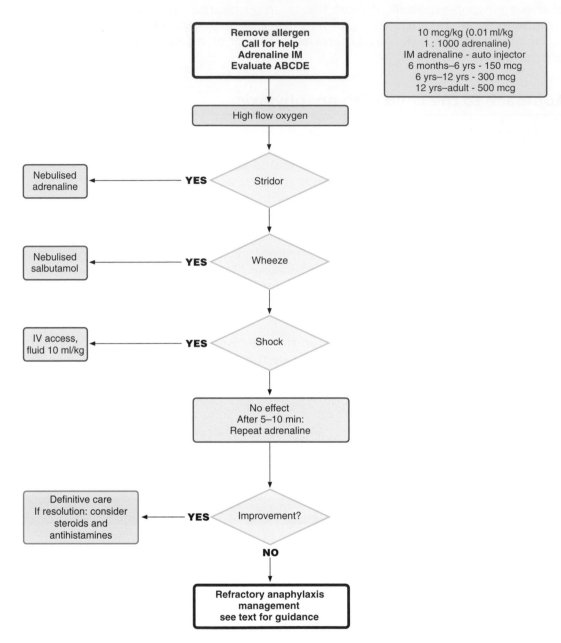

Figure 5.3 Emergency treatment of anaphylaxis algorithm

The management of anaphylactic shock or severe airways involvement (Figure 5.3) requires airway management, administration of adrenaline and aggressive fluid resuscitation. Intubation will be required for severe cases. Note that the intramuscular route is the preferred route for initial doses of adrenaline. IV/IO adrenaline should be reserved for children with life-threatening shock or airway obstruction who have not responded to repeated doses of IM adrenaline, or those in cardiac arrest. The child must be carefully monitored.

Having completed the primary survey and resuscitation and identified by means of the key features that anaphylaxis is the most likely diagnosis, the child is reassessed.

Corticosteroids and/or antihistamines are no longer recommended for the initial acute management of anaphylaxis, although antihistamines can be used to treat (emerging) skin conditions once the patient is stabilised.

Further emergency management

For anaphylaxis features that do not respond to initial IM adrenaline, continue with a bolus of balanced crystalloid and/or ventilatory support, and give a second dose of IM adrenaline 5 minutes after the first. If the reaction does not respond to two doses of IM adrenaline, commence **refractory anaphylaxis management**. Give a rapid fluid bolus and commence an IV/IO adrenaline infusion according to local guidelines and titrate to clinical response. While waiting for the infusion to be prepared, continue IM adrenaline every 5 minutes.

The child should be closely monitored with continuous pulse oximetry, blood pressure and ECG. If the shock is refractory to the adrenaline infusion a second vasopressor, such as noradrenaline, vasopressin or metaraminol, could be considered. Guidance from a paediatric intensive care specialist is vital.

Take a blood sample for mast cell tryptase for future analysis as soon as possible, and a second sample 2–4 hours later.

In addition to this treatment, corticosteroids (e.g. hydrocortisone) are still recommended for refractory reactions. The role these drugs have in acute management is limited, as their onset of action is too delayed to be of much benefit in the first hour.

In cardiac arrest, resuscitation should be aggressive – do not give up too soon. Prolonged cardiopulmonary resuscitation, including extracorporeal membrane oxygenation (ECMO), should be considered as the cause of arrest is potentially reversible and the tissue oxygenation prior to arrest is likely to have been normal.

5.11   Approach to the child with profound anaemia

Severe anaemia exists if the haemoglobin level is less than 50 g/l. The child will be lethargic with severe pallor of the conjunctiva, palms and soles, and there may be signs of heart failure. If acute haemolysis is the cause of anaemia, urine will usually be dark brown. The most usual situation in which a child develops sudden severe haemolysis in high-income western countries is septicaemia associated with sickle cell disease or haemolytic uraemic syndrome (HUS). In children returning from or living in endemic areas, severe malaria may present with severe anaemia, with or without haemolysis. G6PD deficiency may also present with severe haemolytic anaemia following exposure to triggers.

Emergency treatment

- Red blood cell transfusion should be considered when the haemoglobin level is less than 50 g/l
- The presence of heart failure affects the decision to transfuse; diuretics will be required. Fluid overload may exacerbate or lead to cardiogenic shock and pulmonary oedema
- Treatment may also be required as for sepsis with volume support, inotropes and intubation

Management of these children includes early discussion with paediatric critical care services.

> Oxygen saturation monitoring may be falsely reassuring in children who are in profound anaemia

5.12   Approach to the child with sickle cell crisis

Sickle cell disease is characterised by episodic clinical events called 'crises'. A vaso-occlusive crisis is the most common and occurs when abnormal red cells occlude small vessels, causing tissue ischaemia. The other crises are acute chest syndrome, sequestration crisis (severe anaemia and hypotension, resulting from pooling of blood in the spleen and liver), aplastic crisis and hyper-haemolytic crisis. Factors that precipitate or modulate the occurrence of sickle cell crises are not fully understood, but infections, hypoxia, dehydration, acidosis, stress and cold are believed to play some role.

Oxygen therapy, rehydration, antibiotics and analgesia are considered standard treatment in sickle cell crises. Parenteral opioids are essential for relieving pain in severe vaso-occlusive crises and acute chest syndrome.

5.13 Approach to the child with cardiogenic shock

Overview

Cardiogenic shock describes inadequate oxygen delivery to tissues due to failure of the 'pump' (i.e. the heart) to deliver an adequate cardiac output. Whilst the pump failure can be due to primary cardiac disease (e.g. congenital heart disease, cardiomyopathy, myocarditis, arrhythmias or ischaemic heart disease), it is important to recognise that ventricular failure can also be seen secondary to pathologies such as sepsis, and this is more often seen in younger children.

Specific recognition of cardiogenic shock is important as these children often need early positive pressure ventilation, inotropic support and limited use of fluid resuscitation.

Clinical features that may suggest cardiogenic shock include tachycardia, heart murmurs, gallop rhythms, hepatomegaly, weak pulses, narrow pulse pressure, pallor, distended neck vessels and deterioration on administration of fluid boluses. Failure to pick up a SpO_2 trace can suggest poor peripheral perfusion due to low cardiac output. POCUS can be helpful to assess left ventricular function and look for cardiac tamponade (see Appendix I).

Duct-dependent congenital heart diseases

Overview

The ductus arteriosus connects the systemic and pulmonary circulations in fetal life, allowing blood to bypass the pulmonary circulation in utero as gas exchange occurs at the placenta. In the first few days of life the ductus arteriosus (duct) starts closing as part of the transition from fetal to postnatal life. Some neonatal congenital heart lesions are dependent upon a duct to supply either pulmonary or systemic blood flow (Figure 5.4) or to support adequate mixing between parallel circulations (e.g. in transposition of the great arteries). These lesions are known as duct-dependent congenital heart diseases. Anatomical examples are shown in Figure 5.5.

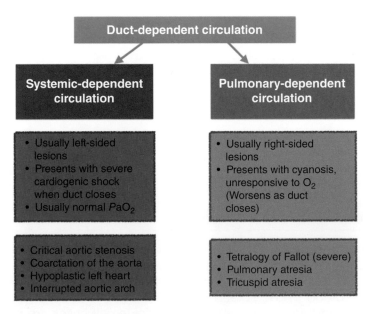

Figure 5.4 **Summary of two main groups of duct-dependent lesions**

(a)

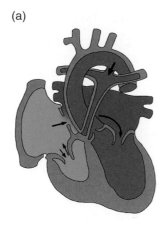

There is no opening in the right ventricular outflow tract so blood cannot exit the small right ventricle to get to the pulmonary circulation for oxygenation. All blood must mix via an intracardiac shunt (atrial or ventricular septal defect) by shunting right to left. In this case, the blood gets to the pulmonary circulation by going via the duct from the aorta to the pulmonary artery (left-to-right shunt). In these cases, the systemic cardiac output is usually good, with the main problem being increasing hypoxia as the duct closes and pulmonary blood flow is reduced. The systemic cardiac output is deoxygenated and as the hypoxia worsens shock can develop

(b)

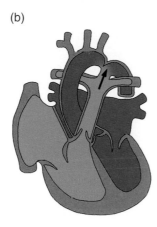

There is obstruction to blood flow within the aorta at the level of the coarctation. Blood flow distal to the obstruction is supplied by the duct by going from the pulmonary artery to the aorta (right-to-left shunt). This means the blood supplying the lower body is at a lower blood pressure and is deoxygenated. As the duct closes, blood flow is maintained to the coronary arteries and brain from the left ventricle, but blood flow to the lower body is reduced or absent, leading to cardiogenic shock

Figure 5.5 Examples of duct-dependent pulmonary circulation. (a) Pulmonary atresia with intact interventricular septum. (b) Coarctation of the aorta

Recognition

The most common time to present with compromise to the systemic or pulmonary circulations due to a closing duct is at 7–10 days of age. However, there should be a high index of suspicion for duct-dependent congenital heart when dealing with any critically unwell neonatal patient. Whilst many are diagnosed antenatally, normal antenatal scans *do not* exclude congenital heart disease.

Clinical features that can suggest duct-dependent lesions include:

- Features of cardiogenic shock (discussed earlier in this chapter)
- Cyanosis (especially if not fully responding to oxygen therapy)
- Weak or absent femoral pulses
- Discrepancy between upper and lower limb blood pressure and oxygen saturations
- Hepatomegaly
- Cardiomegaly
- Abnormal ECGs

Emergency treatment

When neonates present critically unwell, the differential diagnosis is broad. The mnemonic SCAM stands for sepsis, cardiac, abuse and metabolic disorders and is a helpful way of remembering possible causes. However, distinguishing between these can be very difficult during resuscitation and the priority should be the standardised ABCDE approach to resuscitation, with the additional consideration of resuscitating the ductus arteriosus. Some people find it useful to think ABCDDE when resuscitating critically unwell neonates. The additional 'D' standing for duct.

Specific management points for the neonate with suspected duct-dependent circulation include:

- Obtain early support from the local paediatric or neonatal critical care service. In some lesions urgent intervention is needed (e.g. balloon atrial septostomy in transposition of the great arteries)
- Ensure blood pressure and pulse oximetry monitoring is placed on the right arm (preductal circulation) and use this monitoring as your target blood pressure and SpO_2. This is because preductal blood perfuses the coronary arteries and brain. The postductal observations (obtained on the lower limbs) are helpful for diagnosis but not as a target for physiological parameters
- Oxygen therapy should be given to maintain the preductal right arm SpO_2 greater than 75%. Use as much as required to achieve this target. There is no condition in which withholding oxygen improves hypoxia and there are no concerns about oxygen accelerating duct closure when prostaglandin is being used
- Give IV infusion of dinoprostone (prostaglandin E2 or PGE2) or alprostadil (PGE1) urgently:
  - This acts by reopening the duct and restores either systemic or pulmonary blood flow
  - It should be started early if duct-dependent circulation is suspected and can always be stopped later after a detailed echocardiogram
  - The side effects are dose dependent and include apnoea, pyrexia and vasodilatation (leading to hypotension)
  - The impact on the duct is dose dependent. This means low doses of dinoprostone (5–10 ng/kg/min) will keep open a duct that is already open. Higher doses (20–100 ng/kg/min) will reopen a closing or closed duct and therefore the starting dose depends on the clinical situation of the neonate
  - If signs of shock/absent pulses: 20–50 ng/kg/min increasing to 100 ng/kg/min in discussion with paediatric critical care services
  - Lower doses (5–10 ng/kg/min) are only useful in the immediate postnatal period or the very stable neonate
  - Doses can be titrated to saturations and the presence or return of femoral pulses
- Manage preductal right arm hypotension. Whilst a cautious 5 ml/kg of fluid can be tried, it is likely that these children will need inotropic support with an infusion of adrenaline
- The following are indications for intubation and ventilation:
  - Apnoea due to dinoprostone
  - Extreme hypoxia
  - Any degree of hypoxia with respiratory distress
  - Signs of shock
  - Need for interventional procedure
- All neonates presenting shocked should be covered for sepsis with IV antibiotics and aciclovir

Throughout management of this complex patient group ensure early and regular discussions with your local paediatric or neonatal critical care service.

Cardiomyopathy or myocarditis

Overview

Cardiomyopathy is a disease of the heart muscle itself, resulting in pump failure. It is a cause of cardiogenic shock in children. It is usually caused by a genetic pathology, toxins (especially chemotherapy), unrecognised arrhythmias or metabolic disorders. It can also be caused by myocarditis. Myocarditis is an infection of the heart muscle, usually from a viral pathology, and leads to pump failure, and so is a cause of cardiomyopathy. Cardiomyopathy can also be secondary to non-cardiac diseases such as sepsis.

These children can present with varying degrees of heart failure and cardiogenic shock. It can be difficult to distinguish this from other causes of shock. A chest X-ray and 12 lead ECG may help with the diagnosis of cardiomyopathy, while assessment with POCUS can help to differentiate these similar clinical pictures. Fluid resuscitation can often worsen the condition of these children, and this is a clue ventricular function is impaired. If such a patient is in the first few weeks of life, a trial of prostaglandin (PGE1 or PGE2) may be appropriate and would be beneficial for duct-dependent circulations as discussed earlier.

Emergency management

Management depends on whether the child presents with cardiac failure without signs of shock or cardiac failure with signs of shock. Ensure other pathologies (such as sepsis) have been considered and managed as indicated.

Children with cardiomyopathy/myocarditis can be very difficult to manage and can rapidly deteriorate if they develop an arrhythmia. Ensure they are on continuous monitoring. A blood gas is mandatory and a raised lactate should prompt referral to the paediatric critical care service.

Those presenting in heart failure without signs of shock need to be referred to the paediatric cardiologist quickly for treatment of their heart failure, so they do not develop shock. If the child is not shocked consider diuretics to offload the heart, such as furosemide 0.5–1 mg/kg, and consider non-invasive ventilation or high-flow nasal oxygen therapy.

For those already in shock who are suspected to have myocarditis or cardiomyopathy, aggressive fluid resuscitation needs to be avoided and early use of inotropes (e.g. adrenaline infusion) with positive pressure ventilation are likely to be indicated. This should be in close discussion with the paediatric critical care team. Afterload reduction (e.g. with milrinone or dobutamine) may be considered. The availability of ECLS with ECMO and ventricular assist devices (VADs) for the most serious cases needs to be considered, with the focus on the child being stabilised and transferred urgently to the right centre.

Early discussion about transfer to a cardiac centre should take place with your local paediatric critical care service.

5.14   Approach to the child with abnormal rhythm or pulse rate

Overview

Sinus tachycardia and bradycardia can occur in normal physiological states, such as during exercise and sleep. However, they can both also be signs of critical illness from a variety of non-cardiac pathologies. In some situations these rhythms are not sinus, in which case the child may have a primary arrhythmia (Table 5.3). This may be haemodynamically significant and lead to cardiogenic shock. An ECG should be performed in situations of tachycardia or bradycardia when it is not clear that the rhythm is sinus from a rhythm strip.

Table 5.3 Example causes of tachyarrhythmias and bradyarrhythmia	
Causes of tachyarrhythmia	**Causes of bradyarrhythmia**
Supraventricular tachycardias	Pre-terminal event in hypoxia or shock
Ventricular tachycardias	Raised intracranial pressure
Poisoning	Heart blocks (iatrogenic or congenital)
Metabolic disturbance	Poisoning
After cardiac surgery	
Cardiomyopathy	
Primary arrhythmia syndromes (e.g. long QT syndrome, Brugada syndrome)	

Treatment of children with an abnormal rhythm or pulse is highly protocolised and depends on the underlying rhythm. Basic recognition of the arrhythmia is essential. To use the right management protocol, answer three basic questions (Figure 5.6).

Basic recognition of arrhythmia

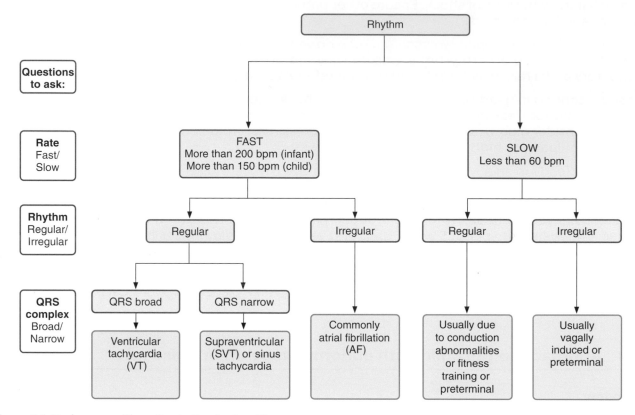

Figure 5.6 Basic recognition of arrhythmia algorithm

Abnormal rhythm or pulse: bradyarrhythmia

Overview

An abnormally slow pulse rate is defined as one less than 60 beats/min or a rapidly falling heart rate associated with poor systemic perfusion.

Most sinus bradycardia in children is a pre-terminal rhythm due to hypoxia and/or myocardial ischaemia from untreated shock but it can sometimes be precipitated by vagal stimulation (e.g. during intubation or airway suctioning). Sinus bradycardia can also be a sign of raised ICP, which could be with or without an altered conscious level (see Chapter 6). Any sinus or non-sinus brady-cardia can also point to poisoning (e.g. with digoxin or β-blockers).

Incidental sinus bradycardia in a clinically well child may be seen in athletic and sporty children and does not require any treatment.

Non-sinus bradycardias usually indicate a type of heart block. Complete heart block is known as third degree heart block. This can be seen as a congenital phenomenon, after cardiac surgery, due to drug overdose or idiopathic. It is recognised as a slow heart rate, with widely spaced QRS com-plexes (which can be broad) with dissociation of P wave activity from the QRS complexes.

Emergency treatment

As described, in paediatric practice bradycardia is predominantly a pre-terminal finding in children with respiratory and/or circulatory insufficiency. Airway, breathing and circulation should be assessed and treated during the primary survey, with particular focus on reversing hypoxia and/or shock. Hypoxia leading to bradycardia results in cardiac arrest if not addressed quickly. Stabilisation of the airway and breathing should be started immediately, and bradycardia will often resolve once oxygenation is restored.

After this basic ABCDE management then pharmacological management of bradycardia can be considered, primarily for the non-sinus bradyarrhythmias and heart block (Figure 5.7).

Management of bradycardia

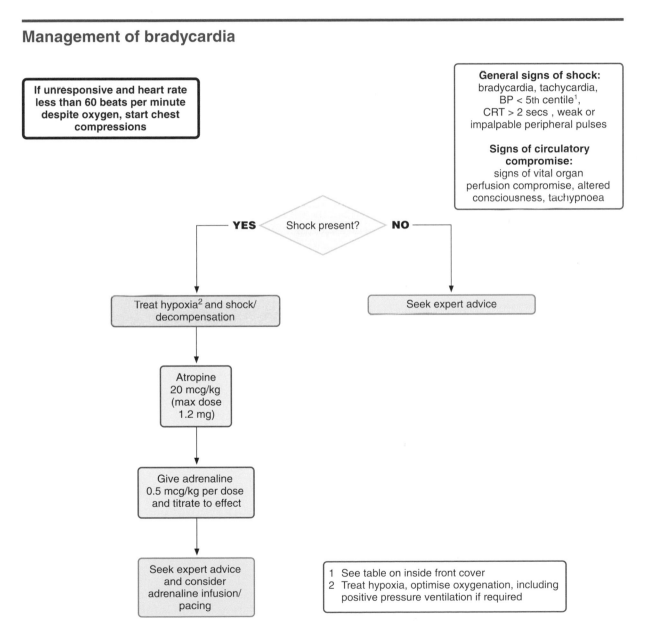

Figure 5.7 Management of bradycardia algorithm
BP, blood pressure; CRT, capillary refill time

If the bradycardia persists following treatment of hypoxia and shock then slowly titrate adrenaline up to 10 micrograms/kg IV/IO. If this is ineffective, consider an adrenaline infusion of 0.05–2 micrograms/kg/min IV/IO.

- In non-sinus bradycardias (e.g. complete heart block), consider giving atropine 20 micrograms/kg IV (maximum dose 1.2 mg). The dose may be repeated after 5 minutes (maximum total dose of 1 mg in a child and 2 mg in an adolescent)
- Consider transcutaneous pacing if the bradycardia is caused by atrioventricular block or abnormal atrioventricular node and arrange more definitive pacing system
- Consider use of isoprenaline infusion (0.02–0.2 micrograms/kg/min in neonates and 1 microgram/kg/min in non-neonatal age groups)
- If there has been *vagal stimulation*, remove the vagal stimulus if possible and stabilise airway and breathing. Atropine can be used at the doses discussed above
- If there has been *poisoning*, seek expert toxicology help
- If bradycardia is due to *raised ICP*, urgent action is needed (see Section 6.3)

Abnormal rhythm or pulse: tachyarrhythmia

Overview

Most tachycardia in children is sinus tachycardia. In infants this may be as high as up to 220 beats/min and in children up to 180 beats/min. Rates over these figures are highly likely to be tachyarrhythmias, but in case of any significant tachycardia (i.e. more than 200 beats/min in an infant and more than 150 beats/min in a child) an ECG rhythm strip should be examined and, if in doubt, a full 12-lead ECG performed.

Recognition of sinus tachycardia is of vital importance as this can be the first sign of critical illness. Causes of sinus tachycardia can include inadequate cardiac output states (e.g. cardiomyopathy, congenital heart diseases), high metabolic demand (e.g. sepsis), hypovolaemia (e.g. gastroenteritis, haemorrhage, third space fluid loss) or situations such as pain, anxiety or exercise.

Clues to suggest a non-sinus tachycardia on a rhythm strip include:

- Extreme tachycardia (more than 200 beats/min)
- Absent P waves, or P waves not before each QRS complex
- Very narrow or wide QRS complex
- Irregular rhythms
- Sudden and abrupt changes in heart rate
- No variability in heart rate when variability would be expected (e.g. child crying versus settled)
- Heart rate fixed despite interventions (e.g. trial of fluid bolus)

There are two main types of tachyarrhythmias to recognise: supraventricular tachycardia (SVT) and ventricular tachycardia (VT).

Approach to the child with supraventricular tachycardia

A SVT is the most common non-arrest arrhythmia during childhood and the most common arrhythmia that produces cardiovascular instability during infancy. SVT in infants generally produces a heart rate more than 220 beats/min, and sometimes much higher. Lower heart rates occur in older children during SVT. SVT is an umbrella term for many types of atrial arrhythmias.

Cardiopulmonary stability during episodes of SVT is affected by the child's age, duration of SVT, prior ventricular function and ventricular conduction rate. Older children can complain of light headedness, dizziness or chest discomfort or they note a racing heart rate. Very rapid rates may be undetected for long periods in young infants until they develop a low cardiac output state and cardiogenic shock. This deterioration occurs because of increased myocardial oxygen demand and limitation in myocardial oxygen delivery during the short diastolic phase associated with very rapid heart rates. The systemic cardiac output is reduced because the ventricular function deteriorates due to ischaemia, the short diastolic filling time reduces the ventricular volumes and the loss of atrioventricular synchrony removes the atrial component of the cardiac output. If baseline myocardial function is impaired (e.g. in a child with a cardiomyopathy), SVT can produce signs of shock in a relatively short time.

It is easy to mistake SVT for a significant sinus tachycardia and vice versa. Careful interpretation of the clinical situation must be undertaken to try and correctly identify which you are dealing with. The following characteristics may help distinguish sinus tachycardia from SVT (Figures 5.8 and 5.9):

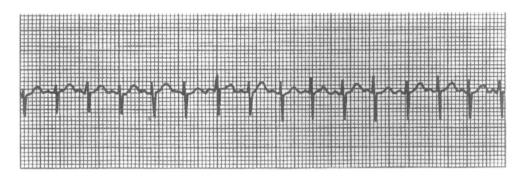

Figure 5.8 Rhythm strip of sinus tachycardia showing upright P waves before each QRS complex

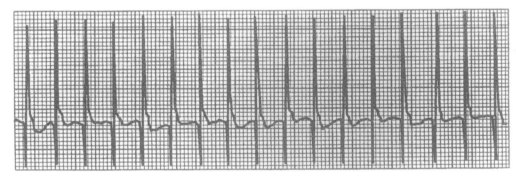

Figure 5.9 Rhythm strip of supraventricular tachycardia showing absent P waves, narrow complex QRS and extreme tachycardia

- *Look at the child's presenting complaint*: a history consistent with high fever or other causes of shock (e.g. gastroenteritis or sepsis) may suggest sinus tachycardia
- *Look at the pattern in heart rate*: SVT starts and ends abruptly, whereas sinus tachycardia changes more gradually
- *Look for heart rate variability*: in sinus tachycardia the heart rate varies from beat to beat and is often responsive to stimulation or interventions such as fluid bolus, but there is no beat-to-beat variability in SVT and the heart rate remains fixed
- *Look carefully for P waves* (they may be difficult to identify at faster heart rates even in sinus tachycardia). P waves in sinus rhythm should be seen before every QRS complex and should be upright in leads I, II, III and aVF and inverted in aVR. If the P waves are inverted in leads I, II, III and aVF then the options are: (i) the ECG leads are not correctly placed; (ii) the child has dextrocardia; or (iii) the child has a form of SVT. The paper speed of the ECG machine may need to be increased to make the identification of P waves easier.

Emergency treatment for SVT

Treatment for SVT should follow the appropriate algorithm (Figure 5.10).

It is important to ensure the child has continuous monitoring applied. IV or IO access should be obtained. Ensure the electrolytes have been checked, including magnesium.

Management of supraventricular tachycardia

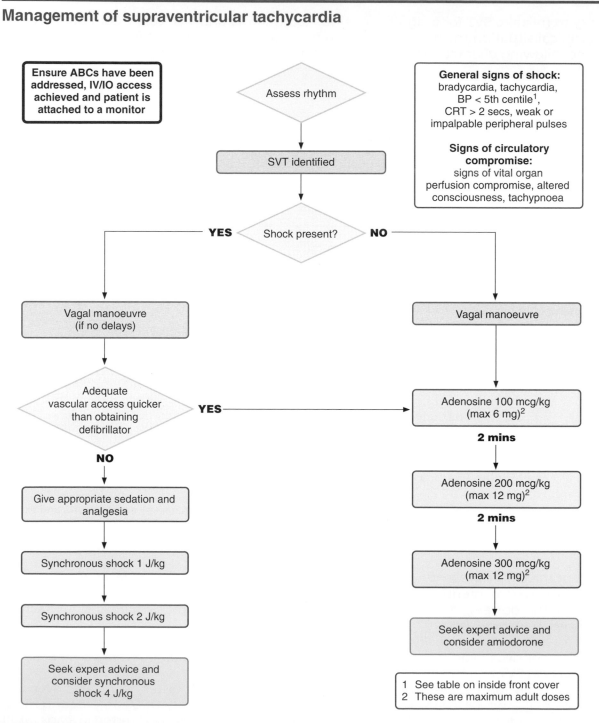

Figure 5.10 Management of supraventricular tachycardia algorithm
BP, blood pressure; CRT, capillary refill time

If the child is **not shocked**, then it is reasonable to consider a vagal manoeuvre whilst adenosine is being prepared. This can be achieved by:

- Eliciting the diving reflex to increase vagal tone by placing a glove with ice cold water over the face
- Performing a Valsalva manoeuvre in older children. This can be done by asking the child to blow into an empty syringe with the plunger pulled back or blowing hard through a straw. If able, ask the child to do a handstand and hold the position for 30 seconds
- Do not use ocular pressure in children because ocular damage may result

If these manoeuvres are unsuccessful or IV/IO access is available then use IV adenosine, which acts by blocking the atrioventricular node and breaking any abnormal electrical conduction pathways, or unmasking an arrhythmia that will require additional treatment. Adenosine has a very short half-life (less than 10 seconds) and is safe for use, even if the rhythm is not SVT. In fact, an adenosine trial can be helpful to distinguish sinus tachycardia from SVT. The only contraindication to adenosine is an irregularly irregular rhythm (incredibly rare in paediatric practice). During adenosine administration the side effects include flushing, nausea, dyspnoea and chest tightness and older children should be warned of this. Due to the short half-life, the side effects wear off quickly.

When giving adenosine, ensure the drug is injected rapidly into the largest possible vein available. Ensure continuous ECG monitoring is recording and printing the rhythm strip. Doses may need to be escalated:

- Start with a rapid bolus of 100 micrograms/kg (max. dose 6 mg)
- If success is not achieved then after 2 minutes use 200 micrograms/kg (max. dose 12 mg)
- If still unsuccesful then after another 2 minutes use 300 micrograms/kg (max. dose 12 mg)
- In older children 500 micrograms/kg may be required

If sinus rhythm is not obtained after adenosine, ensure it is SVT you are managing and not sinus tachycardia and consult your local paediatric critical care service. Some rhythms (e.g. atrial flutter) will require direct current (DC) cardioversion or additional antiarrhythmic medications.

If the child is **shocked** with SVT, do not delay adenosine if IV access is available. If this is not available then a *synchronous* DC shock of 1 J/kg should be delivered, followed by 2 J/kg up to a maximum of 4 J/kg. Ensure anaesthesia/intensive care are involved for appropriate sedation and support for the DC shock. Ventricular function may remain impaired even after successful DC cardioversion, so vasoactive support and intubation may be required. All these cases should be discussed with local paediatric critical care services.

Approach to the child with ventricular tachycardia with a pulse

Ventricular tachycardia is a less common tachyarrhythmia seen in children. It is recognised by a broad complex, rapid QRS with P waves absent or very difficult to see. It can be associated with cardiac arrest or severe haemodynamic instability. All cases should be discussed with your local paediatric critical care services.

VT can be caused by congenital heart disease and cardiac surgery, myocarditis or cardiomyopathy, poisoning with tricyclic antidepressants, procainamide or quinidine, renal disease or other causes of hyperkalaemia or channelopathies (e.g. long QT syndromes).

Torsade de pointes describes a specific type of polymorphic VT, with QRS complexes that change in amplitude and polarity so that they appear to rotate around an isoelectric line. This is seen in conditions characterised by a long QT interval or drug poisoning, such as with quinine, quinidine, disopyramide, amiodarone, tricyclic antidepressants or digoxin.

Sometimes, wide-complex tachycardia can be SVT with bundle branch block and aberrant conduction. This can be very difficult to differentiate from VT by a non-specialist. A dose of adenosine may help identify the underlying aetiology of the arrhythmia but should be used with extreme caution in haemodynamically stable children with wide-complex tachycardia because acceleration of the tachycardia and significant hypotension are known risks. This should not delay definitive treatment in children with shock. A safer approach is to treat it as VT. Seek early advice.

Management of ventricular tachycardia

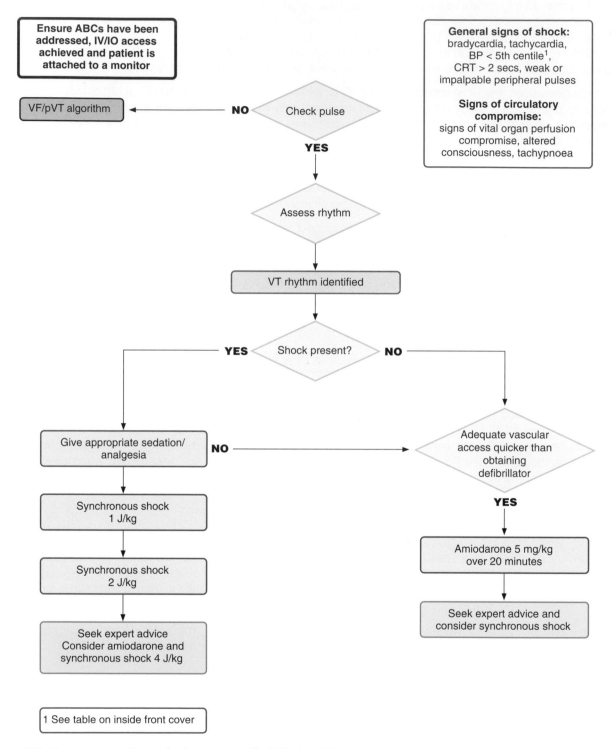

Ensure ABCs have been addressed, IV/IO access achieved and patient is attached to a monitor

General signs of shock: bradycardia, tachycardia, BP < 5th centile[1], CRT > 2 secs, weak or impalpable peripheral pulses

Signs of circulatory compromise: signs of vital organ perfusion compromise, altered consciousness, tachypnoea

VF/pVT algorithm ◄— **NO** — Check pulse

YES

Assess rhythm

VT rhythm identified

YES — Shock present? — **NO**

Give appropriate sedation/ analgesia — **NO** → Adequate vascular access quicker than obtaining defibrillator

YES

Synchronous shock 1 J/kg

Synchronous shock 2 J/kg

Amiodarone 5 mg/kg over 20 minutes

Seek expert advice Consider amiodarone and synchronous shock 4 J/kg

Seek expert advice and consider synchronous shock

1 See table on inside front cover

Figure 5.11 Management of ventricular tachycardia (VT) algorithm
BP, blood pressure; CRT, capillary refill time; pVT, pulseless ventricular tachycardia; VF, ventricular fibrillation

Emergency treatment for VT with a pulse

In the absence of a cardiac output, this is a shockable cardiac arrest and the algorithm for cardiac arrest for ventricular fibrillation/pulseless VT should be followed (see Chapter 18).

If there are any signs of cardiac output, then follow the algorithm for ventricular tachycardia (Figure 5.11). It is important not to delay treatment in VT as the rhythm often deteriorates quite quickly into pulseless VT or ventricular fibrillation.

Ensure IV/IO access is obtained, and electrolytes are checked, including magnesium.

- In the **shocked** child, the treatment is *synchronised* DC cardioversion starting at 1 J/kg, followed by 2 J/kg up to a maximum of 4 J/kg if needed. Ensure anaesthesia/intensive care are involved for appropriate sedation and support for the DC shock, as in these children the ventricular function may still be reduced after DC cardioversion. All these cases should be discussed with your local paediatric critical care service
- If the child with VT is **not shocked**, then early consultation with paediatric critical care services and paediatric cardiology are mandatory. They may suggest amiodarone (5 mg/kg over 20 minutes) that may then need to be followed by a continuous infusion of 5–20 micrograms/kg/min. Other antiarrhythmic drugs may be used.
- Many antiarrhythmic drugs can cause hypotension, which should be treated appropriately
- The use of magnesium sulphate as an IV infusion of 25–50 mg/kg (up to 2 g) is helpful in VT, especially when it is due to torsade de pointes
- In catecholamine-driven VT, IV β-blockers may help calm the adrenergic storm, but this should only be used after discussion with local paediatric critical care services

5.15   After resuscitation and emergency treatment of shock

Following successful restoration of adequate circulation, varying degrees of organ dysfunction may remain, and should be actively sought and managed. The problems are similar but of a lesser degree than those expected following resuscitation from arrest. Thus, after the initial resuscitation and emergency treatment, the child should have a review of ABCDE, as well as a full systems review to ensure stabilisation for safe and effective transfer (see Chapter 23).

5.16   Use of fluids in resuscitation

Which fluid?

For paediatric fluid resuscitation three types of fluid are available:

1. Isotonic crystalloids:
   - 0.9% sodium chloride solution (this can result in hyperchloraemic acidosis)
   - Balanced solutions like Ringer's lactate or Plasma-Lyte (electrolyte composition similar to extracellular fluid)
2. Colloids:
   - Human albumin 4% solution is usually available for fluid resuscitation while 20% is used as a replacement
   - Synthetic colloids become less available but are still used in some countries
3. Blood products:
   - Packed red cells
   - Fresh frozen plasma
   - Cryoprecipitate
   - Platelets
   - Whole blood

Outside trauma there is no conclusive evidence about any benefit of one fluid over the other.

However, there seems to be a consensus on common practice. Fluid resuscitation is started preferably with a balanced crystalloid or, if not readily available, 0.9% sodium chloride. When large volumes of crystalloid are used there is the potential detrimental effect of haemodilution and tissue oedema. In this case, the use of colloids like albumin can be considered. Colloids are suspensions of larger molecules and may provide swifter and more sustained volume expansion of the intravascular space. This is controversial and potential risks of colloids include allergic reactions and renal failure. Packed red cells or clotting products might be used if the haemoglobin is low or there is evidence of coagulopathy. Intravenous fluid resuscitation is difficult to fully protocolise and patient-tailored therapy is appropriate. Consultation with the regional paediatric critical care service can help. Remember that IV fluids (both bolus and maintenance) are drugs: they should be prescribed for the right indication, at the right dose, via the right route and at the right speed/interval.

If blood is needed, a full crossmatch should be undertaken, which takes about 1 hour to perform. For urgent need, type-specific non-crossmatched blood (which is ABO rhesus compatible but has a higher incidence of transfusion reactions) takes about 15 minutes to prepare. In dire emergencies O-negative blood must be given.

How much fluid?

The volume of fluid needed will depend on clinical assessment, and the clinical situation also dictates the rapidity with which boluses are given. Although life-saving capacities of fluid resuscitation are well known, the evidence that fluid overload can be detrimental has become evident in recent literature. So if large volumes are needed, resuscitation is best guided by advanced haemodynamic monitoring such as measurement of the central venous pressure, invasive blood pressure, urine output and/or POCUS. Children requiring large-volume resuscitation need early involvement from and transfer to a paediatric critical care unit. When large volumes are used, fluids should be warmed.

In conclusion, there is no definitive evidence demonstrating which fluid is best for resuscitation. Other important questions about how much and when fluids should be used also remain to be answered. Clinical trials are underway to answer these questions, although they are unlikely to provide simple answers. At present, optimal management should be guided by knowledge of the pathophysiology underlying the disease, and of the different roles of the different fluids.

5.17   Summary

This chapter has discussed how the structured approach should be used in the assessment and management of the child with circulatory failure. Specific conditions and their management have been looked at in greater depth.

CHAPTER 6

Decreased conscious level (with or without seizures)

Learning outcomes

After reading this chapter, you will be able to:

- List the causes of decreased conscious level in infants and children
- Describe the pathophysiology and management of raised intracranial pressure
- Describe how to assess a child with a decreased conscious level
- Describe how to resuscitate a child with a decreased conscious level
- Describe how to assess and treat a child presenting with seizures

---

6.1 Introduction

The conscious level may be altered by disease, injury or intoxication, as well as by cerebral hypoxia or hypoperfusion due to respiratory or circulatory failure. The level of awareness decreases as a child passes through stages from drowsiness (mild reduction in alertness and increase in hours of sleep) to unconsciousness (unrousable, unresponsive).

Because of variability in the definition of words describing the degree of conscious level, the Glasgow Coma Scale (GCS) and the Children's Glasgow Coma Scale (Table 6.1) have been developed as semi-quantitative measures and, more importantly, as an aid to communication between carers. The GCS was developed and validated for use in the head-injured patient but has come to be used as an unvalidated tool for the description of conscious states from all pathologies. Coma occurs when a child is unconscious and unresponsive to painful stimuli and equates to a GCS of 3–8. It represents an acute, life-threatening emergency that requires prompt action to prevent both life-long neurological morbidity and mortality.

In children, causes of coma are either traumatic or non-traumatic. The most common aetiologies are summarised in Box 6.1, with infection being the overall leading cause in all ages.

Children with a decreased conscious level are usually presented by parents who are very aware of the seriousness of the symptom. They may also have noted other features such as fever, headache or exposure to poisoning, which may aid the clinician in making a presumptive diagnosis. In children with neurodevelopmental delay, parents can provide vital information about the child's usual level of responsiveness; deviation from this baseline should be taken as a sign of reduced conscious level.

Advanced Paediatric Life Support: A Practical Approach to Emergencies, Seventh Edition. Edited by Stephanie Smith.
© 2023 John Wiley & Sons Ltd. Published 2023 by John Wiley & Sons Ltd.

Table 6.1 Glasgow Coma Scale and Children's Glasgow Coma Scale

Glasgow Coma Scale (4–15 years)		Children's Glasgow Coma Scale (less than 4 years)	
Response	Score	**Response**	Score
Eye opening		**Eye opening**	
Spontaneously	4	Spontaneously	4
To verbal stimuli	3	To verbal stimuli	3
To pain	2	To pain	2
No response to pain	1	No response to pain	1
Best verbal response		**Best verbal response**	
Orientated and converses	5	Alert, babbles, coos words to usual ability	5
Disorientated and converses	4	Less than usual words, spontaneous irritable cry	4
Inappropriate words	3	Cries only to pain	3
Incomprehensible sounds	2	Moans to pain	2
No response to pain	1	No response to pain	1
Best motor response		**Best motor response**	
Obeys verbal command	6	Spontaneous or obeys verbal command	6
Localises to pain	5	Localises to pain or withdraws to touch	5
Withdraws from pain	4	Withdraws from pain	4
Abnormal flexion to pain (decorticate)	3	Abnormal flexion to pain (decorticate)	3
Abnormal extension to pain (decerebrate)	2	Abnormal extension to pain (decerebrate)	2
No response to pain	1	No response to pain	1

Box 6.1 Disorders causing reduced conscious level in children

- Hypoxic ischaemic brain injury following respiratory or circulatory failure
- Epileptic seizures
- Trauma:
  - intracranial haemorrhage
  - brain swelling
- Infections:
  - sepsis
  - meningitis
  - encephalitis
  - cerebral and extracerebral abscesses
  - malaria
- Intoxication:
  - alcohol
  - drugs, including accidental ingestion
- Metabolic:
  - renal or hepatic failure
  - hypo- or hypernatraemia
  - hypoglycaemia
  - hypothermia
  - hypo- or hypercapnia
  - inborn errors of metabolism
  - hyperammonaemia
- Cerebral tumour
- Stroke or cerebrovascular event (haemorrhagic or ischaemic)
- Cerebral venous sinus thrombosis
- Hydrocephalus, including blocked intraventricular shunts

6.2   Primary survey and resuscitation

ABCDE

The first steps in the management of the child with a decreased conscious level are to assess and, if necessary, support airway, breathing and circulation. This will ensure that the diminished conscious level is not secondary to hypoxia and/or ischaemia and that whatever the cerebral pathology, it will not be worsened by a lack of oxygenated blood supply to the brain.

Follow the algorithm for coma (Figure 6.1).

Initial management of coma

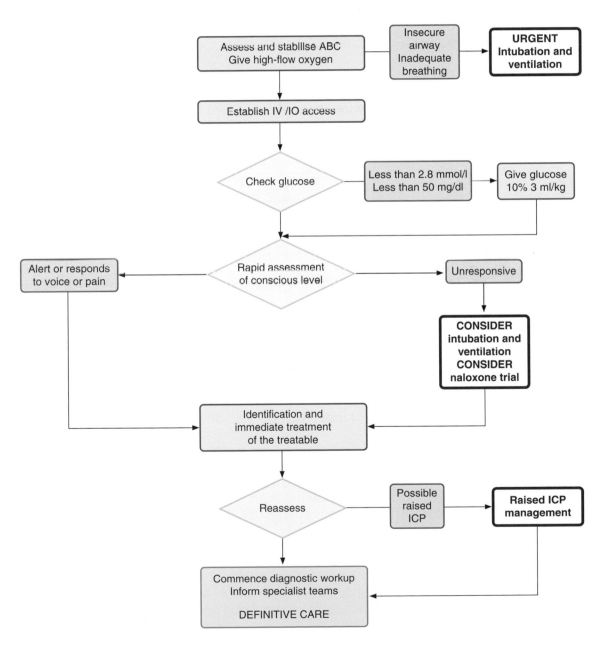

Figure 6.1 Initial management of coma algorithm
ICP, intracranial pressure

Features specific for child with decreased conscious level

Airway

- Ensure the airway is open. Assess the need for airway-opening manoeuvres, airway adjuncts or intubation to secure the airway
- If the child has an AVPU score of 'P' or 'U' or the gag or cough reflex is absent, then the airway is at risk. It should be maintained by an airway manoeuvre or adjunct, and preparations for intubation made as soon as possible

Breathing

- Assess if breathing is adequate and provide appropriate respiratory support
- Some causes of coma may also affect breathing patterns. For example, acidotic sighing respirations may suggest metabolic acidosis from diabetes, an inborn error of metabolism or salicylate/ethylene glycol poisoning

Resuscitation

- All children with a decreased conscious level should receive high-flow oxygen through a face mask with a reservoir or high-flow nasal cannula
- If the child is hypoventilating, respiration should be supported with oxygen via a bag–valve–mask device while preparations are made for intubation and ventilation. Inadequate breathing in coma can lead to a rise in arterial PCO_2, which can cause a dangerous rise in intracranial pressure (ICP)

Circulation

- Hypertension and/or bradycardia indicate critically raised ICP, until proven otherwise. Conversely hypotension and/or tachycardia indicate shock

Resuscitation

- Establish IV/IO access quickly
- Take a blood gas, look at the glucose and send blood urgently for an ammonia level. Correct hypoglycaemia (less than 2.8 mmol/l or 50 mg/dl) with a 3 ml/kg bolus of 10% glucose. Note that if a metabolic condition is suspected, subsequent maintenance rates of 8 mg/kg/min of glucose may be required
- If hypoglycaemia is a new condition for the child, send blood to the laboratory for plasma to be frozen for specific hypoglycaemia investigations as per local protocol. This will allow later investigation of the cause of the hypoglycaemic state. The blood should be taken on initial cannulation before administering glucose but do not delay correcting hypoglycaemia with further attempts
- Blood should also be sent for urea and electrolytes (U&E), liver function test (LFT), full blood count (FBC) and blood culture
- Give a broad-spectrum intravenous antibiotic such as cefotaxime or ceftriaxone. Consider adding amoxicillin to cover *Listeria*. Aciclovir should be given to cover herpes simplex encephalitis if central nervous system infection is suspected. If meningitis is suspected, also consider giving dexamethasone
- Reverse shock with 10 ml/kg boluses of isotonic crystalloid. Reassess and repeat only if fluid responsive
- Vasopressors (noradrenaline, metaraminol, phenylephrine) may be required to maintain blood pressure at a level to ensure cerebral perfusion pressure of 40–60 mmHg, especially if there are concerns about raised ICP. To start, all can temporarily be given through a peripheral vein when a diluted solution is used

Disability

- Abnormal tonic posturing might suggest raised ICP presenting as decerebrate posturing and may be mistaken for seizure activity
- Look for evidence of seizure activity (subtle findings may include fixed eye deviation and nystagmus)
- Look for neck stiffness in a child and a full or tense fontanelle in an infant, which suggest meningitis
- A purpuric rash suggests meningococcal/streptococcal sepsis
- Petechiae or bruising might point to trauma, non-accidental injury or coagulopathy
- Fever is suggestive evidence of an infectious cause (but its absence does not exclude it) or poisoning with ecstasy, cocaine or salicylates. Hypothermia suggests poisoning with barbiturates or ethanol
- Look for evidence of poisoning: history or characteristic smell (see Appendix F)
- Acute focal neurological deficit (e.g. motor weakness, facial palsy) or speech disturbance suggest potential stroke
- Consider a metabolic cause particularly if a prolonged period of poor caloric intake preceded the illness

Resuscitation

- Manage the causes identified above, aiming to reduce secondary insult due to hypoxia or hypoglycaemia

There should be a specific assessment for raised ICP. A history taken from parents might contain evidence of preceding symptoms. The symptoms and signs in Box 6.2 are suggestive of raised ICP. In infants there may be a bulging fontanelle, an increase in head circumference and a high-pitched cry.

Box 6.2 Symptoms and signs of raised intracranial pressure

- Headache (often worse in the morning or on waking the child from sleep)
- Persistent vomiting or history of early morning vomiting
- Seizures
- Abnormal posturing (see Figure 3.4)
- Reduced visual acuity
- Pupillary reaction to light impaired or lost
- Pupillary dilatation, unilateral or bilateral
- Sixth nerve palsy, as a false localising sign
- Hypertension and bradycardia, which together with rapid, irregular breathing form 'Cushing's triad'. This is a late, pre-terminal sign
- Papilloedema, not always present in the acute phase

6.3   Pathophysiology of raised intracranial pressure

Children with a closed fontanelle have a fixed volume cranium, meaning an expansion of intracranial contents due to brain swelling, haematoma or cerebrospinal fluid (CSF) blockage will cause raised ICP. In very young children, before the cranial sutures are closed, considerable intracranial volume expansion may occur if the disease process is slow (e.g. hydrocephalus), but raised ICP can still develop quickly if the process is rapid.

Initially, CSF and venous blood within the cranium decrease in volume. Soon, this compensating mechanism fails and as the ICP continues to rise the cerebral perfusion pressure (CPP) falls and the cerebral arterial blood flow is reduced. CPP is defined as mean arterial pressure (MAP) minus ICP:

$$CPP = MAP - ICP$$

Reduced CPP reduces cerebral blood flow, leading to secondary injury caused by cerebral ischaemia. The aim is to keep CPP above 40–60 mmHg, with infants at the lower end and adolescents at the upper end of this range. In the absence of direct ICP monitoring, an ICP of at least 20 mmHg can be used to calculate the MAP target to maintain CPP.

Increasing ICP will push brain tissue against more rigid intracranial structures. A brain herniation can be classified by where the brain tissue has shifted (Figure 6.2).

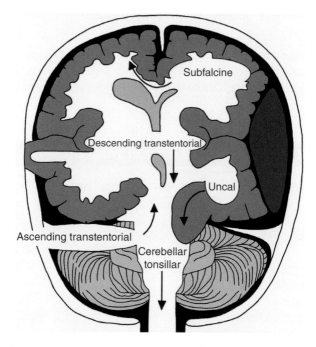

Figure 6.2 Herniations of the brain

1. **Subfalcine.** The brain tissue moves underneath the falx cerebri in the middle of the brain. Brain tissue ends up being pushed across to the other side.
2. **Transtentorial:**
   - **Descending or uncal.** The intracranial volume increase is mainly in the supratentorial part of the intracranial space. The uncus, which is part of the hippocampal gyrus, is forced through the tentorial opening and compressed against the fixed free edge of the tentorium. If the pressure is unilateral (e.g. from a subdural or extradural haematoma), this leads to third nerve compression and an ipsilateral dilated pupil. Next, an external oculomotor palsy appears, and the eye appears deviated 'down and out' and there may be a ptosis. Hemiplegia may then develop on either or both sides of the body, depending on the progression of the herniation
   - **Ascending.** The cerebellum and the brain stem move upward through a notch in a membrane called the tentorium cerebelli

3. **Cerebellar tonsillar.** The whole brain is pressed down towards the foramen magnum and the cerebellar tonsils herniate through it ('coning'). Neck stiffness may be noted. A slow pulse, raised blood pressure and irregular respiration leading to apnoea are seen terminally, usually preceded by significant tachycardia. The presence of hypertension and bradycardia are late signs of raised ICP; their absence should not be taken to mean that the ICP is normal.

It is important to note that there is a widely held misconception that critically rising ICP is always accompanied by a progressive deterioration in conscious level. In fact, a GCS of 15 can be maintained right up until the point of brain-stem herniation and should not be considered reassuring in children with signs and symptoms of critically raised ICP. Immediate medical control of ICP, diagnostic imaging and definitive treatment are required in these circumstances.

6.4   Management of raised intracranial pressure

Management of raised ICP is a time-critical emergency. A full paediatric emergency team should be assembled, and the following actions taken immediately. These actions are collectively referred to as 'neuroprotection'.

- Intubate and ventilate. Initially target normal oxygen saturations and maintain end-tidal carbon dioxide (CO_2) at 3.5–4 kPa (26–30 mmHg), equivalent to $PaCO_2$ 4–4.5 kPa (30–34 mmHg)
- Deeply sedate and fully muscle relax to reduce ICP and cerebral oxygen demand
- Treat seizures to reduce cerebral oxygen demand
- Manage 20° head up
- Give 3% sodium chloride in 3–5 ml/kg boluses IV/IO over 10 minutes
- Mannitol may be used as an alternative if sodium chloride is not available (0.25–0.5 g/kg; i.e. 1.25–2.5 ml/kg of 20% solution IV over 15 minutes)
- Maintain blood pressure at a level to ensure CPP of 40–60 mmHg
- Arrange an urgent computed tomography (CT) scan of the head and contact the neurosurgical centre and the paediatric critical care unit (PCCU)

6.5   Lumbar puncture

Lumbar puncture should not be performed acutely in a child presenting with altered conscious level or signs or symptoms of raised ICP.

There is no benefit in performing an acute lumbar puncture, which carries the risk of coning and death if it is performed in a child with significantly raised ICP. Normal fundi or a normal CT scan do not exclude raised ICP. Treatment for meningoencephalitis should be commenced without delay when infection is part of the differential diagnosis. A blood culture should be taken. If it is considered important, a lumbar puncture can be performed later in the clinical course, when it is safe to do so and polymerase chain reaction (PCR) tests used to look for evidence of specific bacterial or viral infection.

When to defer lumbar puncture

Defer preforming a lumbar puncture if the child has:

- Signs of raised intracranial pressure (see Box 6.2)
- A reduced or deteriorating GCS score
- Focal neurological signs
- Had a prolonged seizure
- Shock
- Clinical evidence of meningococcal/streptococcal sepsis
- A CT or MRI scan suggesting blockage or impairment of the cerebrospinal fluid pathways, e.g. by blood, pus, tumour or coning
- Coagulopathy

From RCPCH (2019)

6.6 Secondary survey and looking for key features

While the primary survey and resuscitation are being carried out, a focused history should be taken of the child's health and activity over the previous 24 hours and of any significant previous illnesses. In a child in a coma, it is often impossible to be certain of the diagnosis in the first hour and so the focus should be on resuscitation and stabilisation while looking for and treating reversible causes.

Specific points for history taking include:

- Recent trauma
- Pre-existing neurological disability
- History of epilepsy
- Poison ingestion: specifically enquire about medicine/agents that the child might have been exposed to
- Known chronic condition (e.g. renal disease, cardiac abnormality, diabetes)
- Known metabolic disorder or family history of one
- Previous episodes of encephalopathy with illness
- Recent foreign travel
- Ear or paranasal sinus infection

Specific additional neurological examination includes:

- Eye examination:
  - Pupil size (may be subjective) and reactivity (Table 6.2)
  - Fundal changes: haemorrhage and papilloedema (trauma, hypertension)
  - Ophthalmoplegia: lateral or vertical deviation
- Reassess posture, tone and power: look for lateralisation
- Assess deep tendon reflexes and plantar responses and look for lateralisation
- Assess for facial palsy or speech disturbance

Table 6.2 Summary of pupillary changes

Pupil size and reactivity	Potential causes
Small reactive pupils	Metabolic disorders, medullary lesion
Pinpoint pupils	Narcotic/organophosphate ingestions, metabolic disorders
Fixed mid-size pupils	Midbrain lesion
Fixed dilated pupils	Hypothermia, severe hypoxia, brain-stem herniation, barbiturates (late sign), during and post seizure, anticholinergic drugs, recent administration of high-dose adrenaline
Unilateral dilated pupil	Rapidly expanding ipsilateral lesion, tentorial herniation, third nerve lesion, epileptic seizures

Lateralisation suggests a localised rather than a generalised lesion, but this is often a false indicator in childhood. The child will need urgent CT or magnetic resonance imaging (MRI) scan for further evaluation.

A general physical examination may add clues to point to a working diagnosis. Specific findings include the following:

- Skin: rash, haemorrhage, trauma and evidence of neurocutaneous syndromes
- Scalp: evidence of trauma
- Ears and nose:
  - Bloody or clear discharge from a base of skull fracture (see Chapter 11)
  - Evidence of otitis media or mastoiditis: can point to meningitis
- Neck tenderness or rigidity: meningitis or cerebrovascular accident
- Odour: alcohol intoxication, ketones in diabetic ketoacidosis or metabolic disorders
- Abdomen: enlarged liver may indicate inherited metabolic disease

The key features, which will be identified clinically, from the history, examination and the initial blood test results, can point the clinician to the likeliest working diagnosis for emergency treatment.

- Coma that develops over several hours, associated with irritability and/or fever and a rash points to meningitis/encephalitis
- A history of drug or poison ingestion and pinpoint pupils point to poisoning with opiates
- Coma occurring in the setting of, or just after, a minor illness presenting with vomiting, hepatomegaly and hypoglycaemia points to metabolic encephalopathy
- A history of travel to a malaria endemic country and splenomegaly might point to malaria
- Coma associated with significant hypertension points to hypertensive encephalopathy
- A vague and inconsistent history and/or suspicious bruising in an infant are suggestive of non-accidental head injury; the presence of retinal haemorrhage is supportive evidence of this
- Hyperglycaemia points to diabetes
- A history of very sudden onset of coma, sometimes with a preceding headache, points to an intracerebral bleed. Speech disturbance or focal deficit might suggest ischaemic stroke

Note that unless meningitis can be excluded by the clear identification of another cause for coma, antibiotics should be given. The consequence of a missed diagnosis is catastrophic and the risk of unnecessary treatment with antibiotics small. This also applies to meningoencephalitis from *Mycoplasma* and herpes, and the use of a macrolide (e.g. azithromycin or erythromycin) and aciclovir, respectively. Early initiation of treatment is important because these have a worse prognosis when treatment is seriously delayed. Senior advice should be sought.

6.7 Approach to the child with meningitis/encephalitis

After the neonatal period, the two most common causes of bacterial meningitis are *Streptococcus pneumoniae and Neisseria meningitidis* (meningococcus). There is still a mortality rate of around 5% and a similar rate of permanent serious sequelae. Infection with *S. pneumoniae* may follow an upper respiratory tract infection with or without otitis media. Long-term morbidity and mortality occur in up to 30% of cases. Widespread Hib vaccination has reduced the incidence of *Haemophilus influenzae* infection. Pneumococcal and meningococcus B vaccines are now part of the childhood immunisation schedule in most countries. A history of weight loss, contact, fever and slow onset of meningeal signs suggests tuberculous meningitis.

For infants presenting at under 1 month of age, the most common causes of bacterial meningitis are group B *Streptococcus* and *Escherichia coli*. This may present some time after delivery, and lead to readmission.

A wide range of infections may also cause encephalitis. The most common viral infection, in infants particularly, is herpes simplex.

Diagnosis of bacterial meningitis

In children of 3 years and under

Bacterial meningitis is difficult to diagnose in its early stages in this age group. The classic signs of neck rigidity, photophobia, headache and vomiting are often absent. A bulging fontanelle is a sign of advanced meningitis in an infant, but even this serious and late sign will be masked if the baby is dehydrated from fever and vomiting. Almost all children with meningitis have some degree of raised ICP, so that, in fact, the signs and symptoms of meningitis are primarily those of raised ICP. The following are signs of possible meningitis in infants and young children:

- Coma
- Drowsiness (often shown by lack of eye contact with parents or doctor)
- High-pitched cry or irritability that cannot be easily soothed by parent
- Poor feeding
- Unexplained pyrexia
- Convulsions with or without fever
- Apnoeic or cyanotic attacks
- Purpuric rash

In children of 4 years and over

These children are more likely to have the classic signs of headache, vomiting, pyrexia, neck stiffness and photophobia. Some present with coma or convulsions. In all unwell children, and children with fever without an apparent source, a careful search should be made for neck stiffness and for a purpuric rash. The finding of such a rash in an ill child is indicative of meningococcal or other bacterial sepsis, for which immediate treatment is required (see Chapter 5).

Emergency treatment of meningitis

Reassess ABCDE

- Specific assessment should be made of the severity of raised ICP, as many of the clinical signs of meningitis arise from this
- Give IV ceftriaxone or cefotaxime (child under 3 months) or another suitable antibiotic if meningitis cannot be excluded and this has not yet been given. Empirically treat a child with raised ICP and meningitis, and defer or do not perform a lumbar puncture. Ensure blood cultures and PCR have been taken, as these may help in the diagnosis
- Treat a febrile child with reduced conscious level or focal neurology with aciclovir and a macrolide to cover herpes simplex virus and *Mycoplasma* encephalitis

It is generally recommended that dexamethasone be administered before or with the first dose of antibiotics and no more than 6 hours later, when bacterial meningitis is confirmed or strongly suspected to reduce the rate of severe hearing loss and other long-term neurological sequelae (150 micrograms/kg up to a max. of 10 mg four times a day).

6.8 Approach to the child poisoned with opiates

These children have usually accidentally ingested oral opioids such as methadone, oxycodone or oramorph. The sedative effect of the drug may reduce the conscious level sufficiently to put the airway at risk and cause hypoventilation.

Emergency treatment of opiate poisoning

Reassess ABCDE

Following stabilisation of the airway, breathing and circulation, the specific antidote is naloxone, with rapid titration to reverse potential life-threatening effects, starting with an initial bolus dose of 100 micrograms/kg IV in children under 12 years. If there is no response, repeat the dose at intervals of 1 minute to the maximum dose of 2 mg, then review the diagnosis. In children over 12 years, the initial dose is 400 micrograms, then 800 micrograms for up to two doses at 1 minute intervals, then one dose of 2 mg if there is still no response. Naloxone has a short half-life, relapse often occurring after 20 minutes. Further boluses, or an infusion of 5–20 micrograms/kg/min, may be required. For older children, intranasal is an alternative route for delivery (1 spray = 1.8 mg).

Adverse events such as ventricular arrhythmias, acute pulmonary oedema, asystole or seizures have incidentally been described, due to the sudden rise in catecholamine (pro-arrhythmogenic) or central neurogenetic responses to narcotic reversal. Assess ABCDE and prepare for resuscitative measures prior to naloxone administration.

6.9 Approach to the child with metabolic coma

The most common metabolic disorders that can result in encephalopathy are hypoglycaemia and diabetic ketoacidosis (see Appendix B). Diabetic ketoacidosis can be associated with cerebral oedema and cerebral venous sinus thrombosis. Nevertheless, metabolic coma can arise from a variety of conditions, including a number of rare, inborn errors of metabolism. These illnesses often present with a rapidly progressive encephalopathy, vomiting, drowsiness and convulsions or coma. There may be associated hepatomegaly, hypoglycaemia, abnormal liver enzymes and/or hyperammonaemia. In a case of otherwise unexplained decreased consciousness, a key urgent investigation is a plasma ammonia, particularly in infants. Ideally, the plasma ammonia sample should be sent rapidly on ice for the most accurate measurement. Interpretation of the concentration can be difficult, as can specific treatment of the hyperammonaemia. Seek advice from a specialist in inherited metabolic disease and the PCCU, as children with hyperammonaemia may need urgent transfer for renal replacement therapy to reduce the ammonia level. Sodium benzoate and sodium phenylbutyrate infusions should be used as the ammonia scavenging agent in the first instance. Carglumic acid can also be used. Encephalopathy secondary to hyperammonaemia commonly presents in the neonatal period but can occur even as late as adulthood.

6.10 Approach to the child with malaria

Plasmodium falciparum causes 95% of deaths and the most severe complications in children with malaria. It is transmitted by the bite of an infected *Anopheles* mosquito, and less commonly by infected blood transfusion, needle stick injuries or by the transplacental route.

The clinical features of severe disease include reduced conscious level, convulsions, metabolic acidosis, hypoglycaemia and severe normocytic anaemia. Cerebral malaria may produce encephalopathy, rapid-onset coma and raised ICP. Diagnosis requires microscopy of a thick film (quick diagnosis) and thin film (species identification). Rapid diagnostic tests also have a high sensitivity and specificity, but always need to be followed by a thick smear. Obtain a complete history, including the likely country or region of origination and get expert advice.

Specific emergency treatment of cerebral malaria

Reassess ABCDE

- Artesunate IV/IO (3 mg/kg if the child weighs less than 20 kg, 2.4 mg/kg if more than 20 kg) is the recommended treatment for severe *P. falciparum* malaria. It is given on admission, then exactly at 12 and 24 hours, then once a day, to get the parasitaemia down as soon as possible in the first 24 hours. Monitor cytology since there is a risk of haemolysis. Consider adding clindamycin when the mortality risk is high (parasitaemia more than 10% or severely ill) after discussion with a specialist. Complete the treatment with artemisinin combined treatment orally, after at least three doses of artesunate IV if the child is clinically better. IV quinine is only an acceptable alternative if artesunate is not available (loading dose 20 mg/kg over 4 hours in glucose 5%, then 10 mg/kg every 8 hours). Use electrocardiogram (ECG) monitoring during administration. Do not give quinine in bolus because of the risk of severe arrhythmia/hypotension. In renal/hepatic failure, reduce the quinine dose by a third after 48 hours. After at least 24 hours or when clinically well enough to switch to oral medication, complete by enteral treatment
- Consider IV antibiotics (e.g. cefotaxime) since the risk of concomitant bacterial (especially Gram-negative) infections is high in children
- Monitor and treat hypoglycaemia as needed
- If there is evidence of life-threatening anaemia (haemoglobin less than 5 g/dl) consider transfusion, especially if there are signs of heart failure. Be cautious with fluid administration, reduce maintenance to 70% of normal and beware fluid overload and cerebral oedema

6.11 Approach to the child presenting with stroke

Stroke is an important childhood disorder, leading to significant mortality and morbidity. However, the condition is often missed due to a low index of suspicion, leading to delayed diagnosis. Better recognition of childhood stroke can facilitate early imaging, assessment and intervention, leading to better outcomes.

Identification of potential stroke

Signs of stroke in children include:

- Acute focal neurological deficit
- Speech disturbance
- Unexplained change in conscious level (GCS of less than 12)

Stroke should also be considered in children with:

- New-onset focal seizures
- New-onset severe headache
- Ataxia
- Vertigo
- Resolved acute focal neurological deficit of unknown cause

Initial management and investigation of suspected stroke

- As with any child with neurological concerns, the priority is to perform a rapid ABCDE assessment and quickly reverse any compromise to airway, breathing and circulation that poses an immediate risk to life. This includes urgent intubation and ventilation if the GCS is less than 8, if the child's airway is not being maintained or if there is suspicion of raised ICP
- Obtain intravenous access and send blood tests for FBC, U&E, LFT, C-reactive protein (CRP), coagulation screen, glucose, blood gas analysis, blood cultures and group and save
- Record time of symptom onset and assess neurological deficit using the PedNIHSS (Paediatric National Institute of Health Stroke Scale) score (https://www.mdcalc.com/calc/10270/pediatric-nih-stroke-scale-nihss, last accessed January 2023) to determine suitability for potential thrombolysis
- Arrange urgent brain imaging. A CT scan **with angiography** (CTA) should be performed within 1 hour of admission to facilitate potential thrombolysis. MRI with stroke-specific sequences may be performed in children in whom there is diagnostic uncertainty after the CT scan; this should be discussed with specialist paediatric neurology services

Management of confirmed stroke

All children with confirmed stroke should be urgently discussed with local paediatric neurology and/or critical care specialists to guide further management. Treatment may need to be initiated locally, but children should subsequently be transferred to a centre with paediatric neurology and critical care expertise on site.

Haemorrhagic stroke

Children with haemorrhagic stroke should be urgently discussed with local paediatric critical care and/or neurosurgical teams and will usually require time-critical transfer for neurosurgical intervention.

Arterial ischaemic stroke

Children with confirmed arterial ischaemic stroke should be considered for emergency intervention, including thrombolysis, thrombectomy or decompressive craniectomy.

Thrombolysis can be considered in children over 2 years old in whom all of the following are true, and if there are no contraindications:

- PedNIHSS score between 4 and 24
- Thrombolysis can be administered within 4.5 hours of symptom onset
- CT has excluded intracranial haemorrhage
- CT demonstrates normal brain parenchyma or minimal early ischaemic change
- CTA demonstrates partial/complete occlusion of the intracranial artery corresponding to the clinical/radiological deficit *or* MRI and magnetic resonance angiography (MRA) show evidence of acute ischaemia on diffusion weighted imaging and partial/complete occlusion of the intracranial artery corresponding to the clinical/radiological deficit

Local protocols and specialist advice should be sought before initiating thrombolysis.

If thrombolysis is not indicated, and there is no evidence of parenchymal haemorrhage, the administration of aspirin (5 mg/kg PO/NG) or anticoagulation should be considered.

Thrombectomy may be considered up to 12 hours after symptom onset (including prior thrombolysis) in children with a PedNIHSS score of more than 6 and favourable brain imaging; this should be discussed by paediatric neurology and interventional radiology specialists.

Decompressive craniectomy may be required in children with vascular infarction caused by stroke and signs of raised ICP or deteriorating conscious level. These children should have immediate raised ICP management as discussed earlier and urgent discussion with neurosurgery.

6.12 Approach to the child with systemic hypertensive crisis

Hypertension is uncommon in children. Renal disorders such as dysplastic kidneys, reflux nephropathy or glomerulonephritis account for most children presenting with severe hypertension. Coarctation of the aorta is another important cause. Blood pressure is rarely measured routinely in otherwise healthy children and therefore hypertension usually presents with symptoms that may be diverse in nature. Neurological symptoms are more common in children than in adults. There may be a history of severe headaches, with or without vomiting. Children may also present acutely with convulsions or in a coma. Some children will present with a facial palsy or hemiplegia, and small babies may even present with apnoea or cardiac failure. Any child presenting with hypertension and neurological signs or symptoms should be assumed to have critically raised ICP and treated accordingly until proven otherwise.

Blood pressure measurement

This may be difficult in small children and misleading if not done correctly. The following guidelines should be observed:

- Always use the biggest cuff that will fit comfortably on the upper arm. A small cuff will give erroneously high readings
- The systolic blood pressure may give a more reliable reading than the diastolic because the fourth Korotkoff sound is frequently either not heard or is audible down to zero
- When using an electronic device, if the result is unexpected recheck it manually before acting on it
- A raised blood pressure in a child who is seizing, in pain or screaming must be rechecked when the child is calm

Blood pressure increases with age – the reading should be checked against normal ranges for the child's age (see the normal ranges table (inside front cover)). Any blood pressure over the 95th centile should be repeated and if persistently raised will need treatment. Blood pressures leading to symptoms will be grossly elevated for the child's age and the diagnosis should not be difficult.

Emergency treatment of hypertension

Reassess ABCDE

Airway, breathing and circulation should be assessed and managed in the usual way and the neurological status assessed and monitored. Convulsions should be managed as per the status epilepticus algorithm (see Figure 6.4) and children with clinical signs of raised ICP should be managed accordingly.

Once the child has been resuscitated, management of the hypertension is urgent, but should only be commenced after discussion with a paediatric nephrologist, cardiologist or intensivist. The aim of treatment is to achieve a safe reduction in blood pressure to alleviate the urgent presenting symptoms whilst avoiding the optic nerve or neurological damage that may occur with too rapid a reduction. Typically, the aim is to bring the blood pressure down to the 95th centile for age (or height) over 24–48 hours, with perhaps one-third of the reduction in the first 8 hours. This must be undertaken in conjunction with close blood pressure monitoring and a titratable infusion of the antihypertensive drug. PCCU admission is mandatory during the initial treatment and children should be cared for in a unit experienced in managing paediatric hypertension. This will usually be the regional paediatric nephrology (or paediatric cardiology) centre. It is essential that adequate consultation takes place before transfer.

Monitoring of visual acuity and pupils is crucial during this time as rapidly lowering the blood pressure may lead to infarction of the optic nerve heads. Any deterioration must be treated by urgently raising the blood pressure by lowering the antihypertensive treatment and/or using IV crystalloids or colloids. Some children may be anuric – renal function (serum creatinine, U&E) should be analysed promptly.

Some drugs commonly used to achieve blood pressure reduction in children are shown in Table 6.3 and the usual starting point would be oral/sublingual nifedipine.

Table 6.3 Drug therapy for severe hypertension

Drug	Dose	Comments
Nifedipine	0.25–0.5 mg/kg oral/ sublingual, emergency dose for hypertensive crisis; may be repeated once	Fluid can be drawn up from capsules and squirted into mouth sublingually Better to bite the capsule and swallow May cause unpredictable and severe reduction of blood pressure – monitor closely
Labetalol	0.25–3 mg/kg/h IV infusion	α- and β-blocker Titratable infusion Do not use in patients with fluid overload or acute heart failure
Sodium nitroprusside	0.5–8 micrograms/kg/min IV infusion (max. 4 micrograms/ kg/min if used for longer than 24 hours)	Vasodilator Very easy to adjust dose Titratable infusion Protect from light Monitor cyanide levels if used at max. dose beyond 48 hours

6.13 Further stabilisation and transfer to definitive care

Children presenting with altered conscious level of unknown cause need an urgent CT scan, especially if there are signs of raised ICP or focal neurological signs, as soon as possible after resuscitation and stabilisation. If the imaging shows evidence of an intracranial bleed or other pathology requiring urgent neurosurgical intervention (e.g. blocked ventriculo-peritoneal shunt), time-critical transfer to a neurosurgical centre may be required. Children shown to have an ischaemic stroke on imaging will need urgent discussion regarding the need for thrombolysis and may also need time-critical transfer to facilitate this. Time-critical transfers are sometimes done by referring teams rather than specialist paediatric critical care transport teams. Early communication is essential.

6.14 Approach to the child with seizures

Some children presenting with reduced conscious level are having seizures. The overall approach should be considered similar to other presentations, but there are some specific considerations.

The Neurocritical Care Society guidelines from 2012 define status epilepticus as a seizure with 5 minutes or more of continuous clinical and/or electrographic seizure activity or recurrent seizure activity without recovery between seizures. In general, seizures that persist beyond 5 minutes are unlikely to stop spontaneously and so it is usual practice to commence anticonvulsive treatment at this point.

Important causes of convulsions in children include fever (usually in a child less than 6 years old), meningitis/encephalitis, epilepsy, hypoxia and metabolic abnormalities. Status epilepticus occurs in approximately 1–5% of patients with epilepsy and up to 5% of children with febrile seizures will present with convulsive status epilepticus (CSE).

Status epilepticus can have a significant morbidity. Adverse neurological outcomes are a recognised complication, which are much more common in patients under 1 year of age. Status epilepticus can also be fatal, with an all-cause mortality rate in children of about 4–6% (i.e. one in 20 children). A proportion of these deaths are caused by the primary pathology and it is therefore important to remember that CSE is not a diagnosis and the treatment algorithm is not necessarily the cure. Potentially reversible primary critical illness must be sought and treated. Death can also occur as a consequence of the known complications of prolonged convulsive seizures. These include airway obstruction, aspiration, respiratory failure, heart failure, cardiac arrhythmias, hypertension, pulmonary oedema and disseminated intravascular coagulation.

Pathophysiology of prolonged seizures

A generalised convulsion increases the cerebral metabolic rate at least threefold. Initially, there is an increased sympathetic activity with the release of catecholamines, which lead to peripheral vasoconstriction and increased systemic blood pressure. There is also a loss of cerebral arterial regulation and, following the increase in systemic blood pressure, there is a resulting increase in cerebral blood flow to provide the necessary oxygen and energy. If convulsions continue, the systemic blood pressure falls and this is followed by a fall in cerebral blood flow. Lactic acid rapidly accumulates and there is subsequently cell death, oedema and raised intracranial pressure resulting in further worsening of cerebral perfusion. Prolonged seizure activity causes downregulation of inhibitory γ-aminobutyric acid receptors in the brain. These changes perpetuate seizure activity and mean that first line anticonvulsants that act on these receptors (benzodiazepines, e.g. lorazepam, midazolam) become less effective as the seizure continues.

Primary survey and resuscitation of children with seizures

ABCDE

Look specifically for any evidence of red flags in a child presenting with prolonged seizures (Figure 6.3). The priority is to assess and quickly reverse any compromise to airway, breathing and circulation that pose an immediate risk to life. Look specifically for any of the following:

A	Airway obstruction not responding to a jaw thrust or airway adjunct
B	Respiratory failure
C	Shock
D	Signs or symptoms of raised ICP, encephalopathy or focal neurology
E	Purpuric rash, puncture marks or signs of head trauma

If any of these red flags are present, then it is likely that the child needs to be intubated and ventilated urgently, while reversible causes are identified and treated. Ketamine is the induction agent of choice due to relative haemodynamic stability. It is anticonvulsant and does not increase ICP as previously thought.

Red flags in the child with seizures

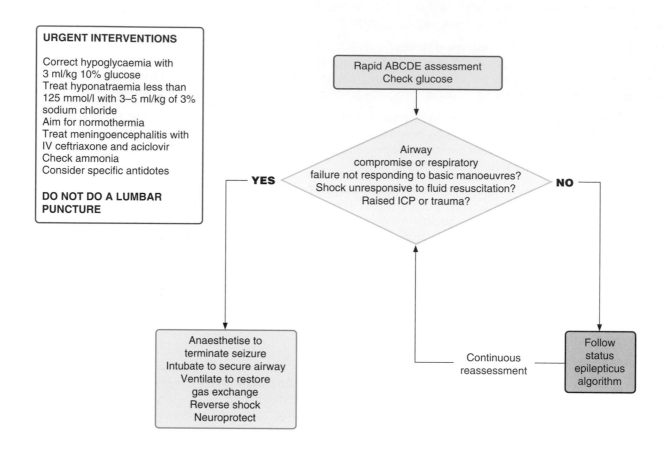

URGENT INTERVENTIONS

Correct hypoglycaemia with
3 ml/kg 10% glucose
Treat hyponatraemia less than
125 mmol/l with 3–5 ml/kg of 3%
sodium chloride
Aim for normothermia
Treat meningoencephalitis with
IV ceftriaxone and aciclovir
Check ammonia
Consider specific antidotes

**DO NOT DO A LUMBAR
PUNCTURE**

Rapid ABCDE assessment
Check glucose

Airway compromise or respiratory failure not responding to basic manoeuvres? Shock unresponsive to fluid resuscitation? Raised ICP or trauma?

YES

NO

Anaesthetise to
terminate seizure
Intubate to secure airway
Ventilate to restore
gas exchange
Reverse shock
Neuroprotect

Continuous
reassessment

Follow
status
epilepticus
algorithm

INDICATIONS FOR CT SCAN

New prolonged seizure
New focal seizure
Refractory seizures
New neurological deficit
Suspected raised ICP
Suspected space occupying
lesion
VP shunt in situ
Trauma
Possible NAI

*Remember to request a
contrast enhanced scan if
suspicion of venous sinus
thrombosis or abscess*

Figure 6.3 Red flags in the child with seizures algorithm
CT, computed tomography; ICP, intracranial pressure; NAI, non-accidental injury; VP, ventriculo-peritoneal

If none of these red flags are present then the algorithm follows the familiar pathway (Figure 6.4), through two doses of benzodiazepines to levetiracetam and finally induction of anaesthesia, intubation and ventilation. Continually reassess for red flags when treating any child with seizures and be ready to intubate and ventilate when it is indicated.

Status epilepticus

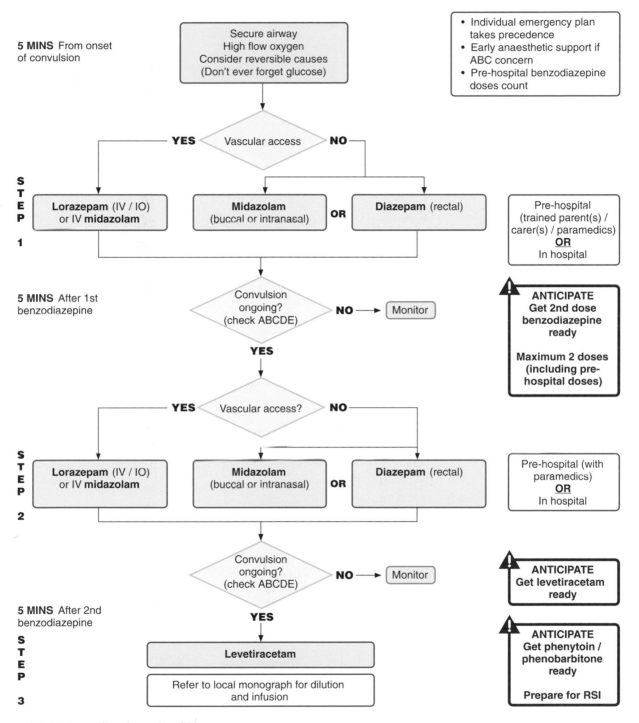

Figure 6.4 Status epilepticus algorithm

(*Continued*)

Status epilepticus (continued)

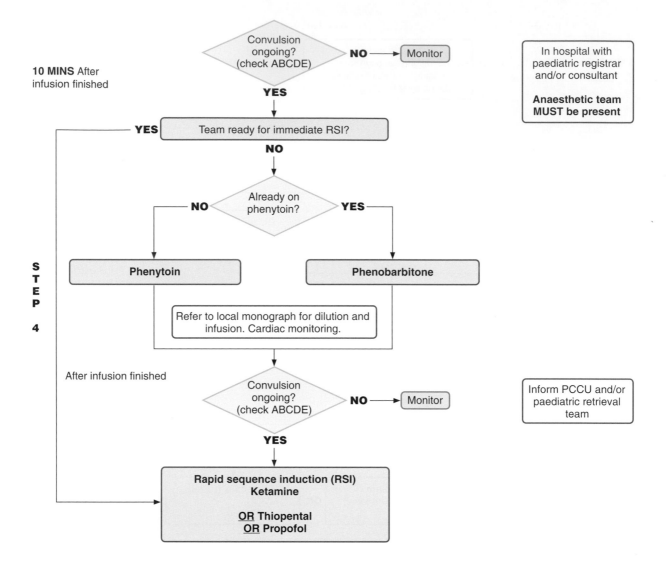

10 MINS After infusion finished

In hospital with paediatric registrar and/or consultant

Anaesthetic team MUST be present

S
T
E
P

4

After infusion finished

Inform PCCU and/or paediatric retrieval team

Lorazepam (IV/IO)	0.1 mg/kg (max 4 mg)
Midazolam (IV/IO)	0.15 mg/kg (max 10 mg)
Midazolam (buccal or intranasal)	3–11 months — 2.5 mg 1–4 years — 5 mg 5–9 years — 7.5 mg 10–17 years — 10 mg ~ 0.3 mg/kg (max 10 mg)
Diazepam (rectal)	1 month–1 year — 5 mg 2–11 years — 5–10 mg 12–17 years — 10–20 mg ~ 0.5 mg/kg (max 20 mg)

Levetiracetam	40 mg/kg IV/IO (max 3 g) Give over 5 minutes
Phenytoin	20 mg/kg IV/IO (max 2 g) give over 20 minutes
Paraldehyde	0.8 ml/kg (max 20 ml) PR of premixed 50:50 solution in olive oil
Phenobarbitone	20 mg/kg IV/IO (max 1 g) give over 20 minutes
Ketamine	1–2 mg/kg
Thiopental (thiopentone)	3–5 mg/kg IV/IO
Propofol	(refer to local monograph)

Figure 6.4 (*Continued*)

This consensus guideline is not intended to cover all circumstances. There are patients with recurrent convulsive status whose physicians recognise that they respond to certain drugs and not to others and for these children an individual protocol is more appropriate. In addition, seizures in neonates are managed differently to those of infants and children.

It is important to recognise that the timings for interventions are listed from the onset of the seizure not from arrival into hospital. Pre-hospital treatment should be noted and not repeated unless there is concern about efficacy of administration. More than two doses of benzodiazepine are associated with an increased risk of respiratory depression.

In all cases

- Continuous ABCDE assessment with immediate treatment if compromised
- Intubate and ventilate immediately if evidence of red flags is identified
- Take blood for glucose, blood gas analysis, U&E and calcium and correct metabolic abnormalities
- Treat hypoglycaemia with 3 ml/kg 10% glucose
- Treat pyrexia with paracetamol or ibuprofen
- Give sodium chloride (3–5 ml/kg of 3% solution) if signs of increased ICP are present, followed by immediate treatment of ICP as described earlier

Five minutes from seizure onset

- If in a pre-hospital setting or when IV/IO access is not established and if the seizure has lasted longer than 5 minutes, give buccal/intranasal midazolam. This can be given by prefilled syringe by age (see later in this section) or 0.3 mg/kg (max. 10 mg). Alternatively, rectal diazepam 0.5 mg/kg (max. 20 mg) can be used
- If IV/IO access is already established or can be established quickly, give IV/IO lorazepam 0.1 mg/kg (max. 4 mg) or IV midazolam 0.15 mg/kg (max. 10 g)

Five minutes after first dose of benzodiazepine

- In the hospital setting, give a second dose of benzodiazepine, and call for senior help
- If the child has received buccal midazolam or rectal diazepam before or in hospital, and is still convulsing, obtain intravenous access to give one dose of IV lorazepam 0.1 mg/kg (max. 4 mg) or IV midazolam 0.15 mg/kg (max. 10 g). Do not give more than two adequate doses of benzodiazepine, including any pre-hospital medication
- If intravenous access still has not been achieved, obtain intraosseous access
- Start to prepare levetiracetam or phenytoin for next step
- Reconfirm it is an epileptic seizure

Five minutes after second dose of benzodiazepine

- At this stage senior help is needed to reassess the child and advise on management. Anaesthetic or intensive care support should be obtained urgently, as the child could need anaesthetising and intubating if this step is unsuccessful
- Give IV levetiracetam 40 mg/kg (max. 3 g) over 5 minutes even if the child usually takes oral levetiracetam
- If the child is still seizing after loading with IV levetiracetam then termination with induction of anaesthesia and intubation is expected. However, if the advanced airway team is not yet prepared and the ABCDE assessment is stable, then either phenytoin (20 mg/kg by IV infusion over 20 minutes, max. 2 g) – or phenobarbitone (20 mg/kg by IV infusion over 20 minutes, max. 1 g) if the child already takes phenytoin – can be given. Continuous ECG, blood pressure and pulse oximetry should be checked throughout
- Rectal paraldehyde (0.8 ml/kg) mixed with an equal volume of olive oil may still appear on individual seizure management plans and should be given accordingly. The maximum single dose of paraldehyde is 20 ml

Ten minutes after finish of infusion

- By this stage, a full paediatric emergency team, including an anaesthetist, paediatric intensivist or other practitioner with advanced paediatric anaesthesia and airway skills must be present
- Emergency induction of anaesthesia should be performed. Ketamine is the safest choice of induction agent. Propofol and thiopentone are sometimes used by experienced practitioners but these drugs can cause profound hypotension and even cardiac arrest. All induction agents should be used with a rapid-onset muscle relaxant (e.g. rocuronium)
- Following induction, commence ongoing analgesia and sedation infusions as per local paediatric critical care guidelines
- Most seizures will stop by this stage. These children can sometimes be safely woken and extubated without transfer to a PCCU, provided seizures are controlled, physiology has normalised and serious reversible causes have been excluded; this should be discussed with local paediatric critical care services
- If seizures continue, commence a midazolam infusion at 100 micrograms/kg/h and arrange transfer to a PCCU
- Further advice on management should be sought from a paediatric intensivist and/or neurologist
- In children under 3 years with a history of chronic, active epilepsy, a trial of pyridoxine should be considered

Post-seizure management

Many children presenting with seizures respond to treatment without the need for intubation and ventilation. There is commonly a post-ictal period which, in combination with antiepileptic drugs, results in a reduced conscious level. This period requires close and continuous monitoring. There is a high risk of airway obstruction and respiratory depression. Potential reversible causes and red flags need to be continually reassessed. Children not protecting their airway after an oro-/nasopharyngeal airway has been put in place, should be intubated and ventilated to keep them safe during this period, even if there is no ongoing seizure activity. There should be a low threshold for a CT scan and other investigations for reduced conscious level for children not showing signs of improving GCS score within 30–60 minutes of seizure termination.

Other post-seizure management includes:

- Maintain normoglycaemia using 5% or 10% glucose, preferably with isotonic crystalloid (e.g. Plasma-Lyte 148 with 5% glucose or 0.9% sodium chloride with 5% glucose)
- Keep serum sodium in the normal range of 135–145 mmol/l
- Consider a nasogastric tube to aspirate the stomach contents
- Regulate temperature, ensuring temperatures above 37.5°C are avoided

Drugs used in status epilepticus

Lorazepam

Lorazepam is equally or more effective than diazepam and possibly produces less respiratory depression. It has a longer duration of action (12–24 hours) than diazepam (less than 1 hour). It appears to be poorly absorbed from the rectal route. Lorazepam is not available in every country. If this is the case, diazepam can be substituted at a dose of 0.25 mg/kg IV/IO or midazolam at a dose of 0.15 mg/kg IV/IO.

Midazolam

This is an effective, quick-acting anticonvulsant that takes effect within minutes but has a shorter lasting effect than lorazepam. It can be given by IV/IO/IM routes or via the buccal or nasal mucosa. Buccal/nasal midazolam may be twice as effective as rectal diazepam, but both drugs produce the same level and degree of respiratory depression. Most children do not convulse again once the seizure has been terminated. All benzodiazepines have the potential to cause significant respiratory depression requiring active management of both airway and breathing.

Buccal midazolam is available in prefilled syringes. The dosing schedule is as follows:

- 1–2 months: 300 micrograms/kg (max. dose 2.5 mg)
- 3–11 months: 2.5 mg
- 1–4 years: 5 mg
- 5–9 years: 7.5 mg
- 10–17 years: 10 mg

The tip of the syringe is inserted into the buccal area between the lower bottom lip and the gum margin at the side of the mouth. If the licensed preparation is not available, draw up the higher dose (0.5 mg) of the intravenous preparation. For nasal application, commercially available nasal spray can be used or the dose (0.3 mg/kg) can be given using a mucosal atomisation device (MAD) on a standard syringe.

Continuous midazolam IV/IO infusion is often used as a treatment in a ventilated patient because of its relative ease of use, its high response rate and low complication rate. The starting dose is 100 micrograms/kg/h, increased in steps of 100 micrograms/kg/h up to a maximum of 1 mg/kg/h.

Diazepam

This is also an effective, quick-acting anticonvulsant with similar characteristics to midazolam. It is widely used but may now be superseded by the more effective midazolam where the latter is available. The rectal dose is well absorbed.

Paraldehyde

The dose is 0.8 ml/kg (max. 20 ml) PR of the premixed 50:50 solution in olive oil or 0.9% sodium chloride. Arachis oil should be avoided because children with peanut allergy may react to it. Paraldehyde can cause rectal irritation, but IM paraldehyde causes severe pain and may lead to sterile abscess formation. Paraldehyde causes little respiratory depression. It should not be used in liver disease.

Paraldehyde takes 10–15 minutes to act and its action is sustained for 2–4 hours. Do not leave paraldehyde standing in a plastic syringe for longer than a few minutes. If paraldehyde is given, this should be at the same time as the levetiracetam is being drawn up or infused. It is also important that the infusion of phenytoin must not be delayed because paraldehyde has been given.

Levetiracetam

Levetiracetam is a newer antiepileptic drug that is now being used as an alternative to phenytoin for second line treatment of CSE. The dose is 40 mg/kg IV/IO (max. 3 g), given over 5 minutes. It has fewer drug interactions and side effects than phenytoin, and the full 40 mg/kg dose can be given even if the child is on regular maintenance levetiracetam.

Phenytoin

The dose is 20 mg/kg IV/IO (max. 2 g), which must be given over at least 20 minutes. The infusion should be made up in 0.9% sodium chloride to a maximum concentration of 10 mg in 1 ml. Phenytoin can cause dysrhythmias and hypotension, therefore monitor the ECG and blood pressure. It has little depressant effect on respiration.

Ketamine

Ketamine is a short-acting dissociative anaesthetic agent that does not cause cardiovascular depression. Recent studies have shown that ketamine administration is safe and effective in cases of refractory status epilepticus, and that it does not raise ICP; therefore, it should be the first line induction agent for most cases of status epilepticus in order to avoid hypotension associated with other agents. The induction dose is 1–2 mg/kg IV/IO.

Propofol

The induction dose is 2.5–4 mg/kg IV and is usually available in dilutions of 1% (10 mg/ml) or 2% (20 mg/ml). It is a white oil-in-water emulsion that commonly causes irritation on intravenous administration. It is very effective for the induction of general anaesthesia, although its use for ongoing sedation for children in critical care has been controversial due to the associated risk of propofol infusion syndrome (potentially fatal effects, including metabolic acidosis, arrhythmias, cardiac failure, rhabdomyolysis, hyperlipidaemia, hyperkalaemia, hepatomegaly and renal failure). Propofol should only be administered by, or under the direct supervision of, experienced staff.

Thiopental (thiopentone) sodium

The induction dose is 3–5 mg/kg IV/IO. It is an alkaline solution, which will cause irritation if the solution leaks into subcutaneous tissues. It is a general anaesthetic agent, with no analgesic effect. Repeated doses have a cumulative effect. It is a potent drug with marked cardiorespiratory effects and must be used only by experienced staff who can intubate a child.

6.15 Summary

This chapter has described how the structured approach should be used in the assessment and management of the child with reduced conscious level with or without seizures. Children presenting acutely with a reduced conscious level should worry treating teams. There are potentially reversible, life-threatening causes and there should be a low threshold for an aggressive approach, especially when the cause is not known. Specifically, this means intubation, neuroprotection, cover for meningoencephalitis and urgent investigations for treatable causes, including glucose, ammonia and CT head. The Royal College or Paediatrics and Child Health (RCPCH) guideline *The Management of Children and Young People with an Acute Decrease in Conscious Level (DECON)* provides an excellent summary of this topic.

CHAPTER 7

Exposure

Learning outcomes

After reading this chapter, you will be able to:

- Complete a full assessment relating to exposure
- Resuscitate dependent on findings
- Describe how to undertake a pain assessment
- Understand the variety and methods of administering analgesia to children

---

7.1   Introduction

As discussed in Chapter 3, the structured approach is:

- **Primary survey**
- **Resuscitation**
- **Secondary survey and looking for key features to aid diagnosis**
- **Emergency treatment**
- **Stabilisation and transfer to definitive care**

Once ABCD have been managed to an optimum stage then progress to E. The E for exposure should encompass a survey of the whole child looking for rashes, bruises, bleeding, etc. At this stage of the assessment it would also be appropriate to do the following if they have not already been done:

- Take a temperature
- Actively seek indicators of chronic conditions
- Look for signs of intoxication
- Consider pain management

It is vital when completing E (exposure) to ensure that the child or young person has their dignity protected throughout and that they feel as comfortable as possible whilst the full examination is undertaken

---

Advanced Paediatric Life Support: A Practical Approach to Emergencies, Seventh Edition. Edited by Stephanie Smith.
© 2023 John Wiley & Sons Ltd. Published 2023 by John Wiley & Sons Ltd.

7.2 Temperature

This is the time to ensure that the temperature is checked if it has not been done previously.

High body temperature

An elevated body temperature can be due to **fever**, as the result of cytokine release causing an increase in the hypothalamic setpoint, in response to various triggers, or to **hyperthermia** due to loss of thermoregulation.

Fever

A fever is one of the most common reasons for parents to seek medical help; in addition, it is one of the commonest causes for admission. Fever is defined as a temperature over 38°C and can be caused by a variety of conditions including infections, inflammatory conditions and a reaction to immunisation.

Symptom relief is with antipyretics, such as paracetamol and ibuprofen, although they should be spaced out correctly and not given persistently without the child being reviewed by a clinical practitioner.

Infections

Infections caused by bacteria, viruses, fungi and atypical organisms often result in a temperature rise as the body mounts an immune response. It is important that the temperature is measured accurately either using a tympanic thermometer or, in extremely unwell children, a rectal thermometer. **A fever in an infant under 3 months is significant and the baby needs a full assessment.** The clinician needs to maintain a low threshold for instigating a full septic screen and starting sepsis treatment. It is important to assess whether the child/baby is unwell and whether there is a significant infection (e.g. meningitis) or mild viral infection which will resolve in a few days. This may require watching for a period of time and repeat observations.

Sepsis can be said to occur when the body's response to infection causes injury to its own tissues and organs. This is a very significant condition and a leading cause of paediatric mortality world-wide. It needs to be identified and treated correctly with intravenous antibiotics and fluids initially and escalating care as required. There are a number of systems to aid in the diagnosis such as the National Institute for Health and Care Excellence (NICE) guidance traffic light system.

Inflammatory conditions

Inflammatory conditions may cause fever. Examples include juvenile chronic arthritis and Kawasaki disease. These conditions will have indicators in the history or other signs visible on examination.

Post immunisation

After immunisation some children can develop a fever, but these are not usually high or prolonged. Reassurance and antipyretic treatments are recommended.

Hyperthermia

Drug ingestion, thyrotoxicosis, central nervous system (CNS) damage and heat stroke are all examples of hyperthermia. Their treatment differs to the management of fever, as antipyretics may not be helpful and specific therapies are often required as well as physical cooling.

Low body temperature

Hypothermia occurs when the temperature is below 35°C. This can be due to a number of factors:

- **Infection**, as described above, especially in young children
- **Exposure** to a cold environment: warm using external warmers, warmed fluids and removal of wet clothes unless there are indications not to warm, for example neuroprotection in significant head injuries or post cardiac arrest
- Secondary to **toxins**
- As a result of **metabolic derangements**
- **Dysfunction of central nervous and endocrine systems**

7.3   Rashes

Rashes take a number of forms and appearances dependent on cause, severity and skin colour.

- Petechiae (less than 2 mm)/purpura (greater than or equal to 3 mm):
  - Meningococcal or any disease that causes coagulation disorders
  - Immune thrombocytopenia (ITP) or any cause of low platelet count
  - Traumatic – accidental or non-accidental
  - Henoch–Schönlein purpura (HSP)
- Specific infectious exanthema:
  - Cold sores – herpes infection has the potential to lead to encephalitis
  - COVID-19 rash
  - Measles, scarlet fever, mumps, chickenpox, rubella and impetigo
- Urticaria relating to allergic reaction

7.4   Indicators of chronic conditions

Look for indicators of chronic conditions especially if the child is unaccompanied and unable to give a history. Examples include:

- Insulin pumps
- Pacemakers
- Ventriculo-peritoneal shunts
- Cochlear implants
- Surgical scars
- Medic alerts bands

7.5   Signs of ingestion

The most obvious indicator of ingestion comes in the history and would be evident in missing medicines, tablets, button batteries or empty packaging (see Appendix F for management). It is also important to look for:

- Discoloration or burns in or around the mouth
- Drooling due to difficulty in swallowing or increased saliva
- Breath smelling of chemicals or alcohol
- Vomiting
- Clinical signs such as drowsiness, confusion or pupillary changes

7.6 Managing pain

The adequate management of pain is integral to all emergency care. Optimising patient comfort not only allows the practitioner to make a more accurate assessment of illness severity, but also minimises the adverse physiological responses to pain that worsen outcome.

It is important that the language used when assessing and improving a child's comfort is carefully selected. The power of the 'nocebo effect', where the use of words describing negative sensations and experiences increases the likelihood of the child actually experiencing these sensations, must be recognised. Enquire about negative experiences such as pain and nausea by using open-ended questions such as 'Do you need something to make you more comfortable?' rather than 'How much pain are you in?' Reassuring the child that they are safe, that they will be made comfortable and that we will help their body to heal can be powerful.

These principles are also important when obtaining consent for procedures. Further information can be found on the Society for Paediatric Anaesthesia in New Zealand and Australia (SPANZA) EPIC website https://www.spanza.org.au/epic (last accessed January 2023).

Recognition and assessment of pain

There are three main ways to recognise that a child is in pain:

- Listening to the child for statements that they are in pain or listening to their parent or carer
- Observing the child's behaviour and physiology for things such as crying, guarding of the injured part, facial grimacing, pallor, stillness and withdrawal, tachycardia and tachypnoea
- Anticipating pain because of the nature of the underlying problem

The purpose of pain assessment is to establish, as far as possible, the degree of pain experienced by the child to allow selection of the right level of pain relief. Reassessment using the same pain tool will indicate whether the pain management has been successful or whether further analgesia is required – the assess, treat and reassess cycle. The use of suitable pain tools and protocols in the emergency setting has been shown to shorten the time to delivery of analgesia.

An observational pain scale overcomes the problems caused by anxiety at presentation and is more appropriate. The Alder Hey Triage Pain Score (AHTPS) is one such tool that has been developed specifically for this situation and is shown to have some validity as well as good levels of inter-rater reliability (Table 7.1). It is an observation-based pain score, which is quick and easy to use.

Table 7.1 The Alder Hey Triage Pain Score: reference scoring chart

Response	Score 0	Score 1	Score 2
Cry/voice	No complaint/cry	Consolable	Inconsolable
	Normal conversation	Not talking/negative interaction	Complaining of pain
Facial expression	Normal	Short grimace or similar less than 50% of time	Long grimace more than 50% of time
Posture	Normal	Touching/rubbing/sparing	Defensive/tense
Movement	Normal	Reduced or restless	Immobile or thrashing
Colour	Normal	Pale	Very pale/'green'

Other commonly used pain scales are self-assessment tools, for example a faces scale or pain ladder (Figure 7.1). Self-assessment tools, however, were primarily developed for use with children where there was the opportunity for explanation of the scale prior to the painful event (e.g. before surgery). This is rarely the case in the emergency department.

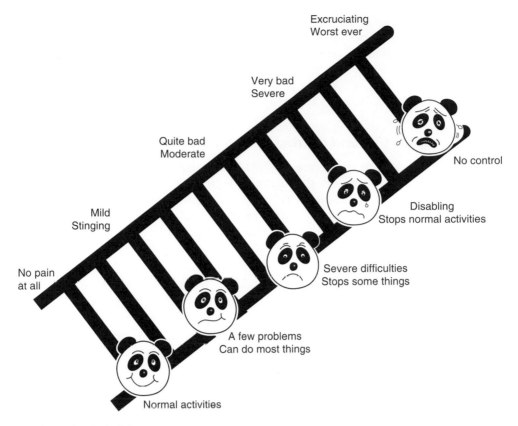

Figure 7.1 Faces scale and pain ladder

Both or either of these tools can be used to assess the pain experienced by the child and help to guide the level and route of analgesia required. The tools can then be used again to assess the efficacy of the intervention and to guide further analgesia.

Assess, treat, reassess

Pain management

There are various strategies for managing pain in the emergency situation that do not require pharmacological interventions.

Environment

The emergency department and the treatment room of the paediatric ward can be frightening places for children. Negative aspects of the environment should be removed or minimised. This includes an overly 'clinical' appearance and evidence of invasive instruments. An attractive environment with toys, themes and colour schemes should be substituted.

Preparation

Approaching the child in a calm, quiet manner, assuring them that they will be looked after well, they will be comfortable and giving them the suggestion that healing can begin immediately, can rapidly settle an anxious child. Simple, age-appropriate explanations about what is happening to them are also important. Except in a life-threatening emergency or when dealing with an unconscious child, an explanation of the procedure to be undertaken and the ways to make it as comfortable as possible should be given to the child and their parents. Words which foretell negative sensations, such as 'pain', 'sharp scratch', 'be brave', 'feel sick' or 'vomit' should be avoided. Studies suggest that, contrary to previous assumptions, these words are more likely to result in a negative experience for the child. Open-ended statements invoking curiosity and suggesting success and the desired outcome are more likely to lead to a comfortable experience. Permission can be given for the child not to be bothered by the procedure. Positive messages such as 'I am going to help you', 'you are doing great' or 'this will make you more comfortable' are helpful. If a play therapist is available they may be able to assist with the preparation and the procedure.

Physical treatments: supportive and distractive techniques

During an invasive procedure, the presence of suitably prepared parents or carers is important. In one study, almost all children between the ages of 9 and 12 years reported that 'the thing that helped most' was to have a parent present during a painful procedure. Parents need some guidance on how to help their child during the procedure beyond just being present. Studies suggest that talking to and touching the child during the procedure is both soothing and anxiety relieving. Other distractive strategies include:

- Looking at pop-up books or interactive toys
- Listening through headphones to stories or music
- Blowing bubbles
- Video or interactive computer games
- Moving images projected onto a nearby wall, such as fish swimming or birds flying
- The presence of transitional objects (comforters), for example a favourite blanket or soft toy
- Lived imagination – have the child imagine a place or an activity that they enjoy. Parents can be helpful with this. Ask them to describe what they are experiencing, using all the senses and taking time for the child to immerse themselves in their imagination. Suggest that they might like to stay and enjoy the place and leave us behind to get the procedure finished

Some emergency departments use hypnosis to manage pain effectively. Hypnosis is a state involving focused attention, reduced peripheral awareness and an enhanced capacity to respond to suggestion. Outpatient-based hypnotherapy to prepare children for unpleasant procedures or to treat other conditions such as enuresis can be very successful. Similar techniques 'on the fly' in emergency settings can also be very effective in reducing the discomfort experienced during procedures. Children are open to new experiences, crave mastery and have powerful imaginations, all of which increase the likelihood of success with hypnosis. With some basic training and practice a child can be helped to tolerate uncomfortable procedures such as venepuncture or reduction of joint dislocations.

Further information can be found on the Society for Paediatric Anaesthesia in New Zealand and Australia (SPANZA) EPIC website https://www.spanza.org.au/epic (last accessed January 2023).

Pharmacological treatment

Local anaesthetics: topical on intact skin

Ametop® gel. This contains tetracaine (amethocaine) base 4%.

- It is used under an occlusive dressing
- Analgesia is achieved after 30–45 minutes
- Anaesthesia remains for 4–6 hours after removal of the gel
- Slight erythema, itching and oedema may occur at the site
- Not to be applied on broken skin, mucous membranes, eyes or ears
- Can cause sensitisation on repeated exposure
- Not recommended for a patient under 1 month of age

Emla®. A mixture of lidocaine 2.5% and prilocaine 2.5% can be used in a similar fashion where sensitivity to Ametop® gel occurs. Emla®, however, takes around 60 minutes to work effectively and tends to cause vasoconstriction rather than vasodilatation.

Alternatively, **ethyl chloride spray** works immediately.

Local anaesthetics: infiltrated

Local anaesthetics are manufactured to a pH of 5 (to improve shelf-life) and are painful for this reason. A buffered solution (i.e. 9 ml of lidocaine with 1 ml of 8.4% sodium bicarbonate) and the use of smaller needles will lessen the pain associated with infiltration, but local adrenaline cannot then be used because the bicarbonate buffer inactivates it.

Overdose or inadvertent injection of local anaesthetics into an artery or vein may result in cardiac arrhythmias and convulsions. Resuscitative facilities and skills must therefore be available wherever and whenever these drugs are injected.

Lidocaine. 1% lidocaine (lignocaine, **contains 10 mg of lidocaine per 1 ml**) is used for rapid and intense sensory nerve block.

- The onset of action is significant within 2 minutes and is effective for up to 2 hours
- It is often used with adrenaline to prolong the duration of sensory blockade and to limit toxicity by reducing absorption (adrenaline concentration 5 micrograms/ml). Adrenaline-containing local anaesthetic should not be used in areas served by an end artery, such as a digit
- **The maximum body dose is 3 mg/kg for plain solutions and 7 mg/kg for solutions that contain adrenaline**

Bupivacaine and ropivacaine. Long-acting local anaesthetics such as bupivacaine or ropivacaine are used – at a concentration of 0.25% or 0.5% (2.5 or 5 mg per ml) – when longer lasting local anaesthesia is required, such as in femoral nerve blocks.

- Onset takes up to 15 minutes, but its effects last up to 8 hours
- Maximum body dosage is 2 mg/kg

Non-opioid analgesics

These drugs exhibit varying degrees of analgesic, antipyretic and anti-inflammatory activity.

Paracetamol. This is probably the most widely used analgesic in paediatric practice. It may be administered by the oral, rectal and intravenous routes. It is thought to work through inhibiting cyclo-oxygenase in the CNS but not in other tissues, so that it produces analgesia without any anti-inflammatory effect. It does not cause respiratory depression. It is very safe when administered at the recommended dose although overdosage in a large single dose, or too frequent smaller doses, may cause hepatotoxicity. Higher loading doses have been shown to improve pain control (see Appendix J).

Non-steroidal anti-inflammatory drugs (NSAIDs). These are anti-inflammatory and antipyretic drugs with moderate analgesic properties. They are less well tolerated than paracetamol, causing gastric irritation, platelet disorders, bronchospasm and renal impairment. They should, therefore, be avoided in children with a history of gastric ulceration, platelet abnormalities and dehydration or renal problems. Their advantage is that they are especially useful for post-traumatic pain because of the additional anti-inflammatory effect. Ibuprofen is given by mouth, and if rectal administration is necessary then diclofenac can be used. Ketorolac can be given intravenously.

Opiate analgesics

Morphine. This produces a rapid onset of excellent analgesia and remains the treatment of choice in many situations. It may be titrated to effect and (temporarily) reversed with naloxone if necessary. The intranasal route for the administration of opiates such as **diamorphine** and **fentanyl** has been shown to be a safe and effective route and is increasingly popular for children. It also has the advantage of being quick and easy, avoiding the trauma of an intravenous cannula.

Side effects include respiratory depression, nausea and vomiting. Cardiovascular effects include peripheral vasodilatation and venous pooling, but in single doses it has minimal haemodynamic effect in a supine child with normal circulating volume. In hypovolaemic patients it will contribute to hypotension but this is not a contraindication to its use and merely an indication for cardiovascular monitoring and action as appropriate. Opioids produce a dose-dependent depression of ventilation primarily by reducing the sensitivity of brain-stem respiratory centres to hypercarbia and hypoxia. This means that a child who has received a dose of an opioid requires observation and/or monitoring and should not be discharged home until it is clear that the effects of the opiate are significantly reduced. The nausea and vomiting produced in adults by morphine seems to be less common in children.

Opiate antagonists

Naloxone. Naloxone is a potent opioid antagonist. It antagonises the sedative, respiratory-depressive and analgesic effects of opioids. It is rapidly metabolised and is given parenterally because of its rapid first pass extraction through the liver following oral administration. Following intravenous administration, naloxone reverses the effects of opiates almost immediately. Its duration of action, however, is much shorter than the opiate agonist. Therefore, repeated doses or an infusion may be required if continued opiate antagonism is wanted.

Inhalational analgesia

Nitrous oxide. This is a colourless, odourless gas that provides analgesia in subanaesthetic concentrations. It is supplied in premixed cylinders at a 50% concentration with oxygen (Entonox®, Kalinox®) or at a concentration of up to 70% with oxygen via a blender. Delivery devices either act on a demand principle (i.e. the gas is only delivered when the child inhales and applies a negative pressure) or via a free-flowing circuit. The latter delivery system requires a scavenger circuit. Generally during nitrous oxide therapy, the child has to be awake and cooperative to be able to inhale the gas; this is an obvious safeguard with the technique.

- Because nitrous oxide is inhaled and has a low solubility in blood, its onset of effect is very rapid. It takes 2–3 minutes to achieve its peak effect. For the same reason, the drug wears off over several minutes, enabling children to recover considerably quicker than if they received narcotics or sedatives. Laryngeal protective reflexes do not always remain intact
- Nitrous oxide is therefore most suitable for procedures where short-lived intense analgesia is required, for example dressing changes; suturing and needle procedures such as venous cannulation; lumbar punctures; and for pain relief during splinting or transport. It is also of benefit for immediate pain relief on presentation until definitive analgesia is effective
- Using a free-flow circuit, nitrous oxide can be used by children as young as 2 years of age, although children will need to be 4 or 5 years of age before they can trigger the demand valve of a premixed cylinder
- Nitrous oxide may cause nausea, vomiting, euphoria and disinhibition. Prolonged exposure to high concentrations can cause bone marrow depression and neuronal degeneration
- Nitrous oxide is contraindicated in children with possible intracranial or intrathoracic air because gas diffusion into the confined space may increase pressure
- As there are no adequate data and the potential risk is unknown, passive exposure to nitric oxide during pregnancy and lactation should be avoided

Sedative and dissociative drugs

In addition to analgesics, psychotropic drugs may also be useful when undertaking lengthy or repeated procedures. Sedatives relieve anxiety but not pain and may reduce the child's ability to communicate discomfort and therefore should not be given in isolation. The problems associated with the use of sedatives are side effects (usually hyperexcitability) and the time required for the child to be awake enough to be allowed home if admission is not necessary. This does not apply to dissociative agents such as ketamine which have a different mode of action, and are widely used for procedures.

Midazolam. Midazolam is an amnesic and sedative drug. It can be given intravenously, intramuscularly, orally or intranasally (although this is unpleasant). It has an onset time of action of 15 minutes after an oral administration and recovery occurs after about an hour. It may cause respiratory depression, necessitating monitoring of respiratory function and pulse oximetry. A few children become hyperexcitable with this drug (paradoxal reaction). Whilst its action can be reversed by flumazenil, intravenously this is rarely necessary and can precipitate seizures.

Ketamine. This is a potent anaesthetic agent that has an established place in paediatric procedural pain relief in many emergency settings. It causes a dissociative anaesthesia, which is amnesic and analgesic, but has little effect on breathing and protective airway reflexes are maintained. Side effects include hypersalivation, tachycardia and hypertension, but previous concerns with regard to increasing intracranial pressure are no longer valid. Laryngospasm is a rare complication that may be precipitated by instrumentation of the upper airway or rapid administration.

Ketamine should be considered as an anaesthetic agent and used with all the precautions generally associated with anaesthesia. Emergence phenomenon (delirium following use of ketamine) can be treated with a low dose of midazolam if necessary but is much less common in paediatric than in adult practice.

Specific clinical situations

Severe pain

Children in severe pain (e.g. major trauma, femoral fracture, significant burns, displaced or comminuted fractures) should receive IV morphine at an initial dose of 0.1–0.2 mg/kg infused over 2–3 minutes (see Appendix J). A further dose can be given after 5–10 minutes if sufficient analgesia is not achieved. The child should be monitored using pulse oximetry and electrocardiography.

Low-dose IV ketamine (0.1 mg/kg) can be additionally given if the pain has not responded to maximal doses of opiates.

Higher doses of ketamine are a safe and alternative initial option for treating severe and acute pain in the emergency room.

Head injuries

There is often concern about giving morphine to a child who has had a head injury and who could therefore potentially lose consciousness secondary to the head injury. If the child is conscious and in pain, then the presence of a potential deteriorating head injury is not a contraindication to giving morphine. First, an analgesic dose is not necessarily a significant sedative; second, if the child's conscious level does deteriorate, then the clinician's first action should be to assess airway, breathing and circulation, intervening where appropriate. If these are stable, then a dose of naloxone will quickly ascertain whether the diminished conscious level is secondary to morphine or (as is much more likely) represents increasing intracranial pressure. There are significant benefits for the head-injured child in receiving adequate pain relief as the physiological response to pain may increase intracranial pressure.

In the common situation of the patient who has an isolated femoral shaft fracture and a possible head injury, a femoral nerve block may be an effective alternative (see Chapter 21).

Emergency venepuncture and venous cannulation

At present, the management of this problem is difficult as topical anaesthetics take up to an hour to be effective. Inhaled nitrous oxide, given by one of the methods described earlier, gives excellent results. Alternatives in an emergency include ethyl chloride spray, an ice cube inside the finger of a plastic glove placed over the vein to be cannulated or local anaesthetic infiltration (1% buffered lidocaine) using a very fine gauge (e.g. 29 gauge) needle. Verbal or other distraction techniques can also be very effective.

7.7 Summary

This chapter gives an outline of the elements that should be considered in the E assessment if they have not yet been assessed and managed in the ABCD primary assessment. Pain management, both pharmacological and non-pharmacological, should be considered.

PART 3
The seriously injured child

CHAPTER 8

Structured approach to the seriously injured child

Learning outcomes

After reading this chapter, you will be able to:

- Identify the importance of injury prevention
- Describe the role of trauma systems
- Describe the team-based, structured approach to the seriously injured child

---

8.1 Introduction

Internationally, unintentional injuries are a leading cause of death in children. The World Health Organization (WHO) estimates 18 000 injury-related deaths in children under 15 years of age each year. The predominant mechanisms are from preventable causes such as road traffic collisions, drownings and fire-related incidents.

In the UK, data from the Trauma Audit and Research Network (TARN) show that pedestrian children suffer the most severe injuries secondary to traumatic brain injury. Mortality is between 8% and 10% of those with major trauma (injury severity score greater than 15), particularly if there is a reduced Glasgow Coma Scale (GCS) score, injury to multiple organ systems or the need for admission to a critical care facility. Infants are more susceptible to severe injuries resulting from suspected physical abuse.

Many more children are injured in accidents that, although not causing death, cause pain, distress and permanent disability. There has been an increase in penetrating injury, particularly knife crime, in the UK over the past decade.

The majority of these events are predictable and preventable. This introduction to the seriously injured child will consider the important role of injury prevention, trauma systems and some specifics about trauma teams.

8.2 Injury prevention

Over the last few decades, injury prevention programmes, together with increased education in schools and public health campaigns, in some countries have succeeded in significantly reducing childhood death rates from injury by introducing key legislation such as child restraints, speed restrictions and laws on the use of motorcycle helmets. This is a remarkable achievement. Injury prevention is a multifaceted, multidisciplinary process that provides many opportunities for clinicians, who are primarily involved in the management of acutely injured children, to play a major role.

8.3　Epidemiology

Circumstances and type of incident

A multitude of injury scenarios are possible, each of which involve the child interacting with their environment. The commonest injuries that cause death are those resulting from motor vehicle accidents, drownings, burns, falls from a height and poisonings. Children in urban environments are at particular risk of motor vehicle collisions and playground falls whilst children in a rural environment are at risk of farm equipment injuries or unintentional chemical exposure. Exposure to different circumstances also varies with age. Children under 5 years of age experience injuries at home, with infants and toddlers at greater risk of inflicted injury. School-age children experience injuries at school, sport and play, and are especially at risk of death as pedestrians and cyclists. Adolescents may unintentionally place themselves at risk of injury, especially where alcohol and drugs may impair their judgement. Self-harm is an increasing cause of death and disability in young people.

Children with major injuries are affected differently – physically, physiologically and psychologically. Initial presentation can be deceptive because the relative elasticity of their tissues allows more energy to be transmitted to other body parts, with less being dissipated at the impact site. This will influence assessment and management.

Understanding the mechanism of injury will help assess how likely it is that a child has major injuries. For example, a fall from above the child's head height is much more significant than a fall from ground level.

Sex

Males are more frequently injured than females. The difference emerges at 1–2 years of age. How much of this difference is innate and how much cultural is a subject for speculation. Females may mature more rapidly in terms of perception and coordination.

Age

The type of injury sustained is closely related to the child's stage of development. Take falls as an example. A newborn baby can only fall if dropped, or if a parent falls holding the baby. An older baby can wriggle and roll off a changing table or a bed. A crawling baby can climb upstairs and fall back. A small child can climb and fall out of a window. An older child can climb a tree or fall in a playground. It is important to the healthcare professionals to know the stages of development of children. This will allow professionals to understand the mechanism of injury and judge whether a given history is plausible when considering non-accidental injury. A child's developmental stage will also influence the clinical assessment and decisions on investigation and treatment.

Social class

It is well-recognised that inequalities in children's environments are linked to health problems. Children in lower socioeconomic groups are twice as likely to die from an injury as children in higher social class groups. For some injury types, the chances of sustaining an injury are increased. Burns, for example, are six times more likely to be sustained by children in lower socioeconomic groups. Pressures such as overcrowding, poor housing or poverty are likely contributory factors.

Psychological factors

Injuries are more common in families where there is stress from mental illness, substance abuse, marital discord, moving home or a variety of similar factors.

8.4 Trauma systems

A trauma system is described as an organised, coordinated effort in a defined geographical area that delivers the full range of care to all injured patients and is integrated with the local healthcare system. After pre-hospital assessment, ambulance crews may bypass hospitals to reach those trauma centres with specialised care, investigations and interventions 24/7.

If a trauma system is in place, then the response to a seriously injured child will be adapted to take into account the pathway for major trauma patients in a certain area. This includes the recognition that secondary transfer of children may become more prevalent. This may also increase the number of time-critical transfers as children are transferred to the place where definitive care for the life-threatening condition can be delivered. Pre-hospital practitioners may consider going directly to a hub trauma centre or moving on at the earliest possibility. The 'moving on' should potentially be seen as an extension of the pre-hospital phase. Clinicians should start planning for transfer as soon as the child arrives and make contact early with the place where definitive care for the life-threatening condition can be delivered. The phrase 'stop/sort/go' emphasises this point.

Trauma systems have an important role in the planning and management of mass casualty events, which are major incidents that present serious threat to the health of the community or cause such numbers or types of casualties as to require special arrangements to be implemented. It is likely that such an event will include children, and indeed some incidents may almost exclusively involve children. **It is essential that all healthcare workers are familiar with their own organisations' major incident plans and procedures**.

Some knowledge of the initial management of blast and ballistic injuries is necessary, and clinical guidelines such as those produced by NHS England (https://www.england.nhs.uk/publication/clinical-guidelines-for-major-incidents-and-mass-casualty-events/; last accessed January 2023) should be immediately available for reference in emergency departments.

Following the terrorist attack at the Manchester Arena in 2017, a number of learning points and recommendations were identified around the initial hospital response, including:

- Casualties may arrive at hospital before a major incident has been recognised or declared
- Re-triage of all casualties on arrival at hospital is essential
- Expect difficulties in identifying children – they will often not carry identification
- Plans should allow for children and their parents/carers to remain together where practical
- Use of improvised tourniquets may be life saving on scene, but need to be specifically looked for on arrival at hospital in order to keep the tourniquet time as short as possible
- Whole-body computed tomography (CT) is essential in blast injuries
- Consider the potential for blood-borne virus transmission if a penetrating wound may have been caused by projectile body matter from another victim, or from a bladed weapon that may have been used on multiple casualties. Hepatitis B vaccination may be indicated
- Antibiotics should be given for penetrating injuries according to local guidelines
- Check carefully for penetrating eye injuries, especially in casualties with a reduced level of consciousness
- A terrorist incident will require a forensic investigation – any removed foreign bodies, etc. need carefully labelling and keeping for the police
- Do not underestimate the psychological impact that critically injured or dying children will have on all levels of staff
- Regular simulation and table-top exercises are essential

> When reading the chapters in this section, it is important that they are placed in the context of your local trauma system

Irrespective of the presence of a trauma system, it is essential that hospitals that receive paediatric traumas should have:

- Specific paediatric guidelines and protocols (Box 8.1)
- Standard operating procedures and pathways (Box 8.1)
- Paediatric equipment and monitoring
- Immediate access to staff with paediatric expertise

Box 8.1 Paediatric guidelines, protocols, procedures and pathways

- Trauma team activation
- Rapid sequence intubation/difficult airway procedures
- Head injury management
- Penetrating cardiac injury management
- Chest drain insertion
- Open fracture management
- Pelvic fracture management
- Drowning pathway
- Burns referral pathway
- Major haemorrhage protocol:
  - tranexamic acid
  - blood products
  - haemostatic agents
  - recombined factor VIIa
  - analgesia
- Imaging:
  - CT guidance
  - X-ray guidance
  - abdominal injury
- Urethrogram and cystogram
- Tetanus prevention
- Safeguarding
- Youth support organisations
- Brain injury pathway

8.5 Trauma teams

Paediatric major trauma happens infrequently, therefore it is important that trauma teams are familiar with all of the elements listed above and that they receive regular training and practice. The roles required in a trauma team are detailed in Box 8.2. Considerations of non-technical skills are to be found in Chapter 2.

Box 8.2 Trauma team and example roles

Actual roles will depend on local processes
- Team Leader – coordinates team actions and communication, directs treatment
- Operating Department Practitioner – assists Airway Specialist in managing airway
- Airway Specialist/Anaesthetist - manages airway
- Assistant 1 – monitors vital signs and administers medication
- Assistant 2 – assists with emergency procedures and checks medications with Nurse 1
- Clinician 1 – conducts primary survey and necessary procedures
- Clinician 2 – gains vascular access and other emergency procedures
- Scribe – liaises closely with Team Leader to maintain an accurate record of assessment, treatments and decisions
- Emergency Department Assistant
- Radiographer – undertakes appropriate trauma imaging
- Radiologist – provides expert review of trauma imaging; may undertake focused point of care imaging and/or interventional procedures
- Lead Nurse
- Specialists – provide expert assessment and relevant interventions and treatments:
  - trauma and orthopaedics
  - surgery
  - paediatric critical care

Trauma alert, team briefing and preparation

Preparation is the key to effective and efficient trauma management. Capturing the information given when the trauma alert is received using a structured approach, for example ATMISTER, enables appropriate briefing and planning prior to the arrival of the child.

A	Age/sex
T	Time of incident
M	Mechanism of injury
I	Injury suspected
S	Signs including vital signs, Glasgow Coma Scale
T	Treatment so far
E	Estimated time of arrival to emergency department
R	Requirements, i.e. bloods, specialist services, tiered response, ambulance call sign

It also allows the team leader to decide on the appropriate response, either a full paediatric trauma team or a targeted specialty response. However, it is important to have an awareness that 30% of children with significant trauma may arrive by car with friends/family without a pre-alert. With less information available another structured approach can be STEP UP.

S	Self	Prepare communication, recognise stresses
T	Team	Plan roles and positions of the team
E	Environment	Prepare equipment
P	Patient/Primary survey	Clear roles/<c>ABCDE
U	Update	Treatment so far
P	Plan	Requirements

After the call has been received from ambulance control, the team leader should complete the following actions (Box 8.3).

Box 8.3 Team leader actions: plan and review

- Remember early management of catastrophic haemorrhage requires urgent blood products so activate the massive haemorrhage protocol early
- Make a plan and back-up plan according to age, mechanism and expected injuries
- Child arrives: 5-second review and adapt plan accordingly

In role allocation consideration must be given to specific roles, including primary survey, airway, breathing and circulation, plus scribe, family support and drug management, taking into account the competencies of the team available.

On arrival, unless the child has a catastrophic haemorrhage, traumatic cardiac arrest or obstructed airway, a controlled 'eyes-on, hands-off' handover occurs. At this point, the team leader completes a 5-second review and adapts the plan accordingly. The form of the structured approach is shown in Box 8.4.

Box 8.4 Structured approach

Immediate
- Primary survey (identify *immediate life threats and act on them*)
- Resuscitation

Focused
- Secondary survey (elicit *key features*)
- Emergency treatment

Detailed review
- Reassessment (system control)
- Further stabilisation and definitive care

8.6 Primary survey and resuscitation

During the primary survey, life-threatening problems should be treated as they are identified (Box 8.5)

Box 8.5 <c>ABCDE

<c>	<Catastrophic external haemorrhage control>
A	Airway (with cervical spine control)
B	Breathing with ventilatory support
C	Circulation with haemorrhage control
D	Disability with prevention of secondary insult
E	Exposure with temperature control

Consider **F** for family and discuss presence of family at the briefing

---

<Catastrophic external haemorrhage>

In major trauma <c>ABCDE has become the established approach. Obvious external exsanguinating haemorrhage becomes the immediate priority.

'Blood on the floor and five more Bs': a life-threatening amount of blood may be lost as a result of traumatic haemorrhage. The haemorrhage may be obvious bleeding outside the body (it can be seen on the 'floor' – remember to check the back and skin folds, including between the buttocks). Or the blood loss may be hidden with the haemorrhage occurring in internal compartments. The most likely areas are:

- Thorax (Breast)
- Abdomen (Belly)
- Pelvis (Buttock)
- Femur (Bone)
- Do not forget that babies can lose significant blood volume into their head (Brain)

These areas are where blood loss should be looked for in the context of ongoing shock without obvious cause, and where initial attempts to control catastrophic haemorrhage should be directed.

- Simple direct pressure, specialised haemostatic dressings or a tourniquet (or indirect pressure on a major artery above the injury) must be applied instantly to stem active external haemorrhage
- Apply a pelvic binder if there is concern for pelvic injury with haemodynamic instability
- Tranexamic acid should be given intravenously 15 mg/kg (max. 1000 mg) as soon as possible

The assessment can then continue with the ABCDE sequence.

Airway and cervical spine

Look for anything compromising the airway.

- Material in the lumen (blood, vomit, teeth or a foreign body)
- Damage to or loss of control of the structures in the wall (the mouth, tongue, pharynx, larynx or trachea)
- External compression or distortion from outside the wall (e.g. compression from a pre-vertebral haematoma in the neck or distortion from a displaced maxillary fracture)

Problems can develop after the primary survey, e.g. bleeding or progressive swelling in facial trauma or burns

A child with a GCS score of 8 or less is unlikely to be adequately protecting their airway

The commonest cause is from occlusion by the tongue in an unconscious, head-injured child

---

Whatever the cause, airway management should follow the structured sequence (see Chapter 17), bearing in mind the need to protect the cervical spine. This is summarised in Box 8.6.

Box 8.6 Airway management sequence

- Jaw thrust
- Suction/removal of foreign body under direct vision
- Oro-/nasopharyngeal airways
- Tracheal intubation
- Surgical airway

Head tilt/chin lift is not recommended following trauma because this manoeuvre can move the cervical spine and may exacerbate an injury. For any mechanism of injury capable of causing spinal injury (or in cases with an uncertain history), the cervical spine is presumed to be at risk until it can be cleared. Children (and adults) can suffer spinal cord injury despite normal plain radiographs (spinal cord injury without radiological abnormality (SCIWORA)). If ignored, ligamentous instability in the absence of radiological evidence of a fracture can have devastating consequences.

If protection is considered necessary, start with manual in-line stabilisation (MILS) by a competent assistant or, if this is not possible, consider using a head block and appropriate strapping. Rigid immobilisation of the head risks increasing leverage on the neck as the child struggles. Minimise anxiety by avoiding unnecessary interventions and encouraging the parents to remain at the bedside.

Vomiting poses an obvious threat to the unprotected airway, especially if there is also a risk of spinal injury. Before providing airway suction, tilt the patient trolley head down, ensuring they are secure.

The child should be taken off the extrication stretcher as soon as possible, using the 20° tilt method (see Chapter 21), and placed directly onto a trauma mattress (Figure 8.1) or an emergency department trolley. If the spine has not been cleared, manual in-line immobilisation will be needed for intubation if indicated. If the child is paralysed, sedated and ventilated the cervical spine cannot be cleared, and spinal immobilisation needs to be maintained until definitive imaging (see Chapter 22) and neurological examinations can take place. A child should not be on a spinal board/scoop for any longer than for the initial survey and transfer to scan.

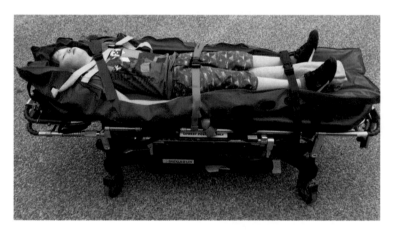

Figure 8.1 Vacuum mattress in use

Breathing

Adequacy of breathing is checked in three domains (see Chapter 3):

- Effort
- Efficacy
- Effects on other organ systems

When examining the chest, look, listen and feel:

Look – remembering asymmetry and asymmetrical movement (flail chest)

Listen – for reduced air entry or crackles

Feel – remember to check for crepitus (surgical emphysema) and tracheal deviation, and percuss to distinguish a tension pneumothorax from a massive haemothorax

Conditions identified

By the end of the primary survey, the following conditions may have been recognised, all of which can have a detrimental effect on respiration, with treatment initiated as soon as they are found:

- **A**irway obstruction
- **T**ension pneumothorax
- **O**pen pneumothorax
- **M**assive haemothorax
- **F**lail chest
- **C**ardiac tamponade
- **D**ecompensating head injury
- **S**hock

If breathing is inadequate, commence ventilation with a bag–valve–mask and prepare for intubation, which is likely to be required. The indications for intubation and mechanical ventilation are summarised in Box 8.7.

Box 8.7 Indications for intubation and ventilation

- Persistent airway obstruction
- Predicted airway obstruction, e.g. inhalational burn
- Loss of airway reflexes (reduced Glasgow Coma Scale (GCS) score and responding to pain or unresponsive)
- Inadequate ventilatory effort or increasing fatigue
- Disrupted ventilatory mechanism, e.g. severe flail chest
- Persistent hypoxia despite supplemental oxygen
- Controlled ventilation required to prevent secondary brain injury (see Chapter 11)

If breath sounds are unequal consider and institute correct management (see Chapter 9):

- Pneumothorax
- Haemopneumothorax
- Misplaced tracheal tube
- Blocked main bronchus or pulmonary collapse
- Diaphragmatic rupture
- Pulmonary contusion
- Aspiration of vomit or blood

Circulation

Circulatory assessment in the primary survey involves the rapid assessment of heart rate and rhythm, pulse volume and peripheral perfusion including colour, temperature and capillary return and blood pressure (Table 8.1). Circulatory assessment must take into account the fact that resting

Table 8.1 Recognition of clinical signs indicating blood loss requiring urgent treatment

Sign	Indicator
Heart rate	Marked or increasing tachycardia or relative bradycardia
Systolic blood pressure	Falling
Capillary refill time (normal less than 2 seconds)	Increasing
Respiratory rate	Tachypnoea unrelated to thoracic problem
Mental state	Altered conscious level unrelated to isolated head injury

heart rate, blood pressure and respiratory rate vary with age (see the normal ranges table (inside front cover)).

Additionally in trauma:

- Check peripheral pulses in limb injury
- Look for internal haemorrhage (chest, abdomen, pelvis and femurs), including consideration of bleeding from multiple sites and progressive deterioration
- Apply pressure to significant external haemorrhage (if appropriate)
- Remember that exposure to cold prolongs the capillary refill time in healthy people
- Check lactate and haemoglobin as early indicators of circulatory compromise
- Consider the possibility of blood loss from a head injury in infants

All seriously injured children require vascular access to be established urgently using two relatively large intravenous cannulae. Peripheral veins are preferred; other options are:

- Intraosseous cannulation of the tibia, femur or humerus
- If there is no suspicion of a cervical spine injury – direct cannulation of the external jugular vein
- Indirect or direct cannulation of the femoral vein using the Seldinger technique ('wire through needle' followed by 'catheter over wire')
- Cut-down onto the cephalic vein at the elbow or the long saphenous vein at the ankle

Vascular access techniques are discussed in detail in Chapter 20. When vascular access is achieved, bloods should be taken, prioritising an urgent cross-match as well as a blood gas for haemoglobin and lactate and a venous sample for clotting. If there are signs of circulatory compromise, uncontrolled bleeding must be considered and appropriate teams summoned, if they are not already part of the trauma team. The initial haemoglobin is unlikely to change in the first instance; be careful not to be reassured by a normal haemoglobin in the first hour. If the child is stable with no signs of shock, an immediate fluid bolus is not required. The principles behind this are '**the first clot is the best clot**'.

There are four key treatments of circulation (Figure 8.2):

1. Stop obvious external bleeding.
2. Replace ongoing blood loss with blood products.
3. Ensure the blood is warm.
4. Give the replacement fast.

Massive haemorrhage following injury is not common in children. Its management requires an understanding of concepts that have become standard in adult trauma care (Figures 8.3 and 8.4):

- Use of tranexamic acid (bolus dose 15 mg/kg; max. 1000 mg followed by an infusion of 2 mg/kg/h)
- Effective use of adjuncts (e.g. tourniquets, pelvic splints)
- Implementation of massive haemorrhage protocols (MHPs)
- Avoidance of hypothermia using heating devices
- Maintenance of an adequate haematocrit used to aid clotting by promoting platelet aggregation in small blood vessels, by use of optimal ratios of red cells to other blood products
- Prompt restoration of perfusion after controlling haemorrhage (monitored by the lactate level returning to normal within a few hours)
- Damage control interventions, involving surgery and interventional radiology
- Massive transfusion can cause an increase in potassium and citrate so careful monitoring of calcium and potassium is necessary as homeostasis will alter significantly

If abdominal haemorrhage is suspected, CT with contrast should be performed. In children, FAST (focused assessment with sonography for trauma) has very limited application and there is limited evidence of its worth in detecting abdominal haemorrhage.

Fluid resuscitation in trauma

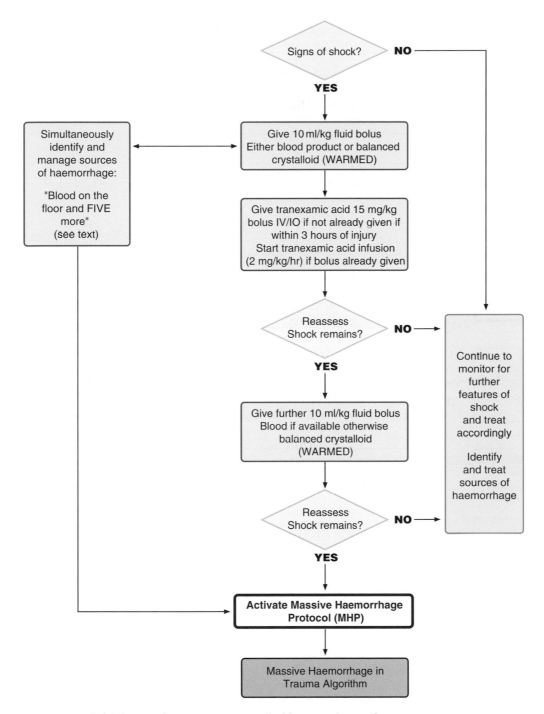

Figure 8.2 Blood and fluid therapy in severe uncontrolled haemorrhage after trauma
FFP, fresh frozen plasma

Massive haemorrhage in trauma

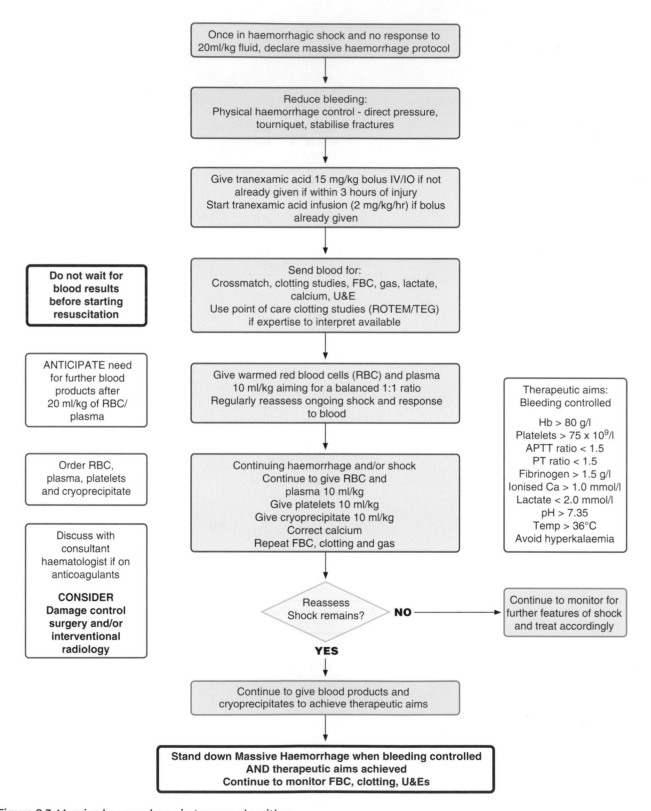

Figure 8.3 Massive haemorrhage in trauma algorithm
APTT, activated partial thromboplastin time; FBC, full blood count; Hb, haemoglobin; PT, prothrombin time; U&E, urea and electrolytes.

Paediatric major trauma

T	Tranexamic acid	• If not administered already 15 mg/kg bolus (max 1 g), followed by • 2 mg/kg/hr over 8 hours (max 125 mg/h)
R	Resuscitation	• Activate MHP and consider: • Rapid infuser • Cell salvage • Normotensive resuscitation (unless post pubertal) • Pelvic binder/splint fractures/tourniquet • Limit crystalloid and colloid use
A	Avoid hypothermia	• Target temperature over 36 degrees Celsius • Remove wet clothing and sheets • Warm fluids • Warming blanket/mattress/external warmer
U	Unstable? Damage control surgery	• If unstable, coagulopathic, hypothermic or acidotic, consider damage control surgery • Aim surgery time less than 90 minutes • Haemorrhage control, decompression, decontamination and splintage
M	Metabolic	• Avoid acidosis • Base excess guides resuscitation • If lactate more than 5 mmol/litre or rising, consider stopping surgery, splint and transfer to PCCU • Monitor blood glucose
A	Avoid vasoconstrictors	• Inappropriate use of vasoconstrictors doubles mortality • However, use may be required in cases of spinal cord or traumatic brain injury
T	Test clotting	• Consider TEG® (thromboelastographic)/ROTEM® • Check clotting every 15 ml PRBC/kg body weight • Aim platelets over 75 x 10/litre • Aim INR & aPTTR less than or equal to 1.5 • Aim fibrinogen more than 1.5 g/litre

I	Imaging	• Consider:
		  • Local guidelines for paediatric trauma
		  • Does this child need imaging at all?
		  • If imaging is required which anatomical area(s) need to be covered?

C	Calcium gluconate	• Maintain ionised calcium more than 1.0 mmol/litre • Administer 0.2 ml/kg 10% calcium gluconate over 10 minutes as required • Give calcium routinely after MHP pack one

Figure 8.4 Paediatric major trauma checklist
Adapted from UHCW NHS Trust Paediatric TRAUMATIC (Copyright (c): L May, A Kelly, M Wyse, K Thies, T Newton)
Contact Laura.May@uhcw.nhs.uk
aPTTR, activated partial thromboplastin time ratio; INR, international normalised ratio; MHP, major haemorrhage protocol; PCCU, paediatric critical care unit; PRBC, packed red blood cells

> The child's condition should be constantly reassessed and immediate damage control surgical intervention to stop the haemorrhage considered

Disability

The assessment of disability (neurological function) during the primary survey consists of a focused neurological examination to determine the conscious level and to assess pupil size and reactivity.

The conscious level is described by the child's response to voice and (where necessary) to pain. The AVPU method describes the child as **a**lert, responding to **v**oice, responding to **p**ain or **u**nresponsive and is a rapid, and simple, assessment.

A	**A**lert
V	Responds to **V**oice
P	Responds only to **P**ain
U	**U**nresponsive to all stimuli

A children's Glasgow Coma Scale (GCS) score should be performed as soon as possible (see Table 6.1), particularly in the context of traumatic brain injury and prior to drugs that alter conscious level such as sedatives and anaesthetics.

> Agitation in a child may suggest cerebral hypoxia

If the primary survey reveals that the child has a decompensating head injury, neurological resuscitation is required. If the GCS score is less than 8 and/or AVPU equivalent of P or U, immediate intervention is necessary. Remember that the GCS is modified in the smaller child (see Table 6.1).

Interventions to be considered whilst organising urgent transfer (if required) include:

- Oxygenation with 15 l/min
- Head up 20°
- Control of carbon dioxide (CO_2) levels (by intubation and controlled ventilation)
- Maintenance of normal blood pressure to support cerebral perfusion including use of inotropes
- Sodium chloride or mannitol osmotic diuretics to help reduce (if indicated) the intracranial pressure
- Anaesthesia/paralysis/sedation/analgesia to reduce cerebral metabolism
- Prompt treatment of any seizures and raised temperature

> As soon as a serious head injury is suspected, a CT scan of the brain should be ordered and the neurosurgical team (which may be off site) alerted

Tranexamic acid (15 mg/kg, max. 1 g) should be considered if within 3 hours of injury and there is suspicion of head injury and evidence of reduced conscious level (GCS less than 15 or V, P, U) or confirmed intracranial bleed on imaging.

See further details in Chapter 11.

If the child is deteriorating neurologically, the child might need urgent transfer to a neurological centre prior to CT.

Exposure

In order to assess a seriously injured child fully, it is necessary to take their clothes off. Children become cold very quickly, and may be acutely embarrassed when undressed in front of strangers. Although exposure is necessary the duration should be minimised, and a blanket provided at all other times.

> Ensure that the child's temperature is maintained and hypothermia is prevented

This is achieved by having a warm resuscitation area and tasking one or more of the nursing team members to keep the child covered with a blanket or hot air warming device at all times and to warm all fluids given.

It is important to examine the child fully. In the context of penetrating injury it is particularly important to ensure that all creases including the perineum and anus are examined as there can be hidden wounds.

Other procedures carried out during the resuscitation phase

Imaging

See Chapter 22.

Investigations

When venous access is achieved and blood is taken for cross-matching, samples for other investigations should be taken at the same time, including full blood count, blood gas, lactate, clotting studies (where available thrombelastograph (TEG®) and thromboelastometry (ROTEM®) analysis may be used), amylase, liver transaminases, urea and electrolytes. Remember to measure the glucose, especially in adolescents (who are prone to both injury and hypoglycaemia after drinking alcohol) and in very small children. Serum β-human chorionic gonadotrophin should also be taken in adolescent females to identify pregnancy.

Oro/nasogastric tube placement

Gastric stasis is a frequent consequence of major trauma and acute gastric dilatation is common in children. If suspected, particularly in the obtunded child, the stomach should be decompressed. If there is evidence or suspicion of base of skull fracture, the tube should not be passed by the nasal route. In the intubated child, the oral route is a simple alternative.

Analgesia

Analgesia can usually be administered just after completing the primary survey and resuscitation. See Chapter 3.

8.7   Secondary survey and looking for key features

Having finished the primary survey and set in place appropriate resuscitative measures, focused care is the next phase of management. The central diagnostic process during this phase is the secondary survey, a systematic clinical examination to identify injuries. It is supplemented by observations, imaging and other investigations. Further information is gathered at this time, especially the history of the events leading up to the injury and the presence of any co-morbid factors. It is important for the team leader to instigate a summary of what the findings are and ensure the team are aware of them.

History

History should be sought from the child, ambulance personnel, relatives and witnesses of the accident. An AMPLE history can be used to obtain relevant information.

A	Allergies
M	Medication
P	Previous medical history (pre-existing medical conditions and immunisations)
L	Last meal
E	Environment and events

In addition, consider the mechanism of injury. The following should alert the team to an increased likelihood of significant injury:

- Fall more than twice the height of the child
- Death or serious injury of another occupant of the vehicle
- Ejection from or trapped under vehicle/prolonged extrication
- Greater than 40 mph head-on collision/bullseye or significant damage to the vehicle
- Stabbing

Secondary survey

The secondary survey is a thorough head-to-toe, front-to-back examination searching for key anatomical features of injury. It is helpful to think in terms of:

- Surface (head to toe, front and back)
- Orifice (mouth, nose, ears, orbits, rectum, genitals)
- Cavity (chest, abdomen, pelvic cavity, retroperitoneum)
- Extremity (upper limbs including shoulders; lower limbs including pelvic girdle)

Occasionally, a full secondary survey may be delayed if immediate life-saving interventions are required. Ensure that this decision is clearly documented and a secondary survey carried out at a later stage.

> Throughout this stage of management, the vital signs and neurological status should be continually reassessed, and any deterioration should lead to an immediate return to the primary survey

Special considerations in injury

- Consider otoscopy (for haemotympanum) and ophthalmoscopy (for retinal haemorrhage)
- Inspect the mouth inside and out – intraoral bruising may represent fractures
- Palpate the teeth for looseness
- Assess for nasal septal haematoma
- Assess for midface stability
- Look for signs of base of skull injury (panda eyes, mastoid bruising)
- Perform a full neurological examination
- Inspect neck veins and pulses if there is a neck injury
- Observe for movement
- Inspect for any external evidence of injury – tyre marks, bruising, lacerations and swelling, including inspection of all creases
- Note unusual injury and bruising patterns suggesting non-accidental injury
- Inspect the perineum
- Inspect the external urethral meatus for blood

Investigations

See Chapter 22 for details on requesting and interpreting trauma imaging. An electrocardiogram (ECG) should be performed in children with chest trauma or unexplained collapse/seizure.

8.8   Emergency treatment

Emergency treatment represents the early response to key findings in the secondary survey and its adjunct investigations. While the interventions are less urgent than those in the resuscitation phase, they will still need to be carried out promptly to minimise the risk of deterioration or unnecessary morbidity. The emergency treatment plan will include treatments for any potentially life-threatening or limb-threatening injuries discovered during the secondary survey. If it does not put the child at undue risk, this plan may be extended to include definitive care of other (more minor) injuries discovered at the same time.

Emergency treatments are discussed in more detail in subsequent chapters.

> In the face of a serious deterioration, return to the primary survey

8.9   Further stabilisation

Further stabilisation and definitive care constitute the final part of the structured approach to trauma care. Good note taking and appropriate, timely referral are essential. If definitive care is to be undertaken in a specialist centre then transfer may be necessary at this stage.

The initial emphasis was on crude physiological assessment (<c>ABCDE) in the primary survey, followed by focusing on the anatomical evaluation of injuries in the secondary survey. From the time of the initial resuscitation, pulse rate, blood pressure, respiratory rate, oxygen saturation and temperature (avoid hypo- and hyperthermia) should be measured and charted frequently (every 5 minutes initially). Beyond these continuing observations, there is now a need to return to overall physiological control by considering the following systems in more detail, especially in a critically injured child:

- Respiration
- Circulation
- Nervous system
- Metabolism
- Host defence

Respiration (A and B)

The airway should be rechecked. If intubated, is the endotracheal tube of an expected length at the teeth (for the size of the child)? Are the breath sounds symmetrical? Could the tube have migrated into a main-stem bronchus?

Arterial blood gas analysis provides essential information in the child with serious head, chest or multiple injuries (arterial oxygen and CO_2 tensions) or in any child who has been intubated. Inserting an arterial line facilitates repeated measurements; in an unintubated child, a venous blood gas should suffice.

Pulse oximetry readings should be displayed continuously. End-tidal CO_2 monitoring is mandatory in the ventilated child. It shows that the breathing circuit is still connected and that the endotracheal tube has not become dislodged. The end-tidal CO_2 should not be regarded as a reliable indicator of arterial CO_2 tension, especially in a shocked child. Ventilation–perfusion mismatch causes it to under-represent the arterial level. It can be regarded as a crude indicator of pulmonary perfusion.

Circulation (C)

This system comprises the three 'haems': haemodynamics, haemoglobin and haemostasis. In a child with serious injuries, the pulse rate and rhythm should be monitored electrocardiographically. Non-invasive blood pressure readings are generally reliable, although in serious head injuries and multiple injuries, it is better to monitor on a beat-to-beat basis using direct arterial measurements via an arterial line usually at the radius. This also allows estimation of the haemoglobin (or haematocrit) at hourly intervals to help detect ongoing bleeding and to determine the requirement for further transfusion. Base deficit (or lactate) measurements indicate the adequacy of tissue perfusion, although it is still important to reassess the child clinically. Other invasive techniques, such as central venous pressure monitoring, may be considered at this stage, but should only be undertaken by appropriately trained personnel.

After major blood loss, plasma, platelets and cryoprecipitate may be needed to correct coagulopathy following the measurement of clotting times and platelet count. Remember that hypothermia affects clotting. Also consider using viscoelastic assays such as TEG® or ROTEM® which may give a more rapid assessment of clotting at the bedside. If not available, recheck coagulation profile frequently.

Urinary catheterisation

In a child, a urinary catheter should only be inserted if the child cannot pass urine spontaneously or if continuous accurate output measurement is required to achieve stabilisation after a serious physiological insult. The route (urethral or suprapubic) will depend on factors related to signs of urethral, bladder, intra-abdominal or pelvic injury (such as blood at the external meatus, or bruising in the scrotum or perineum; see Chapter 10). If a boy requires urethral catheterisation, urethral damage must be excluded first. The smallest possible silastic catheter should be used in order to reduce the risk of subsequent urethral stricture formation. If any doubt exists then the decision to catheterise the child can be left to the responsible surgeon. Urine should have dipstick urinalysis and sent for microscopy.

In seriously injured children, the urinary output serves as an indicator of systemic perfusion and should be recorded hourly. It should be maintained at 1–2 ml/kg/h, or higher if there has been a major crush injury or electrical burn with a high risk of myoglobinuria. If it is low, hypovolaemia is the likely cause, although other causes should be considered. If it is high, it may reflect excessive fluid therapy, but remember that diabetes insipidus can occur within a few hours of a serious head injury.

Nervous system (D)

Pupil size and reactivity and the GCS score should be checked and recorded every 15 minutes initially. Any deterioration should prompt the need to discuss the case with a neurosurgeon or consider a CT scan (or repeat one). Intracranial pressure (ICP) monitoring is an important means of identifying life-threatening rises in pressure. In conjunction with invasive blood pressure measurements, it provides a means of tracking cerebral perfusion pressure. ICP monitoring can be established in the operating theatre or the critical care unit. Its use should be confined to hospitals with appropriately skilled personnel, but the importance of cerebral perfusion pressure should be understood by all those who deal with critical head injuries in children. See further details in Chapter 11.

Metabolism (electrolytes, fluid balance, gut and hormones)

This system refers to biochemical processes and includes renal, hepatic, gastrointestinal and endocrine problems. Glucose ('don't ever forget glucose') monitoring and control, is important in both young children and in adolescents who may have have taken alcohol or unknown drugs. Monitor urine output and check serum biochemistry (see Circulation section above).

Host defence (injury, infection, immunity, intoxication)

Host defence represents the interaction between the body as a whole and external influences. As such, it encompasses injury (including injury from poor positioning and thermal injury), infection (including wound care), immunity (including need for tetanus prophylaxis) and intoxication (including alcohol and drugs that may be present in the circulation).

Thermal injury is an important concern: hypothermia hinders blood clotting and predisposes to infection, while fever increases metabolic demand and must be avoided in the severely head-injured child. Wound care, antibiotic prophylaxis for open fractures, and checking that tetanus immunisations are up to date (has the child been immunised at all?) are all considered at this stage, as is careful positioning to avoid problems such as pressure injury from a poorly fitted splint. Consider tetanus toxoid and tetanus immunisation in a heavily contaminated wound (soil or faeces) as per national guidelines.

'Tertiary survey'

In addition to physiological system control, it is essential for transport escorts, intensive care staff or receiving unit medical staff, who may take over care at this stage, to re-examine the child and review the investigations (especially the imaging) from an anatomical viewpoint to seek out any missed injuries.

Returning to the primary survey

Any sudden deterioration in the child's condition should trigger an immediate reassessment of the airway, breathing, circulation and disability so resuscitation can once more be undertaken.

Note taking

The structured approach discussed in this chapter can provide a framework for the writing of notes. It is recommended that these should be set out as shown in Table 8.2. Many trauma centres have dedicated trauma booklets.

Table 8.2   Template for note taking
History
Mechanism of injury and pre-hospital/pre-major trauma centre interventions
Past history
Primary survey and resuscitative interventions
<c>
A
B
C
D and E
Secondary survey and emergency treatment of injuries
Head
Face
Neck
Chest
Abdomen
Pelvis
Spine/back
Extremities
Further stabilisation
Respiration
Circulation
Nervous system
Metabolism
Host defence

Referral

Many teams may be involved in the definitive care of a seriously injured child. It is essential that referrals are made appropriately, clearly and early. Guidance about which children to refer to which team is given in subsequent chapters.

Transfer

Injured children may require transfer either within the hospital or to another centre to deliver life-saving and definitive care. In either case, thorough preparation of the equipment, patient and documentation is essential. A careful balance must be achieved between delaying such care and setting off with an inadequately stabilised child. Transport of children is discussed in more detail in Chapter 23.

8.10 Summary

This chapter has described how the structured approach to initial assessment and management allows the clinician to care effectively for the seriously injured child. Life-threatening issues should be treated when found, before progressing to secondary survey, emergency treatment and definitive care. Knowledge of local major incident guidance is important and needs to be practised regularly.

CHAPTER 9

The child with chest injury

Learning outcomes

After reading this chapter, you will be able to:

- Identify the chest injuries that pose an immediate threat to life and those that are discovered later
- Describe how to manage these injuries

9.1 Introduction

Isolated chest injuries are uncommon in children; they are usually associated with multisystem injury. Problems may result directly from chest injury or may be secondary to other injuries. Consequences of severe trauma, such as gastric dilatation or pulmonary aspiration after vomiting or regurgitation, may further compromise respiratory function.

Children have relatively elastic tissues. Substantial amounts of kinetic energy may be transferred through a child's chest wall to deep structures with little or no external sign of injury and without rib fractures. A lack of evident rib fractures on the chest radiograph does not exclude major thoracic visceral disruption; conversely, the presence of rib fractures indicates high-energy transfer.

Children have relatively little respiratory reserve. Their high metabolic rate and small functional residual capacity allow them to desaturate more rapidly when their oxygen supply is curtailed. Their horizontal ribs and underdeveloped musculature make them tolerate chest wall disruption badly. Flail chest, for example, is poorly tolerated.

The risk of iatrogenic chest problems must be appreciated. The child's relatively short trachea allows the endotracheal tube to become easily displaced into a main-stem bronchus or into the oesophagus. Mask ventilation can cause inadvertent gastric distension and overinflation of the lungs can result in a pneumothorax (especially after intubation if the endotracheal tube has migrated beyond the carina). If a traumatic pneumothorax already exists, ventilation will cause it to increase in size and may turn it into a tension pneumothorax.

Thoracic injuries must be considered in all children who suffer major trauma. Some may be life threatening and require immediate resuscitative therapy during the primary survey and resuscitation. Others may be discovered during the secondary survey (and its associated investigations) and be dealt with by emergency treatment. Some situations will need prompt, specialist surgical intervention, but most chest injuries can be managed in the first hour using general advanced life support skills. Practical procedures are described in detail in Chapter 21. During subsequent detailed review, attention will be redirected to the chest to maintain respiratory control and to search for missed injuries. See Box 9.1 for Imaging in chest trauma.

Advanced Paediatric Life Support: A Practical Approach to Emergencies, Seventh Edition. Edited by Stephanie Smith.
© 2023 John Wiley & Sons Ltd. Published 2023 by John Wiley & Sons Ltd.

Box 9.1 Imaging in chest trauma

Chest X-ray (CXR)

The primary investigation for blunt chest trauma is the chest X-ray. This will detect pneumothorax, haemothorax, gross mediastinal injuries, flail chest and may show rib fractures

Point of care ultrasound (POCUS)

Focused ultrasound used in the emergency situation to identify pneumothorax, haemothorax or cardiac tamponade

Computed tomography (CT)

CT chest should be performed for penetrating chest injuries

CT chest in blunt trauma should be dictated by the nature of the trauma, the clinical condition of the child and the initial CXR findings

---

9.2 Thoracic Injuries posing an immediate threat to life

The following conditions are life threatening. They should be identified during the primary survey and treated immediately. They do not need to be confirmed by adjunct investigations.

A	Airway obstruction
T	Tension pneumothorax
O	Open pneumothorax
M	Massive haemothorax
F	Flail chest
C	Cardiac tamponade

Airway obstruction

The management of airway obstruction is discussed in Chapter 17.

Tension pneumothorax

This is a life-threatening emergency that can be rapidly fatal if not treated promptly. Air accumulates under pressure in the pleural space. This pushes the mediastinum across the chest and kinks the great vessels, compromising venous return to the heart and reducing cardiac output (Figure 9.1). The diagnosis is a clinical one.

Signs

- The child will be hypoxic and may be shocked
- Unless the child is deeply unconscious, there will be signs of respiratory distress
- There will be decreased air entry and possible asymmetrical air movement on inspection, with hyper-resonance to percussion on the side of the pneumothorax
- Distended neck veins may be apparent in some children
- The trachea deviates away from the side of the pneumothorax, although this is not always easy to identify clinically
- Point of care ultrasound (POCUS) (see Appendix I) mid-axillary of the chest may be useful

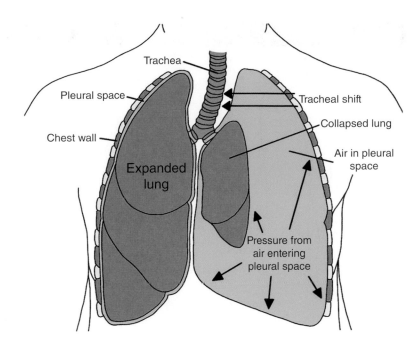

Figure 9.1 Tension pneumothorax

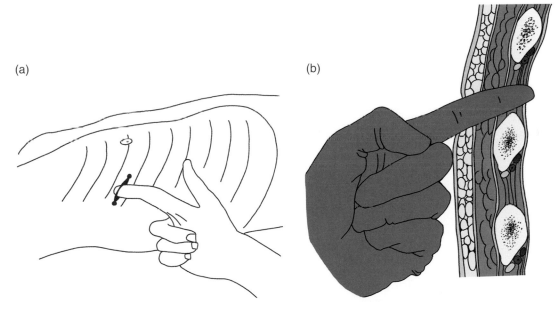

Figure 9.2 (a, b) Finger thoracostomy

Resuscitation

- High-flow oxygen should be given through a reservoir mask
- Immediate finger thoracostomy (an incision to allow continuous drainage (Figure 9.2)) or needle thoracocentesis should be performed to relieve the tension (Figure 9.3)
- A chest drain should be inserted urgently to prevent recurrence or progression to a tension pneumothorax

Air may be forced into the pneumothorax by positive pressure ventilation. If the child is ventilated, a simple pneumothorax is very likely to progress rapidly into a tension pneumothorax

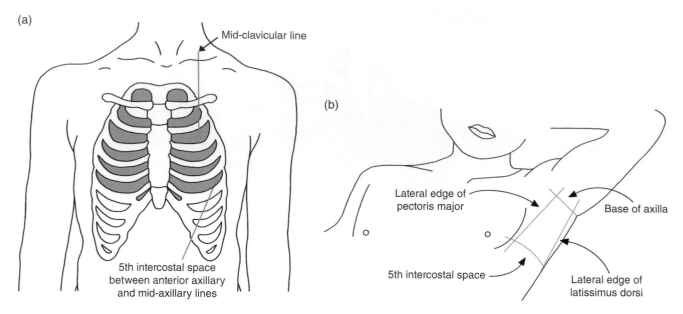

Figure 9.3 (a, b) Landmarks for chest decompression

Open pneumothorax

In this situation there is a penetrating wound in the chest wall with associated pneumothorax. The wound may be obvious, but if it is on the child's back it will not be seen unless actively looked for. If the diameter of the defect is greater than about one-third of the diameter of the trachea, air will preferentially enter the pleural space via the defect rather than be drawn into the lungs via the trachea when the child takes a breath. It is then referred to as a sucking chest wound.

Signs

- Air may be heard sucking and blowing through the wound
- The other signs of pneumothorax will be present
- There may be an associated haemothorax (i.e. a haemopneumothorax)
- POCUS of the chest may be useful

Resuscitation

- High-flow oxygen should be given through a reservoir mask
- The immediate treatment for a sucking wound is to occlude the wound site by using a ported chest seal, provided that the defect is not larger than the base of this device (Figures 9.4 and 9.5). If a ported seal is unavailable, use a three-sided occulsive dressing (Figure 9.4)
- A chest drain will be required as part of emergency treatment. It should not be inserted through the defect itself as this may spread contamination and restart bleeding

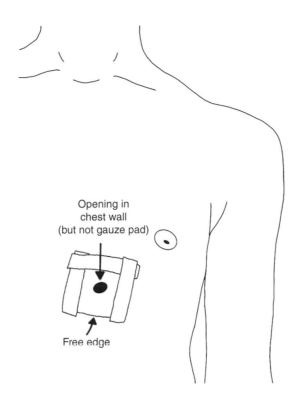

Opening in
chest wall
(but not gauze pad)

Free edge

Figure 9.4 Occlusive dressing (taped on three sides)

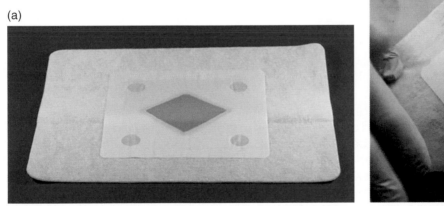

(a)

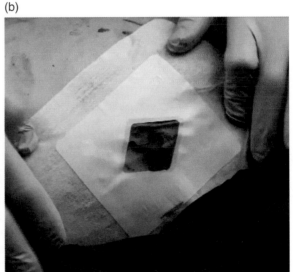

(b)

Figure 9.5 (a) Ported chest seal, and (b) Russell chest seal
Reproduced by permission of Safeguard Medical Technologies

Massive haemothorax

A massive haemothorax will be identified during the B (breathing) stage of the primary survey, although it is even more of a circulatory problem than a respiratory one.

Blood accumulates in the pleural space. This may result from damage to blood vessels (arteries or veins from the pulmonary or systemic vessels) within the lung, the mediastinum or the chest wall (or from a combination). The hemithorax can contain a substantial proportion of a child's blood volume, causing haemorrhagic shock as well as local pressure effects.

Signs

- The child will show signs of shock and may be hypoxic despite added oxygen
- There will be decreased chest movement, decreased air entry and dullness to percussion on the side of the haemothorax
- POCUS of the chest may be helpful to confirm if a haemothorax is present

Resuscitation

- High-flow oxygen should be given through a reservoir mask
- Intravenous access ×2 should be established and blood volume replacement commenced
- A relatively large chest drain should be inserted urgently

Flail chest (or chest wall instability or deformity)

If a number of adjacent ribs are fractured in two or more places, a segment of the chest wall may be free-floating, moving inwards with inspiration and outwards with expiration (paradoxical movement). Such a flail segment is rare in children because of the elasticity of the child's chest wall. When it does occur, we expect major force to have been involved and serious underlying lung (and mediastinal) injury should be anticipated. If the reported mechanism does not involve significant force, suspect an erroneous history (remember non-accidental injury) or, more rarely, osteogenesis imperfecta.

Flail segments may not be noticed on initial examination for three separate reasons: firstly, severe pain on breathing will cause the child to splint the chest wall (this may be unmasked by analgesia); secondly, a child who has already been intubated will be receiving positive pressure ventilation, which moves the floating segment in unison with the rest of the chest wall; or thirdly, the flail segment may be posterior and unnoticed if the back of the chest is not examined carefully. Rib fractures do not always show up well on the chest radiograph, so imaging should not be relied upon in making the diagnosis.

Signs

- The child may be hypoxic despite added oxygen and in considerable pain
- Paradoxical chest movement is characteristic but may not be obvious as indicated above. A high index of suspicion should be retained
- Other evidence of rib fractures (e.g. crepitus on palpation) may be seen

Resuscitation

- High-flow oxygen should be given through a reservoir mask
- Tracheal intubation and ventilation should be considered immediately if the child is compromised. If ventilation is necessary, it may need to be continued for up to 2 weeks before the flail segment becomes 'sticky' and stabilises. On the other hand, minor cases may do well simply with good pain relief and with oxygen by face mask. Nasal or facial continuous positive airway pressure (CPAP), combined with pain relief, may be effective in intermediate cases
- Pain relief should be given using titrated intravenous opioids in the first instance. Local or regional neural blockade avoids the respiratory depressant effects of opioids and should be considered. However, intercostal blocks and epidural catheters are hazardous in the uncooperative child and sedation may be needed to achieve safety – the risks and benefits of the decision must be carefully considered. Epidural analgesia in children should be carried out by an expert and only after injury to the spine has been ruled out formally

Cardiac tamponade

Cardiac tamponade can occur after both penetrating and blunt injury, although it is much more common after penetrating trauma. The blood that accumulates in the fibrous pericardial sac reduces the volume available for cardiac filling during diastole. As more blood accumulates, the cardiac output is progressively reduced.

Signs

- The child will be in shock
- The heart sounds may be muffled
- The neck veins may be distended, although this will not be apparent if the child is also hypovolaemic
- The child may present with a history of syncope and altered mental status
- POCUS may confirm the pericardial fluid and the signs of cardiac tamponade

Resuscitation

- High-flow oxygen should be given through a reservoir mask
- Large-bore Intravenous access should be established, and blood volume replacement commenced. This may temporarily increase cardiac filling
- An emergency thoracotomy will generally be required. A cardiothoracic surgeon (or a paediatric or general surgeon in centres without cardiothoracic surgery) should be involved as soon as the diagnosis is suspected

If personnel are not available to carry out an emergency thoracostomy, an emergency needle pericardiocentesis should be considered. Removing even a small volume of fluid from within the pericardial sac can dramatically increase cardiac output. If available, this should be done with ultrasound guidance.

9.3   Serious injuries discovered later

These conditions will generally be discovered during the secondary survey and its associated investigations, but delayed presentation and masking by other injuries can occur, demanding continual vigilance into the detailed review phase and beyond.

Pulmonary contusion

Children have a high incidence of pulmonary contusion. Energy is readily transmitted to the lungs as the ribs are elastic and do not easily dissipate energy by fracturing. If the ribs do fracture, the degree of force is such that pulmonary contusion is likely too. Pulmonary contusion usually results from blunt trauma, although the shock wave from a high-speed bullet can also cause it. At the microscopic level, pulmonary contusion manifests itself as oedema and interstitial and intra-alveolar haemorrhage.

Clinical features include hypoxia, dyspnoea and haemoptysis, but are not specific. Initially, there may be little to show on the chest radiograph, although an area of non-segmental opacification may be clearly visible from the outset. The appearance on the plain chest film is not specific and may be confused with aspiration, other causes of consolidation/collapse and even with haemothorax (on a supine film). It is important to realise that the clinical features and radiological findings may progress over the next few hours. Bedside ultrasound may be useful to identify peripheral lung contusions.

A computed tomography (CT) scan is not usually indicated for confirming simple pulmonary contusion as contusions are self-limiting and usually resolve by 48 hours. A CT scan, when indicated for other reasons, can help to distinguish pulmonary contusion from other diagnoses, but it is not warranted for this purpose alone.

Treatment consists of the administration of high-flow oxygen, and mechanical ventilation may be necessary. Uncomplicated contusions will largely resolve within the next 36 hours. Physiotherapy plays an important role in reducing the risk of pulmonary collapse and secondary infection.

Cardiac contusion

This is the most common cardiac injury in children, usually resulting from motor vehicle collisions. Clinical features are chest pain, arrhythmias and unexplained tachycardia or hypotension. Symptoms may not present for 24–48 hours. However, clinically significant injury is unlikely if the child is haemodynamically stable with a normal 12-lead electrocardiogram (ECG) at presentation. Sinus tachycardia, ST segment changes, premature beats or atrial arrhythmias in a stable child indicate the need for admission and cardiovascular monitoring. Cardiac troponins may be useful in identifying myocardial injury, with some studies showing 100% sensitivity for cardiac contusion in the context of trauma. Deterioration warrants an echocardiogram. Inotropic support may be required.

More severe trauma may result in cardiac rupture and mortality is high. Diagnosis is made on echocardiogram and operative repair is necessary.

Tracheal and bronchial rupture

Tracheobronchial disruption has a high mortality and requires prompt referral to a specialist cardiothoracic surgeon. It presents as a pneumothorax or haemopneumothorax, typically with a persistent (and often vigorous) air leak after the insertion of a chest drain. Subcutaneous emphysema is frequently present.

Emergency care may involve the insertion of more than one chest drain (with suction applied). When intubation is required, the passage of the endotracheal tube may further disrupt a tracheal tear. When mechanical ventilation is needed, it is important to limit the pressure applied to the airway. This requires specialist ventilation techniques. Unless the leak is small enough to seal spontaneously, definitive surgical repair will be needed.

Disruption of the great vessels

This is usually due to a high-speed motor vehicle crash and is generally fatal at the scene. A child with aortic rupture who survives and arrives at hospital likely has a tear that has tamponaded itself within an intact adventitial (outermost) layer and will require urgent specialist intervention.

The child may be shocked and peripheral pulses may be poorly palpable. On the other hand, if the leak has (temporarily) sealed itself with little blood loss, relative hypertension can occur. Symptoms are generally non-specific. The diagnosis should be suspected on chest X-ray if the mediastinum is widened or has an abnormal profile on chest radiograph, there is tracheal or oesophageal deviation, or if there are upper rib fractures. Remember that a supine anteroposterior film will increase the apparent width of the mediastinum and that the thymus is shown as a prominent mediastinal mass in small children. Sternal and spinal fractures can also cause apparent mediastinal widening.

Contrast CT is important to make the diagnosis. It is important to avoid surges in blood pressure that could precipitate rebleeding. Definitive repair requires interventional radiology or cardiothoracic surgery.

Ruptured diaphragm

Diaphragmatic rupture is a rare blunt injury in children. It is generally thought to be more common on the left side, although some recent studies have questioned this. Penetrating trauma may also involve the diaphragm, usually in the form of knife stab wounds entering the chest or abdomen. Unless other structures are damaged at the same time, such knife wounds may be asymptomatic, only to present many years later as diaphragmatic hernias.

The child with a ruptured diaphragm may be hypoxic due to diaphragmatic dysfunction and to pulmonary compression from a herniated viscus. Shock may result from mediastinal distortion that affects venous return or result from haemorrhage from adjacent structures. The plain chest radiograph may show an apparently raised hemidiaphragm or evidence of abdominal contents within the chest, for example bowel shadowing or a nasogastric tube. Surgical referral should be made. Most ruptures can be repaired from the abdomen, without the need for thoracotomy.

9.4   Other injuries

Simple pneumothorax

Air is present in the pleural space with some degree of lung collapse, but it is not yet under pressure (tension). Signs of hypoxia with decreased chest wall movement, diminished breath sounds and normal or increased resonance to percussion on the side of the pneumothorax may be found, but the signs may be subtle or barely perceptible compared with tension pneumothorax. The diagnosis is usually made on the plain chest radiograph as a lung edge with no lung markings beyond it. However, an anterior pneumothorax is often difficult to recognise. The increasing use of thoracic CT scanning in severe blunt trauma is picking up injuries that may have been missed on plain films.

As traumatic pneumothoraces may not resolve spontaneously, a chest drain should be considered, even if the child is relatively asymptomatic. If the child needs to be ventilated, a chest drain must be inserted as a matter of urgency to avoid a simple pneumothorax developing into a tension pneumothorax.

9.5   Practical procedures

Needle thoracocentesis, chest drain insertion and pericardiocentesis are described in Chapter 21. Clamshell thoracotomy should only be performed by those with expertise and therefore it is not described in detail within the practical procedures. It is not a procedure that is recommended for the non-expert.

9.6   Referral

A competent clinician, trained in advanced life support skills, can provide immediate management for most of the life-threatening injuries discovered during the primary survey. Emergency cardiothoracic surgical involvement will be needed if cardiac tamponade is diagnosed. Other serious injuries discovered during the secondary survey will need cardiothoracic referral.

Indications for cardiothoracic surgical referral
- Continuing massive air leak after chest drain insertion
- Continuing haemorrhage after chest drain insertion
- Cardiac tamponade
- Disruption of the great vessels

Children who require ventilation as part of the treatment of their chest injury (such as those with significant pulmonary contusion) will need transfer to a paediatric intensive care unit. Critical care management will be needed for transfer and as part of continuing stabilisation in general. Appropriate medical and nursing referrals should be made.

9.7 Further stabilisation

In serious chest injuries, the oxygen saturation and pulse rate must be continuously monitored through to the detailed review stage and beyond. The respiratory rate and blood pressure need to be checked frequently. Chest drains must be well secured. Arterial blood gas monitoring is invaluable in severe cases for confirming adequate oxygenation and adjusting carbon dioxide tensions (particularly if there is a concomitant head injury). Remember that many conditions worsen with time, especially pulmonary contusion. An arterial line will also allow the haemoglobin, base deficit and lactate to be monitored.

Continual clinical review is required. Changes in the respiratory pattern and in the apparent degree of illness, in conjunction with trends in the monitoring data, will alert the vigilant clinician to new problems and missed injuries.

Penetrating chest injury

Penetrating thoracic injuries may cause a range of serious conditions which should be picked up within the assessment of breathing and circulation in the primary survey. Thoracic gunshot wounds are more destructive in children under 12 years of age and these children are more likely to require a thoracotomy.

Management of pneumothorax and haemothorax remains the same as for blunt injury, with the insertion of a large-bore chest drain. Thoracotomy is usually not required for haemothorax after penetrating injury unless there is a massive haemothorax (more than 20 ml/kg) or ongoing bleeding of more than 2–4 ml/kg/h from the chest tube.

Emergency department thoracotomy should only be undertaken by senior clinicians, when all necessary equipment is available and in specific clinical circumstances. These circumstances include:

- Children with penetrating cardiac trauma who have a suspected cardiac tamponade scan with unsuccessful pericardiocentesis or loss of signs of life. This is most commonly seen with anterior mediastinal penetrating injury
- Children who are pulseless with witnessed cardic arrest within 10 minutes

Diaphragmatic injury occurs in approximately 15% of patients and is not always immediately evident in the primary survey. A low threshold for consideration should occur when the penetrating object has entered the victim's body between the level of their nipples and the costal margin. Injury to the oesophagus and the thoracic duct often do not present until after the primary survey. Clinical signs include finding saliva or food in the chest drain or the presence of chyle in the drain.

Initial imaging of a child who has suffered from penetrating chest trauma includes a plain chest radiograph which may demonstrate the position of any penetrating instruments that remain in situ and gives information on the conditions described earlier. However, if a patient is stable enough to undergo a helical CT scan then this gives substantially more detailed information on the trajectory and position of any injuries and the status of the major vessels.

9.8 Summary

This chapter has emphasised the important emergency management of chest injuries in children. Cardiothoracic surgical referral may be necessary once the immediate management of life-threatening conditions has been carried out.

CHAPTER 10

The child with abdominal injury

Learning outcomes

After reading this chapter, you will be able to:

- Describe how to assess the injured abdomen
- Identify the options for definitive care

10.1 Introduction

Blunt trauma causes the majority of abdominal injuries in children. Most occur because of accidents on the roads, although a significant number happen during recreational activities. It is important to consider non-accidental injury. A high index of suspicion is necessary if some injuries are not to be missed.

The abdominal contents are susceptible to injury in children for a number of reasons:

- The abdominal wall is thin and offers relatively little protection
- The diaphragm is more horizontal than in adults, causing the liver and spleen to lie lower and more anteriorly
- The ribs, being very elastic, offer less protection to these organs
- The bladder is intra-abdominal, rather than pelvic, and is therefore more exposed when full

> The management of children with abdominal injury may be complicated by respiratory compromise because of diaphragmatic irritation or splinting

10.2 History

A precise history of the mechanism of injury may help in diagnosis. Rapid deceleration, such as experienced during road accidents, causes abdominal compression or shearing of fixed organs. The solid organs and duodenum especially are at risk from such forces. Direct blows, such as those caused by punching (consider non-accidental injury if the history is not compatible) or impact with bicycle handlebars, readily injure the underlying solid organs. Injury to the pancreas or duodenum is a particular feature of handlebar injury due to their fixed position anterior to the spine. Finally, straddling injuries associated with a significant perineal haematoma or urethral bleeding suggests urethral injury.

Advanced Paediatric Life Support: A Practical Approach to Emergencies, Seventh Edition. Edited by Stephanie Smith.
© 2023 John Wiley & Sons Ltd. Published 2023 by John Wiley & Sons Ltd.

10.3   Assessment of the injured abdomen

Initial assessment and management must be structured and directed to the care of the airway, breathing and circulation as discussed in Chapter 8.

Examination

If shock is not responsive to fluid replacement during the primary survey and resuscitation, and no obvious site of haemorrhage exists, then intra-abdominal injury may be the cause of blood loss. The abdomen should be assessed urgently to establish whether early surgical or interventional radiological management is necessary.

The abdomen should be inspected for bruising, lacerations and penetrating wounds. Although major intra-abdominal injury can occur without obvious external signs, visible bruising increases the likelihood of significant injury. A high index of suspicion and frequent, repeated clinical assessment is appropriate in such cases. The external urethral meatus should be examined for blood. The child may require logrolling to examine the back.

Gentle palpation should be carried out. This will reveal areas of tenderness and rigidity. Care should be taken not to hurt the child because their continued cooperation is important during the repeated examinations that form an important part of management.

Aids to assessment

Rectal and vaginal examinations are rarely required in the injured child. Internal digital examination therefore should be limited to the surgeon who has overall responsibility for the child. Adequate analgesia and both gastric and urinary bladder drainage may help the assessment by decompressing the abdomen.

Gastric drainage

Air swallowing during crying with consequent acute gastric dilatation is common in young children. Early passage of a nasogastric/orogastric tube of an appropriate size is beneficial. If there is a possibility of a basal skull fracture this should be by the oral rather than nasal route. The tube should be aspirated regularly and left on free drainage at other times. A massively distended stomach can mimic intra-abdominal pathology needing laparotomy, and cause serious diaphragm splintage with consequent respiratory compromise.

Urinary catheterisation

Catheterisation of a child should only be performed if the child cannot pass urine spontaneously or if continuous accurate output measurement is required. The route (urethral or suprapubic) will depend on factors related to signs of urethral, bladder, intra-abdominal or pelvic injury (such as blood at the external meatus, or bruising in the scrotum or perineum). If a child requires urethral catheterisation, urethral damage must be excluded first. The catheter should be silastic and as small as possible in order to reduce the risk of subsequent urethral stricture formation.

Investigations

Blood tests

Intravenous access will have already been secured during the primary survey and resuscitation, and at that time blood will have been drawn for baseline blood counts, urea and electrolytes and cross-matching. Amylase and liver function tests should be requested and can usually be performed on the sample sent for urea and electrolytes. Repeated monitoring of blood parameters may be appropriate in some patients.

Imaging

See Chapter 22 for guidelines on requesting and interpreting trauma imaging.

10.4   Definitive care

Many children can be managed without surgical intervention. For surgery to be avoided, the following are essential:

- Adequate observation and frequent monitoring
- Precise fluid management
- The immediate availability of a paediatric surgeon (a good interventional radiology service may limit the requirement for surgery). This may necessitate transfer to a paediatric surgical facility

As well as avoiding the morbidity associated with laparotomy, this approach also reduces the number of children at risk of overwhelming, potentially fatal sepsis following splenectomy.

Indications for surgical intervention

In the face of uncontrolled or significant haemorrhage despite appropriate resuscitation, damage control surgery should be undertaken by a paediatric trained surgeon. The purpose of this is to reduce the progression of acidosis, hypothermia and coagulopathy, the main causes of death in trauma. Children with penetrating injuries or evidence of intestinal perforation should also be considered for urgent surgery. The majority of solid organ injuries should be managed conservatively in an appropriately staffed, paediatric area. This has lower morbidity, mortality and blood use than an operative approach.

Penetrating abdominal injuries

Children with penetrating abdominal injuries should be assessed using the primary survey. Penetrating injury between the nipples and the costal margin have an increased risk of diaphragmatic injury and careful assessment of both the thorax and abdomen is necessary. Unlike blunt abdominal injuries, in penetrating injuries the hollow viscera are more likely to be injured than the solid viscera, with up to 70% of children having injury to the gastrointestinal tract. Impalement injuries are notorious for affecting the perineum and can cause significant damage to the rectum, lower urinary tract and pelvic floor muscles.

Helical computed tomography (CT) imaging can give a substantial amount of information on the potential trajectory of the penetrating implement(s) and their association with vessels and solid organs, and, in the case of perineal injuries, the lower urinary tract and rectum. The presence of free air in the abdomen is an indication of perforation of a hollow viscus but its absence does not rule out this injury. Generally, a formal laparotomy is indicated in all patients with penetrating injury to their abdomen to assess for injury to the stomach, small bowel and large bowel, although in selected cases laparoscopy is being increasingly used.

Penetrating perineal injuries require examination under anaesthetic and repair of the damaged tissue when possible. If rectal or anal injury has occurred, a colostomy is often required to protect the healing tissue. If a urethral or bladder injury has occurred, the child may require a urinary or suprapubic catheter, or both, usually inserted in theatre under direct vision.

10.5 Summary

This chapter has described how the assessment and management of airway, breathing and circulation should be carried out before assessing the abdomen. Abdominal injuries may be a cause of shock and will be identified as part of the circulatory assessment. The majority of children with solid organ injury can be managed non-operatively.

CHAPTER 11

The child with traumatic brain injury

Learning outcomes

After reading this chapter, you will be able to:

- Describe the structured approach to the child with traumatic brain injury
- Implement neuroprotective strategies

11.1   Introduction

Epidemiology

Head injury is the most common single cause of trauma death in children aged 1–15 years. Head injury deaths in children most commonly result from road traffic collisions – pedestrians are the most vulnerable, followed by cyclists and then passengers in vehicles. Falls are the second most common cause of fatal head injuries. In infancy, the most common cause is suspected physical abuse.

Pathophysiology

Primary traumatic brain injury is the damage incurred as a direct consequence of the impact. Neurones, axonal sheaths and blood vessels may be physically disrupted at the moment of impact, often with irreversible cell damage. **Secondary** brain injury represents further damage to central nervous system tissue by secondary insults, and adverse physiological events that can occur minutes, hours or days after the initial injury. Such insults include hypotension, hypoxia, raised intracranial pressure (ICP) and seizures. A key aim of head injury management is to prevent or minimise secondary brain injury.

Primary damage

- Injury to neural tissue:
  - Focal cerebral contusions and lacerations (direct impact and contrecoup)
  - Diffuse axonal injury (shearing injury)
- Injury to intracranial blood vessels:
  - Extradural haematoma (especially the middle meningeal artery)
  - Subdural haematoma (especially dural bridging veins)
  - Intracerebral haematoma
  - Subarachnoid haemorrhage

Advanced Paediatric Life Support: A Practical Approach to Emergencies, Seventh Edition. Edited by Stephanie Smith.
© 2023 John Wiley & Sons Ltd. Published 2023 by John Wiley & Sons Ltd.

Injury to the cranium and to the dural sac may be associated with the above neural and vascular injuries. Open skull fractures, where there is a breach in the skull (vault or base) and in the dural membrane, allow brain tissue to come into contact with the external environment (directly or via the sinuses), with consequent risk of infection.

Secondary damage

This may result from either the direct effects of cerebral injury or from the cerebral consequences of associated injuries and stress.

- Ischaemia from poor cerebral perfusion secondary to raised ICP:
  - Expanding intracranial haematoma (exacerbated by coagulopathy)
  - Cerebral swelling/oedema
- Ischaemia secondary to hypotension and anaemia:
  - Haemorrhage with hypovolaemia or dilutional anaemia
  - Other causes of hypotension (spinal cord injury, drug-induced vasodilatation or later sepsis)
- Hypoxia:
  - Airway obstruction
  - Inadequate respiration (loss of respiratory drive or mechanical disruption of chest wall or diaphragm)
  - Shunt from pulmonary contusion or later respiratory failure
- Hypoglycaemia and hyperglycaemia
- Fever
- Convulsions
- Later infection

Raised intracranial pressure

Once the sutures have closed at 12–18 months of age, the child's cranial cavity behaves like an adult's with a fixed volume. If cerebral oedema worsens or if intracranial haematomas increase in size, the pressure within the cranium increases. Initial compensatory mechanisms include diminution in the volume of cerebrospinal fluid and venous blood within the cranial cavity. When these mechanisms fail, ICP rises, compromising cerebral perfusion:

$$\text{Cerebral perfusion pressure} = \text{Mean arterial pressure} - \text{Mean intracranial pressure}$$

Normal cerebral blood flow is 50 ml of blood per 100 g brain tissue per minute. A fall in cerebral perfusion pressure decreases cerebral blood flow. A flow below 20 ml/100 g brain tissue/min will produce ischaemia. This in turn increases cerebral oedema, causing a further rise in ICP. A cerebral blood flow of below 10 ml/100 g brain tissue/min leads to electrical dysfunction of the neurones and loss of intracellular homeostasis.

A generalised increase of ICP in the supratentorial compartment initially causes transtentorial (uncal) herniation, leading to transforaminal (central) herniation and death. In uncal herniation, the third nerve is nipped against the free border of the tentorium, causing ipsilateral pupillary dilatation secondary to loss of parasympathetic constrictor tone to the ciliary muscles. In central herniation, also known as *coning*, the cerebellar tonsils are forced through the foramen magnum.

In childhood, the most common cause of raised ICP following head injury is cerebral oedema. Children are especially prone to this problem. They may, of course, also have expanding extradural, subdural or intracerebral haematomas that require prompt surgical treatment. Depending on the aetiology of the raised ICP, treatment is either aimed at preventing ICP rising further or removing its cause (by surgical evacuation of haematomas).

There are special considerations in infants with head injuries. Unfused sutures allow the cranial volume to increase initially. Large extradural or subdural bleeds may occur before neurological signs or symptoms develop. Such infants may show a significant fall in haemoglobin concentration.

In addition, the infant's vascular scalp may bleed profusely, causing shock. In children aged over 1 year with shock associated with head injury, serious extracranial injury should be sought as the cause of the shock.

11.2   Triage

Head injuries vary from the trivial to the fatal. Triage is necessary in order to give more seriously injured patients a higher priority. Factors indicating a potentially serious injury are shown in Box 11.1.

Box 11.1 Factors indicating a potentially serious injury

- A history of substantial trauma such as involvement in a road traffic collision or a fall from a height
- A history of loss of consciousness
- Children who are not fully conscious and responsive
- Any child with obvious neurological signs/symptoms such as convulsions or limb weakness

---

11.3   Primary survey and resuscitation

The first priority is to assess and stabilise the airway, breathing and circulation as discussed in Chapter 8. Head injury may be associated with cervical spine injury, and stabilisation must be achieved as previously described.

Pupil size and reactivity should be examined and a rapid assessment of conscious level should be made. In the first place, the AVPU classification may be used.

A	**A**lert
V	Responds to **V**oice
P	Responds only to **P**ain
U	**U**nresponsive to all stimuli

In a time-limited situation, it is not essential to work out the numerical Glasgow Coma Scale (GCS) score immediately, although the EVM (eye, verbal, motor) responses will have been noted. But it is important to note the response to voice or pain (if not responding to voice) in more detail using the GCS before proceeding with neurological resuscitation. The assessment serves as a baseline for continuing care and as a key indicator of the need to intervene immediately.

Resuscitation of a child with a traumatic brain injury requires good coordination and you should have a low threshold for calling the trauma team. Immediate control of the airway, breathing and circulation should be carried out in response to the primary survey findings, according to the general approach in Chapter 8. This support will help to prevent secondary cerebral damage caused by hypoxia and shock arising from both the head injury and other coexistent injuries. Throughout the resuscitation process, the team leader must be aware of the need for urgent neurosurgical intervention or the timely transfer to a neurosurgical centre (within the first hour of a child's attendance).

During the primary survey assessment of disability, any evidence of decompensating head injury will have been recognised. In the severely injured child, extra information from blood gas sampling will be obtained during the resuscitation phase or ongoing monitoring. In the UK, the National Institute for Health and Care Excellence (NICE) has produced evidence-based guidelines for treatment, imaging and referral of head-injured children. On the basis of simple clinical evaluation, supported when necessary by blood gas data, recommended indications for immediate intubation and ventilation in severe head injury are given in Box 11.2.

Box 11.2 Indications for immediate intubation and ventilation

- Coma – not obeying commands, not speaking, not eye opening (equivalent to a GCS score of less than 9)
- Loss of protective laryngeal gag reflexes
- Ventilatory insufficiency as judged by blood gases: hypoxaemia (PaO_2 less than 9 kPa (68 mmHg) on air or less than 13 kPa (98 mmHg) with added oxygen) or hypercarbia ($PaCO_2$ more than 6 kPa (45 mmHg))
- Spontaneous hyperventilation (causing $PaCO_2$ less than 3.5 kPa (26 mmHg))
- Respiratory irregularity

Other indications
- Significantly deteriorating conscious level
- Unstable facial fractures
- Copious bleeding into the mouth
- Seizure

Penetrating brain injuries

Penetrating brain injuries (PBIs) are less prevalent than blunt trauma but are considered to carry a worse prognosis. Gun shot wounds (GSWs) are the predominant cause of PBI although perforation from other sharp objects may occur. When a GSW penetrates the vault the projectile crushes the soft brain tissue in its path, creating a permanent tract of injury. The brain compresses around this with the transfer of energy, with a shock wave that reverberates resulting in cavitation and compression. This mechanism can create significant injury around the permanent tract and can result in shearing injuries or can result in haematomas and contusions. In comparison, a stab wound to the head has a more favourable outcome due to the absence of the indirect injuries sustained with a GSW.

Injuries to the head can be hidden within the hair and thus meticulous inspection is required following immediate resuscitation. All orifices should be inspected. The initial GCS score should be documented as it may help determine prognosis. In penetrating brain injuries a decreased level of consciousness particularly a GCS score of less than 9 should prompt securing the airway with intubation.

Imaging should be completed. Non-contrast computed tomography (CT) is the primary modality used to assess the injury, characterise the tract and identify foreign bodies to inform neurosurgical management. Magnetic resonance imaging is NOT recommended due to the potential hazard of intracranial metallic objects.

Unlike blunt traumatic brain injuries, massive bleeding may occur rapidly with injury PBI. In GSWs, coagulopathy may ensue due to the release of factors including thromboplastin by injured brain cells. Early and continued monitoring of coagulation is warranted.

An early neurosurgical opinion should be sought as almost all of those with survivable PBI will require some neurosurgical intervention. Goals of surgery are control of bleeding, evacuation of haematomas, wound management and creating a watertight closure. If there is a significant mass effect, necrotic brain tissue may require debridement. Routine removal of bone or missile fragments distal from the wound is not recommended as mortality is increased.

It is good practice to administer prophylactic antibiotics especially when any cerebrospinal fluid (CSF) leak is identified. The risk of infection is considered to be higher in paediatric PBI, being about 40%.

About 30–50% of patients with a PBI will develop seizures, with 10% appearing within 7 days post injury. Some studies recommend prophylactic anticonvulsants in the first week but this should be guided by specialist involvement.

Penetrating neck injuries

Penetrating neck injury is defined as an injury that breaches the platysma muscle. The neck is a vulnerable area with unprotected vascular, aerodigestive and neurological structures with arterial injuries occurring in about 25%, and aerodigestive injuries in 30%. Both are associated with high mortality. The neck is classified into three anatomical zones: zone 1 from the clavicles to the cricoid; zone 2 from the cricoid to the angle of the mandible; and zone 3 from the angle of the mandible to the skull base (Figure 11.1).

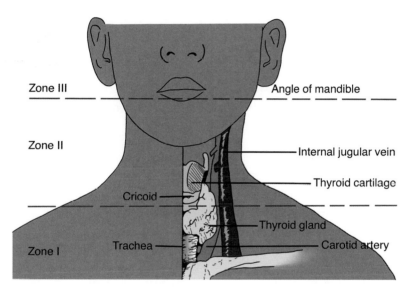

Figure 11.1 Zones of the neck

During resuscitation, immediate consideration should be given to the airway including full examination. Any airway manipulation should be under direct vision. Early anaesthetic and surgical (ENT) review is recommended.

Impaled objects should be kept in place for surgical removal. Early inspection is crucial to determine where the injury has occurred and whether the platysma has been breached. Surgical exploration should be considered dependent on physiological status and clinical examination findings. Signs suggesting the need for surgical exploration are:

- Shock
- Pulsatile bleeding or expanding haematoma
- Audible bruit or palpable thrill
- Airway compromise
- Wound bubbling
- Subcutaneous emphysema
- Stridor
- Hoarseness
- Difficulty or pain when swallowing secretions
- Neurological deficits

These signs may be associated with major injury in up to 90–100% of cases and it may be appropriate for the child to bypass imaging, instead taken directly to theatre. In the absence of 'hard' signs in a stable patient, CT with angiography may be appropriate. This has a low sensitivity for detecting pharyngo-oesophageal injuries and therefore a contrast swallow ± endoscopy may be required in addition.

This approach is in contrast to the traditional zone-based algorithm with mandatory exploration for zone 2 injuries. It is important to understand the zones, as injuries happening in zone 1 may require the presence of cardiothoracic surgeons along with ENT surgeons. A more selective approach based on clinical and radiological findings avoids operative morbidity and is considered safe in children.

Vascular injury is independently predictive of mortality in penetrating neck injuries. Direct external pressure should be applied in the <c> (catastrophic haemorrhage) part of the primary survey. If direct external compression does not stem the flow, Foley balloon catheter tamponade may help. A Foley catheter is inserted into the wound tract, and the balloon is inflated and withdrawn until resistance is met and the catheter clamped. This may allow time for surgical review and resuscitation.

Prophylactic antibiotics should be considered for all penetrating neck injuries.

11.4 Secondary survey and looking for key features

History

The history of the injury itself and the child's course since the injury should be established from bystanders and pre-hospital personnel. Other history should be obtained from parents or carers.

Examination

The head should be carefully observed and palpated for bruises and lacerations to the scalp and for evidence of a depressed skull fracture. Look for evidence of a basal skull fracture, such as blood or CSF from the nose or ear, haemotympanum, panda eyes or Battle's sign (bruising behind the ear over the mastoid process).

The conscious level should be reassessed using the modified GCS if the child is less than 4 years old, or using the standard scale in older children. These scales are shown in Table 11.1. It should be noted that the coma scales reflect the degree of brain dysfunction at the time of the examination. Assessment should be repeated frequently – every few minutes if the level is changing. Communication with the child's care-givers is required to establish the child's best usual verbal response. A 'grimace' alternative to verbal responses should be used in pre-verbal or intubated children (Table 11.2).

The pupils should be re-examined for size and reactivity. A dilated, non-reactive pupil indicates third nerve dysfunction due to an ipsilateral intracranial haematoma until proven otherwise.

The fundi should be examined using an ophthalmoscope. Papilloedema will not be seen in acute raised ICP, but the presence of retinal haemorrhage may indicate non-accidental injury in a young infant.

Motor function should be assessed. This includes examination of extraocular muscle function and facial and limb movements. Limb tone, movement and reflexes should be assessed and any focal or lateralising signs noted.

Table 11.1   Glasgow Coma Scale and Children's Glasgow Coma Scale

Glasgow Coma Scale (4–15 years)		Children's Glasgow Coma Scale (under 4 years)	
Response	**Score**	**Response**	**Score**
Eye opening		**Eye opening**	
Spontaneously	4	Spontaneously	4
To verbal stimuli	3	To verbal stimuli	3
To pain	2	To pain	2
No response to pain	1	No response to pain	1
Best verbal response		**Best verbal response**	
Orientated and converses	5	Alert; babbles, coos words to usual ability	5
Disorientated and converses	4	Less than usual words, spontaneous irritable cry	4
Inappropriate words	3	Cries only to pain	3
Incomprehensible sounds	2	Moans to pain	2
No response to pain	1	No response to pain	1
Best motor response		**Best motor response**	
Obeys verbal command	6	Spontaneous or obeys verbal command	6
Localises to pain	5	Localises to pain or withdraws to touch	5
Withdraws from pain	4	Withdraws from pain	4
Abnormal flexion to pain (decorticate)	3	Abnormal flexion to pain (decorticate)	3
Abnormal extension to pain (decerebrate)	2	Abnormal extension to pain (decerebrate)	2
No response to pain	1	No response to pain	1

Table 11.2   The best grimace response

Grimace response	Score
Spontaneous normal facial/oromotor activity	5
Less than usual spontaneous ability or only response to touch stimuli	4
Vigorous grimace to pain	3
Mild grimace to pain	2
No response to pain	1

Investigations

Blood tests

Blood for full blood count, clotting, glucose and urea and electrolytes should already have been taken during the immediate care phase, and blood for cross-matching sent off at the same time. Blood gases should be taken in head-injured children to allow careful control of $PaCO_2$ and PaO_2, as well as to check pH and base deficit or lactate. End-tidal carbon dioxide (CO_2) should also be monitored.

Imaging

Refer to Chapter 22.

11.5   Emergency treatment

> The initial aim of management for a child with a traumatic brain injury is prevention of secondary brain damage. The key aims are to maintain oxygenation, ventilation and circulation, and to institute neuroprotective measures, to avoid rises in intracranial pressure

The indications for performing an emergency head CT scan are given in Box 11.3.

Box 11.3 Indications for performing an emergency head CT scan within 1 hour

For children who have sustained a head injury and have any of the following risk factors, perform a CT head scan within 1 hour of the risk factor being identified:
- Suspicion of non-accidental injury
- Post-traumatic seizure but no history of epilepsy
- On initial emergency department assessment a GCS score of less than 14, or for children under 1 year a GCS (paediatric) score of less than 15
- At 2 hours after the injury, a GCS score of less than 15
- Suspected open or depressed skull fracture or tense fontanelle
- Any sign of basal skull fracture (haemotympanum, panda eyes, cerebrospinal fluid leakage from the ear or nose, Battle's sign)
- Focal neurological deficit
- For children under 1 year, presence of bruise, swelling or laceration of more than 5 cm on the head

For children who have sustained a head injury and have more than one of the following risk factors, perform a CT head scan within 1 hour of the risk factors being identified:
- Loss of consciousness lasting more than 5 minutes
- Abnormal drowsiness
- Three or more discrete vomiting episodes
- Dangerous mechanism of injury
- Amnesia retrograde or antegrade lasting more than 5 minutes

The key aims of management can best be achieved by paying attention to <c>ABCDE. If the airway is at risk, it should be secured. Children with a GCS score of 8 or less or who appear agitated/combative should be intubated and ventilated without delay. Ketamine (2 mg/kg) and rocuronium (1 mg/kg) are the induction agents of choice as they offer a degree of neuroprotection and avoid the risk of sudden hypotension (see Chapter 19). Capnography must be used immediately after intubation to confirm endotracheal tube placement, to serve as a disconnection monitor, and to help maintain normocapnia or mild hypocapnia if there is evidence of a raised ICP. Remember that the end-tidal CO_2 level may differ significantly from the arterial level, especially in the shocked child–**it is essential to check the PCO_2 level with a blood gas sample. The PaO_2 should be maintained at a level greater than 13 kPa (98 mmHg), aiming for an oxygen saturation between 94% and 98%.** Routine hyperventilation has not been shown to improve outcome and arterial PCO_2 levels should be maintained between 4.5 and 6 kPa (35–45 mmHg). Lower levels may adversely affect cerebral perfusion in the areas of brain still responsive to changes in PCO_2. However, in the presence of an acutely rising ICP, lowering the PCO_2 to 4–4.5 kPa (30–35 mmHg) is considered an appropriate temporary measure until signs of herniation are reversed. Hypotension should be treated vigorously to avoid hypoperfusion of the brain. Adequate intravascular volume should be ensured by the administration of a fluid bolus initially with balanced crystalloid, unless head injury is part of polytrauma when blood products should be considered. If further support is necessary, consider early inotropic support and the use of blood products. The aim is to maintain cerebral perfusion pressure between 40 and 50 mmHg. Assuming a raised ICP, mean arterial blood pressure (which is a measure of the average arterial blood pressure through a cardiac cycle) should be monitored and maintained above target thresholds to ensure adequate cerebral pressure.

Mean arterial pressure targets (age specific)

Under 1 year	More than 50 mmHg
1–5 years	More than 60 mmHg
5–14 years	More than 70 mmHg
Over 14 years	More than 80 mmHg

To avoid an increase in raised ICP, further neuroprotective measures must be undertaken. The child's bed must be tilted to 20° elevation, maintaining the head and neck in a midline position. Sodium chloride 2.7–3% (3 ml/kg) should be administered, maintaining the serum sodium greater than 140 mmol/l but usually less than 150 mmol/l. The use of mannitol 0.25–0.5 g/kg may be indicated to reduce the level of intracranial oedema. Immediate transfer to a neurosurgical unit must be organised and the child transferred without any unnecessary delay. A loading dose of levetiracetam or phenytoin may be useful to avoid any risk of convulsion or seizure activity. It is important to keep the child normothermic throughout, avoiding any dramatic changes in core temperature.

The CRASH 3 study suggests that there is a beneficial effect in adults if tranexamic acid is given within 3 hours of mild and moderate traumatic brain injury. As with CRASH 2, it seems plausible that the same effect could be seen in children and tranexamic acid may be useful in preventing progressive intracranial haemorrhage in traumatic brain injuries without an increase in adverse effects. Tranexamic acid 15 mg/kg IV/IO should be given to children with suspected head injury and reduced conscious level or those with intracranial bleed confirmed on imaging if started within 3 hours of the injury.

Analgesia

Following initial assessment, sufficient analgesia should be administered by careful titration. There have been concerns that opioid analgesic agents will lower the conscious level, cause respiratory depression and conceal pain in the abdomen and elsewhere. However, withholding analgesia may contribute to deterioration of the child's condition by leading to a rise in ICP. Failing to control pain will leave the child agitated and uncooperative, making any assessment of the pain more difficult, rather than easier.

It is important to appreciate that head-injured children are often more sensitive to opioids. If the child's conscious level is normal, despite other evidence of head injury, IV morphine in an initial standard dose of 100–200 micrograms/kg (less than 1 year of age: 80 micrograms/kg), administered in increments, is appropriate. In obtunded children, particularly if the GCS score is less than 9, intubation and ventilation will have a higher priority than analgesia alone. In intermediate cases, a useful rule of thumb is to expect that half the standard dose may be sufficient in the first instance.

Remember that opioids can be rapidly reversed with naloxone if necessary, although it is clearly better to avoid overadministration by cautious titration. Alternative opioids such as fentanyl that act more quickly when given intravenously or that can be given by an alternative route (e.g. mucosal) may be considered, as described in Chapter 7. Local anaesthetic techniques such as femoral nerve block may also be used to good effect, avoiding opioid side effects.

Management of specific problems

Deteriorating conscious level

If airway, breathing and circulation are satisfactory and hypoglycaemia has been excluded, then a deteriorating conscious level is assumed to be due to increased ICP, resulting from an intracranial haematoma or cerebral oedema. A CT scan and urgent neurosurgical referral are indicated, and the temporising manoeuvres shown in Box 11.4 may be instituted.

Box 11.4 Measures to increase cerebral perfusion temporarily

- Nurse in the 20° head-up position and head in midline to help venous drainage
- Ventilation to maintain **end-tidal** CO_2 (**ETCO$_2$**) 3.5–4.0 kPa (equivalent to arterial $PaCO_2$ 4.0–4.5 kPa (30–35 mmHg)*
- Infusion of IV 2.7–3% sodium chloride (3 ml/kg) or mannitol 0.25–0.5 g/kg (i.e. 1.25–2.5 ml/kg of 20% solution IV over 15 minutes)
- Combat hypotension if present with crystalloid/blood infusion and inotropes if necessary
- Ensure adequate analgesia and sedation

*Note this level is lower than normal because it is a temporary, short-term, urgent intervention

---

Signs of uncal or central herniation

These signs (see Chapter 5) should lead to immediate institution of the measures in Box 11.2 and emergency neurosurgical referral.

Convulsions

A focal seizure should be regarded as a focal neurological sign of considerable concern. A generalised convulsion, while also worrying, has less prognostic significance in children. Seizure activity raises ICP in both non-paralysed and paralysed patients, as well as causing an acidosis and increased cerebral metabolic demand. The lack of limb or facial movement makes it more difficult to recognise a seizure if the child has been paralysed, but fitting should still be suspected if there is a sharp increase in heart rate and blood pressure, with dilatation of the pupils.

Seizures due to head injury should be controlled promptly. Hypoglycaemia should be excluded, especially in small children and in adolescents who have been drinking alcohol. Levetiracetam or phenytoin should be used to control the seizure.

Neurosurgical referral

Agreed indications for neurosurgical referral are shown in Box 11.5 (NICE guidelines).

Box 11.5 Indications for referral to a neurosurgeon

- Persisting coma (GCS score less than 9) after initial resuscitation
- Unexplained confusion lasting for more than 4 hours
- Deteriorating conscious level (especially motor response changes)
- Focal neurological signs
- Seizure without full recovery
- Definite or suspected penetrating injury
- Cerebrospinal fluid leak

Other cases may be discussed to consider referral and to ensure optimal management, such as when there is evidence of a depressed or basal skull fracture or if the initial GCS score is between 8 and 12. In general, the care of all children with new, surgically significant abnormalities on imaging should be discussed with a neurosurgeon.

11.6   Detailed review and further stabilisation

Review anatomical injuries and physiological system control. It is easy to miss injuries in the context of an altered conscious level. A high index of suspicion is essential. Reconsider the mechanism of injury, review the physical and radiological findings, and make sure that the appropriate specialists have been involved. Document your secondary survey findings and communicate requirement for further assessment, such as completion of secondary survey and a tertiary survey, when clinical condition allows.

In the severely head-injured child, physiological system control is of critical importance in preventing secondary insults. The airway and ventilation have been dealt with as part of emergency treatment. The position of the endotracheal tube should now be checked on a chest radiograph and the tube fixation adjusted and re-secured, if necessary. Attention to detail in adjusting the ventilator settings, according to repeated arterial blood gas sampling, is vital. A systolic blood pressure above the 95th centile for age should be maintained to ensure adequate cerebral pressure. Sedation and paralysis play an important role in tolerating the endotracheal tube and in suppressing rises in ICP, but must not be allowed to cause hypotension. A morphine and midazolam infusion should be initiated immediately after intubation. Bleeding from other injuries should already have been stopped and the blood volume restored. Normoglycaemia and a normal or slightly reduced temperature help to guarantee an optimal outcome.

Vigilance is needed to recognise any significant deterioration in the child's condition. If any of the following examples of neurological deterioration are present, this should prompt urgent reappraisal by the supervising medical team (NICE, 2014).

Examples of neurological deterioration prompting urgent reappraisal

- Development of agitated or abnormal behaviour
- A sustained (over 30 minutes) drop of 1 point in the GCS (especially in the motor score)
- Any drop of 2 points in the GCS
- Severe/increasing headache/vomiting
- New neurological signs

11.7   Transfer to definitive care

Children with a traumatic brain injury often require time-critical transfers for timely surgical intervention. In such circumstances, the delay in waiting for a retrieval team to arrive may be unacceptable, so that the responsibility for transfer may revert to the primary hospital. Where this timely surgical intervention is not required there may be time to wait for a team from the receiving hospital. For further details information on transfer see Chapter 23.

11.8   Summary

This chapter has emphasised the importance of initial management of traumatic brain injury to prevent secondary damage. Attention should be paid to airway, breathing, circulation and neuroprotective strategies.

CHAPTER 12

The child with injuries to the extremities or the spine

Learning outcomes

After reading this chapter, you will be able to:

- Identify the extremity injuries that pose an immediate threat to life and limb
- Describe how to manage these extremity injuries
- Recognise the incidence of spinal cord injury
- Identify the steps necessary to prevent exacerbation of an underlying cord injury
- Describe the structured approach to the stabilisation of the spine

---

12.1 Extremity trauma: introduction

Skeletal injury accounts for 10–15% of all childhood injuries – of these, 15% involve physeal disruptions. It is uncommon for extremity trauma to be life threatening in the multiply injured child. It is crucial to recognise and treat associated life-threatening injuries before assessing and managing extremity skeletal trauma as it is uncommon for this to be life threatening in the multiply injured child. However, although rarely life-threatening, fractures and associated extremity trauma must be managed well or they can have devastating implications for subsequent rehabilitation. This chapter deals with problems from the perspective of multiple injuries; the principles apply equally to individual injuries. It should be remembered that children's bones can absorb more force than adults and this may result in an underestimation of the degree of trauma to associated soft tissues.

12.2 Assessment of extremity trauma

Unless extremity injury is life threatening, evaluation is carried out during the secondary survey and treatment commenced during the definitive care phase. Single, closed extremity injuries may produce enough blood loss to cause hypovolaemic shock, but this is not usually life threatening. Pelvic fractures are relatively uncommon in children – the energy that would have fractured a pelvis in an adult may have been transmitted to vessels within the pelvis of a child, leading to disruption and haemorrhage. Closed fractures of the femur may cause loss of approximately 20% of the intravascular volume into the thigh, and blood loss from open fractures can be even more significant. This blood loss begins at the time of the injury, and it can be difficult to estimate the degree of pre-hospital loss.

Advanced Paediatric Life Support: A Practical Approach to Emergencies, Seventh Edition. Edited by Stephanie Smith. © 2023 John Wiley & Sons Ltd. Published 2023 by John Wiley & Sons Ltd.

12.3 Primary survey and resuscitation of extremity trauma

All multiply injured children should be approached in the structured way discussed in Chapter 8. Relevant history should be sought from relatives and pre-hospital staff. Extremity deformity and perfusion prior to arrival at hospital are especially important, and information concerning the method of injury is helpful.

Life-threatening injuries

These include the following:

- Massive haemorrhage
- Crush injuries of the abdomen and pelvis
- Traumatic amputation of an extremity

They should be dealt with immediately and take precedence over any other extremity injury.

Crush injuries to the abdomen and pelvis

The pelvic bones of a child are much more cartilaginous and thus more flexible than those of an adult; therefore if fractures occur it will only be after significant impact. A child's pelvis tends to be narrower than that of an adult and thus does not offer the same protection to the internal structure and organs. The significance of a fracture in itself is not important but the subsequent damage caused to the associated organs and structures can be life threatening and must be treated accordingly. Pelvic disruption can lead to life-threatening blood loss. The child will present with hypovolaemic shock; this may remain resistant to treatment until either the pelvic disruption is stabilised or the injured vessels are occluded.

Initial treatment during the primary survey and resuscitation phase consists of splinting of the pelvis with a pelvic splint (or improvised device), tranexamic acid administration (15 mg/kg) and initiation of the massive haemorrhage algorithm (see Figure 8.3). The diagnosis may be obvious if disruption is severe or if fractures are open. More often this cause of resistant hypovolaemia is discovered on pelvic imaging. If a pelvic fracture or injury is suspected, manual handling should be kept to the minimum (using the 20° tilt if necessary) and computed tomography (CT) should be considered for first line imaging rather than X-ray. Emergency orthopaedic opinion should be sought, and interventional radiology considered if no laparotomy is indicated for abdominal injuries.

Traumatic amputation

Traumatic amputation of an extremity proximal to the wrist or ankle may be partial or complete. Paradoxically, it is usually the former that presents the greatest initial threat to life. This is because completely transected vessels go into spasm, whereas partially transected vessels may not. Blood loss can be large and the pre-hospital care of these injuries is critical; an exact history of this should be sought.

Once in hospital, exsanguinating haemorrhage must be controlled. Two wide-bore cannulae should be inserted and pneumatic tourniquets applied to the injured limb. If the child is in shock, but the bleeding points are well controlled, vigorous fluid therapy may be instituted. If the bleeding is still uncontrolled, fluid boluses should be commenced in 10 ml/kg boluses, and the massive haemorrhage algorithm should be initiated as soon as possible (see Chapter 8).

On the basis of experience from land-mine injuries, an elasticated compression bandage and dressing, if applied carefully, may help stem the haemorrhage and better preserve tissue viability. Emergency orthopaedic and plastic surgical opinions should be sought. If no active bleeding is taking place, the stump should be dressed with a sterile dressing soaked in sodium chloride and the limb splinted and elevated. The child should receive intravenous antibiotic prophylaxis within an hour of their arrival to hospital and their tetanus status should be checked.

Reimplantation techniques are available in specialist centres. The success rate is improving, particularly in children. Urgent referral and transfer are necessary – the amputated part will only remain viable for 8 hours at room temperature, or for 18 hours if cooled. The amputated part should be cleaned, wrapped in a moist, sterile towel, placed in a sterile, sealed plastic bag and transported in an insulated box filled with crushed ice and water in the same vehicle as the child. Care should be taken to avoid direct contact between the ice and tissue. If, after discussion with the specialist centre, it is decided that reimplantation is not appropriate, the amputated part should still be saved because it may be used for grafting of other injuries.

Massive, open, long-bone fractures

The blood loss from any long-bone fractures may be significant; open fractures bleed more than closed ones because there is no tamponade effect from surrounding tissues. As a general rule, an open fracture causes twice the blood loss of a corresponding closed fracture. Thus a single, open, femoral shaft fracture may result in 20–30% loss of circulating blood volume. This in itself is life threatening. On arrival at hospital during the initial resuscitation phase, two relatively large-bore cannulae should be inserted and fluid boluses should be commenced according to the child's overall circulatory state (see Chapter 8). Exsanguinating haemorrhage should be controlled both by application of pressure at the fracture site, and by correct splinting of the limb; in certain cases the use of tourniquets may be indicated. The child should receive prophylactic antibiotics within the hour and their tetanus status checked.

Emergency orthopaedic opinion should be sought. Angiography may be necessary to examine whether any major vessel rupture has occurred, and if such an injury is considered likely then a vascular surgical opinion should be obtained immediately.

12.4   Secondary survey and looking for key features of extremity trauma

The viability of a limb may be threatened by vascular injury, compartment syndrome or open fractures. These situations are discussed below.

Vascular injury

Assessment of the vascular status of the extremity is a vital step in evaluating an injury. Vascular damage may be caused by traction (resulting in intimal damage or complete disruption), or by penetrating injuries caused by either a missile or the end of a fractured bone. Brisk bleeding from an open wound or a rapidly expanding mass is indicative of active bleeding. Complete tears are less likely to bleed for a prolonged period due to contraction of the vessel. It should be remembered that nerves usually pass in close proximity to vessels and are likely to have been damaged along with the vessel.

The presence of a pulse, either clinically or on Doppler examination, does not rule out a vascular injury. A diminished pulse should not be attributed to spasm.

The signs of vascular injury are shown in Box 12.1.

Box 12.1 Signs of vascular injury

- Abnormal pulses
- Impaired capillary return
- Decreased sensation
- Rapidly expanding haematoma
- Bruit

If these signs are present, urgent investigation and emergency treatment should be commenced. The fracture should be aligned and splints checked to ensure that they are not restrictive. If no improvement occurs, a vascular surgeon should be consulted and angiography considered. Vascular damage may not always be immediately apparent so constant reassessment is essential.

Compartment syndrome

If the interstitial pressure within a fascial compartment rises above capillary pressure, then local muscle ischaemia occurs. If this is unrecognised, it eventually results in Volkmann's ischaemic contracture. Compartment syndrome usually develops over a period of hours and is most often associated with crush injuries. It may, however, occur following simple fractures and also as a result of misplaced intraosseous infusions. The classic signs are shown in Box 12.2.

Box 12.2 Classic signs of compartment syndrome

- Pain, accentuated by passively stretching the involved muscles
- Decreased sensation
- Swelling
- Pallor of limb
- Paralysis
- Pulselessness

Distal pulses only disappear when the intracompartmental pressure rises above arterial pressure; by this time irreversible changes have usually occurred in the muscle bed. Initial treatment consists of releasing any constricting bandages and splints. If this is ineffective, then urgent surgical fasciotomy should be performed.

Open fractures

Any wound within the vicinity of a fracture should be assumed to communicate with the fracture. Open wounds are classified according to the degree of soft tissue damage, the amount of contamination and the presence or absence of associated neurovascular damage. Initial treatment includes removal of gross contamination and covering the wound with a sterile, sodium chloride-soaked dressing. A photograph of the wound should be taken to reduce the number of times the dressing is removed. No attempt should be made to ligate bleeding points because associated nerves may be damaged as this is done. Bleeding should be controlled by direct pressure. Broad-spectrum antibiotics should be given, and tetanus immunisation status checked. (Consult local guidance for antibiotic choice.) Further management is surgical debridement, which should be carried out within 6 hours by orthopaedic and plastic surgeons under operating theatre conditions.

Non-accidental injury must always be considered if the history is not consistent with the injury pattern. It is discussed in detail in Appendix D.

12.5 Emergency treatment of extremity trauma

Life-threatening problems identified during the primary survey in the multiply injured child are managed first. Only then should attention be turned to the extremity injury. The specific management of complications such as vascular injury, compartment syndrome, traumatic amputation and open wounds have been discussed earlier in this chapter.

Spinal

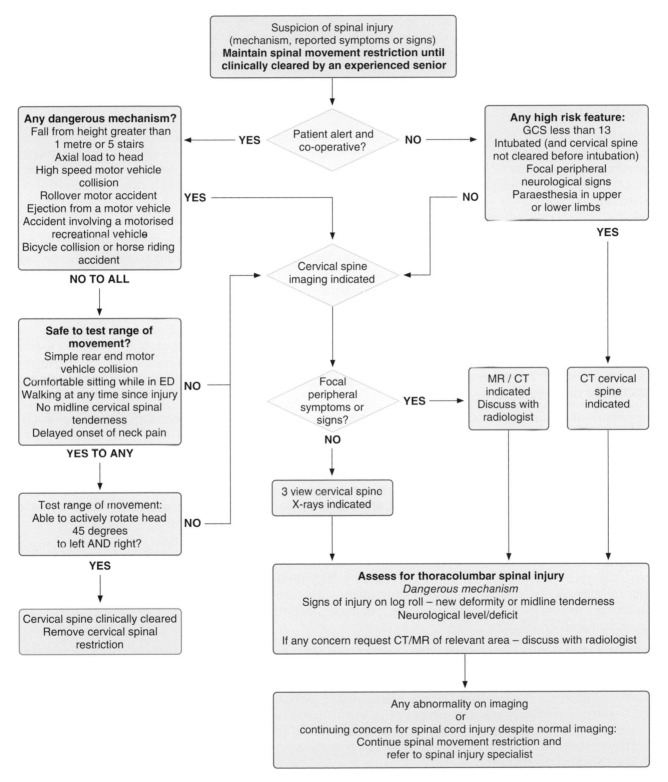

Figure 12.1 Spinal imaging, referral and clearance
CT, computed tomography; ED, emergency department; GCS, Glasgow Coma Scale; MR, magnetic resonance

12.6 Spinal trauma: introduction

Severe spinal injuries are rare in children (5 children between 2019 and 2020 in the UK according to UK TARN data). For any mechanism of injury capable of causing cervical spine damage (or in cases with uncertain history), the cervical spine is presumed to be at risk. A high index of suspicion, correct management and prompt referral are necessary in order to prevent exacerbation of underlying cord injury (Figure 12.1).

Immobilisation

If the child is unconscious, uncooperative or has had a significant mechanism of injury that makes it possible to have a spinal injury, spinal movement should be restricted until a comprehensive assessment can be completed. Significant mechanisms include high-speed road traffic collisions, falls or jumps from height especially with axial loading, mechanisms with rapid acceleration or deceleration, blunt trauma resulting from crush or impact, multiple trauma or penetrating injury to the back, or trauma where there has been loss of consciousness.

The head and neck should be stabilised initially by manual immobilisation. Do not try to straighten a head that is held in an abnormal posture (torticollis) – support the child to maintain the head position they have adopted. Head blocks and tape should be considered to assist with stabilisation of the neck and to provide staff and carers with a visual indicator that the cervical spine has not been cleared. An infant may require a pad under the shoulders to elevate the body and prevent neck flexion because of a large head.

Some situations are particularly difficult. An injured child may be uncooperative for many reasons including fear, pain or hypoxia. Manual immobilisation should be maintained and the contributing factors addressed. Too rigid immobilisation of the head in such cases may increase leverage on the neck as the child struggles.

The remainder of the spine should be protected from excessive movement using measures such as keeping the child flat on a firm mattress, minimising bending and twisting of the spine during transfers by using specialised equipment and tilting to 20°.

Children being transported between institutions may require additional measures to restrict spinal movement. This may involve head blocks, sand bags or a vacuum mattress, where possible axial loading must be avoided. **Spinal boards should only be used in the short term for extrication**; scoop stretchers should be used to assist with transportation and transfer.

Once a child has been immobilised, a member of staff must remain with the child at all times for reassurance, to ensure there is minimal movement and that the airway remains patent. Immobilisation of the cervical spine can be very frightening and disorientating to a child and thus must be carried out supportively and sensitively with careful explanation appropriate to the child's age and cognitive level throughout the procedure. Parents and carers may be very helpful in calming an agitated child.

Assessing spinal injury in children can be complex, with a number of anatomical, physiological and psychological factors contributing to the challenge. A thorough history, including as much information as is available on the mechanism of injury as well as a systematic assessment including focused trauma neurological examination, are necessary to evaluate a child suspected of having sustained spinal trauma. It is important to protect the entire spine until it can be cleared clinically, supported by appropriate radiological investigations. Decision algorithms can be helpful. However, in some situations, such as where there is a dangerous mechanism of injury, the expertise of an experienced clinician should be sought.

Indications for CT imaging of cervical spine in children suspected to have cervical spine injury include:

- Glasgow Coma Scale (GCS) score less than 13 on initial assessment
- The child has been intubated
- Focal neurological signs
- Paraesthesia in the upper or lower limbs

- A definitive diagnosis of cervical spine injury is needed urgently (e.g. before surgery)
- The child is having other body areas scanned for head injury or multiregion trauma
- There is strong clinical suspicion of injury despite normal X-rays
- Plain X-rays are technically difficult or inadequate
- Plain X-rays identify a significant bony injury

Care should be taken when assessing children who may be distressed because of anxiety, painful distracting injuries or intoxication. If there is concern that a reliable assessment cannot be made, it is safer to continue to restrict spinal movement and organise appropriate imaging.

If guidelines for clinically clearing the cervical spine are met (Box 12.3), indicating a low risk of cervical spine injury, the child should be asked to rotate their neck to the left and right. If the child is unable to actively rotate the head to 45° on each side because of pain or mechanical restriction, the neck should be immobilised again and the spine imaged. If there is no pain or limitation on movement, immobilisation is no longer required.

Box 12.3 Guidelines for clinically clearing a cervical spine

- Is there a high risk mechanism of injury? (yes to any requires imaging as per guidance in imaging (see Chapter 22))
  - Fall from a height of greater than 1 metre or five stairs
  - Axial load to the head (e.g. a diving injury)
  - High-speed motor vehicle collision (more than 40 mph), especially head-on collisions
  - Rollover motor accident
  - Ejection from a motor vehicle or ejection from car seat in infants
  - Accident involving motorised recreational vehicles such as quad bikes
  - Bicycle collision
- Can the range of movement be safely assessed? (yes to any means you can gently test range of movement)
  - Involved in simple rear-end motor vehicle collision
  - Is comfortable in a sitting position in the emergency department
  - Has been ambulatory at any time since injury
  - Has no midline cervical tenderness
  - Presents with delayed onset of neck pain

After a high-energy mechanism of injury, if there is evidence of a serious trunk injury or cardiorespiratory instability, a CT scan from the occiput to the pelvis should be considered, irrespective of the conscious level. This will encompass the entire spine. Plain spinal films are not then required.

If there are features suggestive of cord or nerve root injury a magnetic resonance imaging (MRI) scan is indicated. The timing is a matter of clinical judgement by a spinal injury specialist.

12.7 Injuries of the cervical spine

Cervical spine injury in children is very rare, and becomes increasingly rare the younger the child; however, they are associated with substantial levels of impact. The cervical spine attains its adult form from the age of about 8 years, and so injuries of the cervical spine in children aged over 8 years tend to be in the adult pattern, that is mainly of the lower cervical vertebrae (C5–C7). However, in children of 7 years and under, involvement of the atlas and axis with injuries is more common. These injuries are normally characterised by distraction of the osseous ring rather than the compression or comminution seen in older children and adults. Fractures at one level should prompt a search for fractures elsewhere in the whole spinal column. High-level cervical fractures are often fatal at the scene, so they may be under-represented in children who reach hospital. A high index of suspicion for these serious injuries should be maintained. Relative bradycardia for age and measured blood pressure might be a clue to upper cervical spinal cord injury.

Cervical spine imaging

Imaging must be undertaken in all children who cannot have their spine cleared clinically. The development of the cervical vertebrae is complex. There are numerous physeal lines (which can be confused with fractures), and a range of normal sites for ossification centres. Pseudosubluxation of C2 on C3 and of C3 on C4 occurs in approximately 9% of children, particularly those aged 1–7 years. Interpretation of cervical radiographs can therefore be difficult even for the most experienced (50% sensitivity). Even with normal plain radiographs, a spinal cord injury without radiographic abnormality (SCIWORA) may be present. For spinal cord injuries, MRI is the preferred imaging modality. However, CT may be the most practical imaging to obtain in an emergent situation and will demonstrate bony and ligamentous injuries adequately.

Indirect evidence of cervical fracture can be detected by assessing retropharyngeal swelling. At the inferior part of the body of C3, the pre-vertebral distance should be one-third the width of the body of C2. This distance varies during breathing and is increased in a crying child. Cervical spine X-rays are discussed in more detail in Chapter 22. Some children will require further imaging and specialist consultation depending on their clinical and radiological features.

Injury types

Atlantoaxial rotary subluxation is the most common injury to the cervical spine. The child presents with torticollis following trauma. Radiological demonstration of the injury is difficult, and CT or MRI may be necessary. Other injuries of C1 and C2 include odontoid epiphyseal separations and traumatic ligament disruption. It should be noted that significant cervical cord injuries have been reported without any radiological evidence of trauma.

Immediate treatment

Despite the rarity of fractures, a severely injured child's spine should be protected until spinal injury has been excluded. If in any doubt, the child should continue to be protected and senior help sought.

Spinal cord injury may be suggested by cardiovascular derangement, which may include hypotension or hypertension with inappropriate bradycardia. In these instances, immediate treatment includes neuroprotective measures. Inotropic support may be required. Corticosteroids are not standard but may be advised by neurosurgical specialists.

12.8   Injuries of the thoracic and lumbar spine

Injuries to the thoracic and lumbar spine are rare in children; they are most common in the multiply injured child. In the second decade, 44% of reported injuries result from sporting and other recreational activity. Some spinal injuries may result from non-accidental injury. When an injury does occur, it is not uncommon to find multiple levels of involvement because the force is dissipated over many segments in the child's mobile spine. This increased mobility may also lead to neurological involvement without significant skeletal injury.

The most common mechanism of injury is hyperflexion, and the most common radiographic finding is a wedge- or beak-shaped vertebra resulting from compression. This type of injury can be associated with motor vehicle collisions and injuries associated with seat belts. Evidence of seat belt bruising or associated abdominal or thoracic injury should prompt evaluation for thoracolumbar trauma.

Symptoms and signs include pain in the back, bruising, deformity/step or point tenderness elicited during examination of the back (during log roll). The most important clinical sign is a neurological level identified on a systematic examination of dermatomes and myotomes. A spinal cord injury assessment chart (Figure 12.2) can be used to determine at what level sensory or motor deficit occurs. Neurological assessment is difficult in children, and such a level may only become apparent

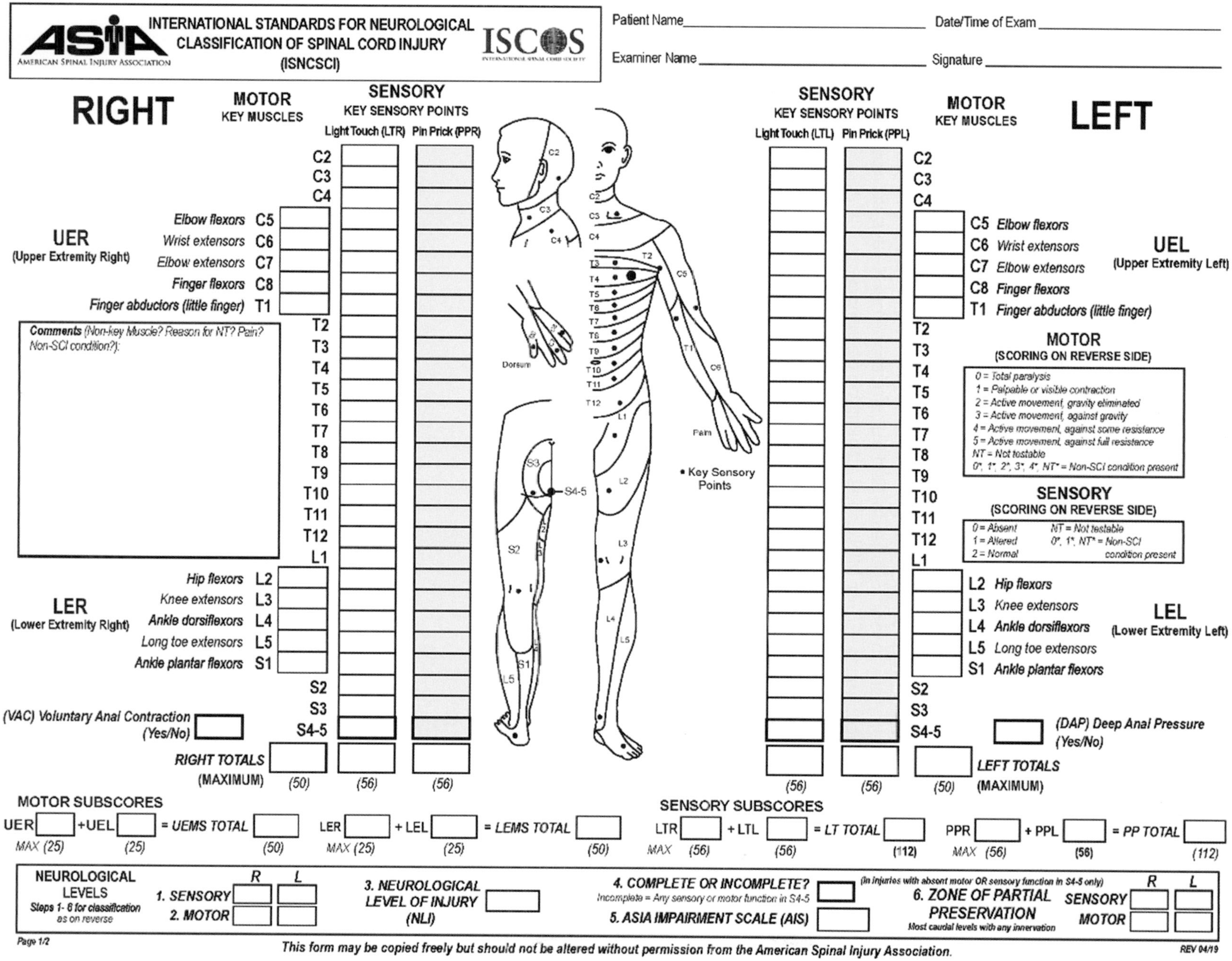

ASIA — AMERICAN SPINAL INJURY ASSOCIATION

INTERNATIONAL STANDARDS FOR NEUROLOGICAL CLASSIFICATION OF SPINAL CORD INJURY (ISNCSCI)

ISCOS

Patient Name ______ Date/Time of Exam ______

Examiner Name ______ Signature ______

RIGHT

MOTOR — KEY MUSCLES

SENSORY — KEY SENSORY POINTS: Light Touch (LTR), Pin Prick (PPR)

C2, C3, C4

UER (Upper Extremity Right): Elbow flexors C5; Wrist extensors C6; Elbow extensors C7; Finger flexors C8; Finger abductors (little finger) T1

T2, T3, T4, T5, T6, T7, T8, T9, T10, T11, T12, L1

Comments (Non-key Muscle? Reason for NT? Pain? Non-SCI condition?):

LER (Lower Extremity Right): Hip flexors L2; Knee extensors L3; Ankle dorsiflexors L4; Long toe extensors L5; Ankle plantar flexors S1

S2, S3, S4-5

(VAC) Voluntary Anal Contraction (Yes/No)

RIGHT TOTALS (MAXIMUM) (50) (56) (56)

• Key Sensory Points

LEFT

SENSORY — KEY SENSORY POINTS: Light Touch (LTL), Pin Prick (PPL)

MOTOR — KEY MUSCLES

C2, C3, C4

UEL (Upper Extremity Left): C5 Elbow flexors; C6 Wrist extensors; C7 Elbow extensors; C8 Finger flexors; T1 Finger abductors (little finger)

T2, T3, T4, T5, T6, T7, T8, T9, T10, T11, T12, L1

MOTOR (SCORING ON REVERSE SIDE)

0 = Total paralysis
1 = Palpable or visible contraction
2 = Active movement, gravity eliminated
3 = Active movement, against gravity
4 = Active movement, against some resistance
5 = Active movement, against full resistance
NT = Not testable
0*, 1*, 2*, 3*, 4*, NT* = Non-SCI condition present

SENSORY (SCORING ON REVERSE SIDE)

0 = Absent; 1 = Altered; 2 = Normal; NT = Not testable; 0*, 1*, NT* = Non-SCI condition present

LEL (Lower Extremity Left): L2 Hip flexors; L3 Knee extensors; L4 Ankle dorsiflexors; L5 Long toe extensors; S1 Ankle plantar flexors

S2, S3, S4-5

(DAP) Deep Anal Pressure (Yes/No)

LEFT TOTALS (MAXIMUM) (56) (56) (50)

MOTOR SUBSCORES

UER ___ + UEL ___ = UEMS TOTAL ___ — MAX (25) (25) (50)

LER ___ + LEL ___ = LEMS TOTAL ___ — MAX (25) (25) (50)

SENSORY SUBSCORES

LTR ___ + LTL ___ = LT TOTAL ___ — MAX (56) (56) (112)

PPR ___ + PPL ___ = PP TOTAL ___ — MAX (56) (56) (112)

NEUROLOGICAL LEVELS — Steps 1-6 for classification as on reverse — R / L

1. SENSORY
2. MOTOR
3. NEUROLOGICAL LEVEL OF INJURY (NLI)
4. COMPLETE OR INCOMPLETE? — Incomplete = Any sensory or motor function in S4-5
5. ASIA IMPAIRMENT SCALE (AIS)
6. ZONE OF PARTIAL PRESERVATION — (In injuries with absent motor OR sensory function in S4-5 only) — Most caudal levels with any innervation — SENSORY / MOTOR — R / L

Page 1/2

This form may be copied freely but should not be altered without permission from the American Spinal Injury Association.

REV 04/19

Figure 12.2 Spinal cord injury assessment chart

Reproduced with kind permission of American Spinal Injury Association (ASIA): International Standards for Neurological Classification of Spinal Cord Injury, revised 2019; Richmond, VA

after repeated examinations. Because of the difficulties of assessment, a child with multiple injuries should be assumed to have spinal injury, and therefore their spines should remain protected. If injury is confirmed, further treatment is similar to that in adults. Unstable injuries may require open reduction and stabilisation with fusion.

12.9   Spinal cord injury without radiographic abnormality

The low incidence (0–2% of all children's fractures and dislocations) of bony injury is explained by the mobility of the cervical spine in children, which dissipates applied forces over a greater number of segments. This explains the relatively higher incidence of SCIWORA seen in children. Excessive movements in trauma can damage the cervical spinal cord without an accompanying injury to the vertebral column that is obvious on X-rays. The cervical spine is affected more frequently than the thoracic spine. Because the upper segments of the cervical spine have the greatest mobility, the upper cervical cord is most susceptible to this injury.

Children who are seriously injured should have immobilisation of the spine maintained until such time as a full neurological assessment can be carried out since normal X-rays do not exclude a cord injury. If there is any doubt, helical CT or MRI scans should be obtained.

12.10   Summary

This chapter has described that extremity trauma is rarely life threatening unless there is exsanguinating haemorrhage. It is important to consider spinal injuries when there has been a significant mechanism of injury. Spinal immobilisation must be applied until the definitive assessment is complete.

CHAPTER 13

The burned or scalded child

Learning outcomes

After reading this chapter, you will be able to:

• Describe how to use the structured approach to assess and manage a child with a burn

13.1 Introduction

Epidemiology

Worldwide, burns are the fifth most common cause of non-fatal childhood injuries. The number of deaths from burns has decreased because of a combination of factors; the move away from open fires, safer fireguards, increased use of smoke alarms and more stringent low-flammability requirements for night clothes all playing a part. Non-fatal burns often involve clothing and are associated with flammable liquids. Despite burn death rates decreasing in many high-income countries, the rate of child deaths from burns is currently over seven times higher in low- and middle-income countries than in high-income countries (WHO, 2018).

Scalds are usually caused by hot drinks or contact burns, but bath water and cooking oil scalds are not uncommon. The improvement in survival following scalding (which followed improvements in treatment) has reached a plateau. There is a strong link between burns to children and low socio-economic status. Family stress, poor housing conditions and overcrowding are implicated in this.

Non-accidental injury should be considered if there are inconsistencies in the history given as to how/when a burn occurred, a delay in seeking medical help, the history being incompatible with the pattern of burn, certain patterns of burn, and the pattern of burn being consistent with forced immersion. Local safeguarding procedures must be followed.

Pathophysiology

Two main factors determine the severity of burns and scalds – these are the temperature and the duration of contact. The time taken for cellular destruction to occur decreases exponentially with temperature: at 44°C contact would have to be maintained for 6 hours, at 54°C for 30 seconds and at 70°C epidermal injury happens within a second. This relationship underlies the different patterns of injury seen with different types of burn. Scalds generally involve water at below boiling point and contact for less than 4 seconds. It is important to also remember that skin in infants is thinner compared with adults, and is functionally still developing; consequently contact times for injuries in

Advanced Paediatric Life Support: A Practical Approach to Emergencies, Seventh Edition. Edited by Stephanie Smith.
© 2023 John Wiley & Sons Ltd. Published 2023 by John Wiley & Sons Ltd.

this group are even shorter. Scalds that occur with liquids at a higher temperature (such as hot fat or steam), or in children incapable of minimising the contact time (such as young infants and the handicapped), tend to result in more serious injuries. Flame burns involve high temperatures and consequently produce the most serious injuries of all.

It must be emphasised that the most common cause of death within the first hour following burn injuries is due to smoke inhalation. Smoke-filled rooms not only contain soot particles, hot gases and noxious substances but are also depleted of oxygen; inhalation of all or any of these can lead to cardiac arrest. Thus, as with other types of injury, attention to the airway and breathing is of prime importance.

13.2   Primary survey and resuscitation

When faced with a seriously burned child it is easy to focus on the immediate problems of the burn, and forget the possibility of other injuries. The approach to the burned child should be the structured one advocated in Chapter 8.

Airway and cervical spine

The airway may be compromised either because of inhalational injury and oral scalds or because of severe burns to the face. The latter is usually obvious, whereas the former two may not be and a high index of suspicion is required. The presence of inhalation injury is directly related to mortality – an observational study carried out in the USA found that there was a 15% higher mortality rate where inhalation injury was present. The indicators of inhalational injury are shown in Box 13.1.

Box 13.1 Indications of inhalational injury

- History of exposure to smoke in a confined space
- Deposits around the mouth and nose
- Carbonaceous sputum

Because oedema occurs following thermal injury, the airway can deteriorate rapidly. Thus even suspicion of airway compromise, or the discovery of injuries that might be expected to cause problems with the airway at a later stage, should lead to immediate consideration of tracheal intubation by an appropriately experienced practioner. This procedure increases in difficulty as oedema progresses; it is therefore important to perform it as soon as possible. All but the most experienced should seek expert help urgently, unless apnoea requires immediate intervention.

If there is any suspicion of cervical spine injury, or if the history is unobtainable, appropriate precautions to immobilise the neck should be taken until such injury is excluded (see Chapters 8 and 12).

Breathing

Once the airway has been secured, the adequacy of breathing should be assessed. Signs that should arouse suspicion of inadequacy include abnormal rate (high or low), abnormal chest movements and cyanosis (a late sign). Circumferential burns to the chest or abdomen (the latter in infants) may cause breathing difficulty by mechanically restricting chest movement.

All children who have suffered significant burns should be given high-flow oxygen. If there is evidence of increased work of breathing, then senior anaesthetic help should be sought and intubation and ventilation should be considered.

Circulation

In the first few hours following injury signs of hypovolaemic shock are rarely attributable to burns. Therefore, any such signs should raise the suspicion of bleeding from elsewhere, and the source should be actively sought. Intravenous access should be established with two cannulae during resuscitation, and fluids started. If possible, drips should be put up in unburnt areas, but burned skin (eschar) can be perforated if necessary. Remember that the intraosseous route can be used to administer fluid and drugs. Blood should be taken for blood glucose, carboxyhaemoglobin level, haemoglobin, electrolytes and urea and cross-matching at this stage.

Disability

Reduced conscious level following burns may be due to hypoxia (remember smoke-filled rooms may contain little oxygen), head injury or hypovolaemia. It is essential that a quick assessment is made during the primary survey as described in Chapter 8 because this provides a baseline for later observations.

Exposure

Exposure should be complete, remembering that burned children lose heat particularly rapidly, and should be kept in a warm environment and covered with blankets when not being examined. Children may well present in a hypothermic state if first aid has involved placing the whole child under a shower/running cold water. Remove all jewellery including piercings as soon as possible prior to digit and/or limb swelling.

13.3   Secondary survey and looking for key features

As well as being burned, children may suffer the effects of blast, be injured by falling objects or may fall while trying to escape from the fire. Thus other injuries are not uncommon and a thorough head-to-toe secondary survey must be carried out. This is described in Chapter 8. Any injuries discovered, including the burn, should be treated in order of priority.

Assessing the burn

The severity of a burn depends on its relative surface area and depth. Burns to particular areas require special attention.

Surface area

The surface area is usually estimated using burns charts. It is particularly important to use a paediatric chart when assessing burn size in children because the relative surface areas of the head and limbs change with age. This variation is illustrated in Figure 13.1 and the table accompanying it.

Another useful method of estimating relative surface area relies on the fact that the child's palm and adducted fingers cover an area of approximately 1% of the body surface. This method can be used when charts are not immediately available, and is obviously already related to the child's size. Note that the 'rule of 9s' cannot be applied to a child who is less than 14 years old. There are a number of apps available to help assess burned surface area and these include the Mersey Burns app. An example of this is shown in Figure 13.2 where there has been a 13% total body surface area (TBSA) scald in a 2-year-old child (weighing 15 kg) that happened about 2 hours previously.

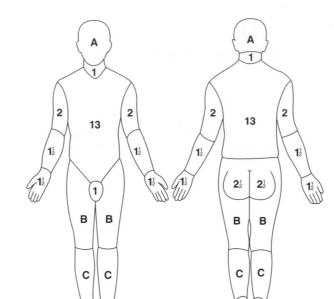

	Surface area at				
Area indicated	0	1 year	5 years	10 years	15 years
A	9.5	8.5	6.5	5.5	4.5
B	2.75	3.25	4.0	4.5	4.5
C	2.5	2.5	2.75	3.0	3.25

Figure 13.1 Differences in body surface area (per cent) in children
Reproduced from Artz (1969) with permission of Elsevier

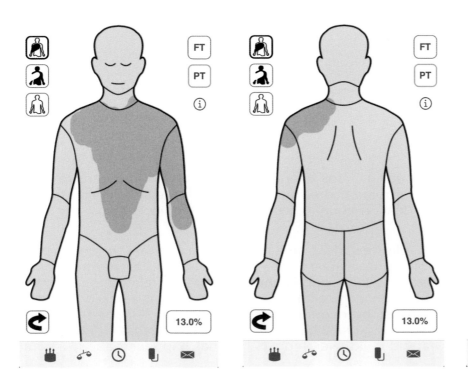

Figure 13.2 Mersey app (example screen-shots)

Depth

Burns are classified as being superficial epidermal, superficial dermal, mid-dermal, deep dermal, partial thickness or full thickness. Superficial dermal burns present with pale pink skin with blisters; mid-dermal burns have sluggish capillary refill, are dark pink in colour and sensation to touch may be decreased; deep dermal burns have blotchy, red skin and may or may not have blisters and the hallmark of these burns is the loss of the capillary blush phenomenon. Partial-thickness burns cause some damage to the dermis, blistering is usually seen and the skin is pink or mottled. Deeper, full-thickness burns damage both the epidermis and dermis, and may cause injury to deeper structures as well. The skin looks white or charred, and is painless and leathery to the touch.

Special areas

Burns to the face and mouth have already been mentioned with regard to airway concerns. Burns involving the hands or feet can cause severe functional loss if scarring occurs. Perineal burns are prone to infection and present particularly difficult management problems. Circumferential, full- or partial-thickness burns of the limbs or neck may require urgent incision to relieve distal ischaemia. Similarly, circumferential burns to the torso may restrict ventilation and also require urgent incision. This procedure is called escharotomy and usually needs to be done before transfer to a burns centre. All burns in any of these special areas should be discussed with a specialist burns centre.

13.4   Emergency treatment

Analgesia

Most children with a burn will be in severe pain, and this should be dealt with urgently. Older children may manage to use Entonox®, but most will not. Any child with more than a minor burn should be given intranasal diamorphine or fentanyl initially and then further pain can be controlled with intravenous morphine at a dose of 100 micrograms/kg (under 1 year: 80 micrograms/kg), if needed, as soon as possible. Further doses are often required but must be titrated against pain and sedation.

> There is no place for the administration of intramuscular analgesia in burns because it is painful and absorption is unreliable

Fluid therapy

Two cannulae should already have been sited during the primary survey and resuscitation and therapy for shock (10 + 10 ml/kg) commenced if indicated. Children with burns of 10% body surface area or more will require intravenous fluids as part of their burns care. This fluid is in addition to their normal maintenance fluid requirement. The additional fluid (in ml) required per day to treat the burn can be estimated using the following modified Parkland formula:

$$\text{Percentage burn} \times \text{Weight(kg)} \times 3 = \text{Total fluid replacement for burn in 24 hours}$$

Half of this should be given in the first 8 hours following the time of their burn. The fluid given is usually crystalloid. Remember that this is only an initial guide; subsequent therapy will be guided by urine output, which should be kept at 1–2 ml/kg/h. Urethral catheterisation should be considered early to help with fluid management (especially if the burn injury is more than 15% TBSA).

Wound care

Infection is a significant cause of mortality and morbidity in burns victims, and wound care should start as early as possible to reduce this risk. Furthermore, appropriate wound care will reduce the pain associated with air passing over burned areas. The burned area should be cooled immediately for 20 minutes. Although cold compresses and irrigation with cold water may reduce pain and can be useful for several hours after the injury, it should be remembered that burned children lose heat rapidly. Children should never be transferred with cold soaks in place.

Burns should then be covered with non-adhesive sterile towels or cling film. Cling film is often used as a sterile dressing, and can be applied loosely onto the burned area. No additional ointments or creams should be applied. Unnecessary re-examination should be avoided and blisters should be left intact. Photographs taken prior to applying the dressing can aid this process and allow others to assess the burn without disturbing the child. Provide tetanus prophylaxis if required.

Management of carbon monoxide poisoning

During a fire, burning of organic compounds in a low-oxygen environment produces carbon monoxide. Inhalation by the victim induces the production of carboxyhaemoglobin, which has a 200-fold greater affinity for oxygen molecules than haemoglobin. A high level will therefore cause cellular hypoxia as oxygen will not be given up to cells. Children who have been in house fires should have their blood carboxyhaemoglobin measured. (Note: most pulse oximeters show the oxygen saturation, regardless of haemoglobin concentration, i.e. normal SpO_2 does not exclude carbon monoxide poisoning.)

Levels of blood carboxyhaemoglobin of 5–20% are treated with oxygen (which speeds up the removal of carbon monoxide). Levels over 20% should prompt consideration of hyperbaric oxygen chamber treatment – discuss with the paediatric burns service.

In some environments the burning of plastics, wool and silk can produce cyanide. Assessment and treatments are complex. Be aware of the possibility of cyanide poisoning and consider it in a child from a house fire who is in a coma or presents with a severe metabolic acidosis without apparent cause. In general, antidotes are used when blood levels of cyanide are greater than 3 mg/l. Discuss treatment immediately with a poisons centre if cyanide poisoning is suspected as other factors such as the concomitant presence of carboxyhaemoglobin are contraindications for some antidotes.

13.5   Further stabilisation and transfer to definitive care

Definitive care requires transfer to a paediatric burns service. Criteria for transfer are shown in Box 13.2.

Box 13.2 Initial indication for referral to a specialised burns service

1. A child with a partial-thickness burn greater than 2% total body surface area (TBSA)
2. In addition, any child with a burn injury regardless of age and % TBSA who presents with any of the following should be discussed with the local burns service and consideration given for the need for referral:
   - Inhalation injury (defined as either visual evidence of suspected upper airway smoke inhalation, laryngoscopic ± bronchoscopic evidence of tracheal/bronchial contamination/injury or suspicion of inhalation of products of incomplete combustion)
   - Full-thickness burn greater than 1% TBSA
   - Burns to special areas (hands, face, neck, feet, perineum)
   - Burns to an area involving a joint that may adversely affect mobility and function
   - Electrical burns
   - Chemical burns
   - Any burn with suspicion of non-accidental injury should be referred to a specialised burns service for an expert assessment within 24 hours
   - Burns associated with major trauma
   - Burns associated with significant co-morbidities
   - Circumferential burns to the trunk or limbs

If in doubt, discuss the child with the specialist paediatric burns service team who will advise the level of care required (at a centre, unit or facility).

As with any injury in childhood, consider the possibility of non-accidental injury. Note the timeliness of presentation, and assess whether the history given to account for the burn or scald fits in with the clinical appearance of the injury in size, shape, age and location. Consider whether the injury is consistent with the child's development. If concerned or in doubt, consult with a safeguarding specialist.

13.6   Toxic shock syndrome

Toxic shock syndrome (TSS) is a toxin-mediated disease that can occur in children, usually following relatively small burns. It causes significant mortality, and therefore any child presenting unwell within a few days post burn who has a fever and a rash or diarrhoea and vomiting should be urgently investigated and treated if TSS is suspected. Urgent senior help should be sought for children suspected of having TSS. Any child discharged home with a small burn should be given written information about TSS.

13.7   Summary

This chapter has described the initial assessment and management of the burned child which should be directed towards care of the airway, breathing and circulation. Assessment of the area and depth of the burn should be undertaken during the secondary survey.

CHAPTER 14

The child with an electrical injury

Learning outcomes

After reading this chapter, you will be able to:

- Demonstrate the assessment and management of the child with an electrical injury using the structured approach

14.1 Introduction

Epidemiology

Many minor electrical injuries do not require medical treatment and the incidence of this sort of injury is unknown. Only a small percentage of electrical injuries requiring hospital attention occur in children. Electrical injuries usually occur in the home and involve relatively low currents and voltage. The mortality from electrical injuries from high-power external sources such as electrified railways is high. Electrical burns are still one of the main injuries to result in amputations of limbs and can have devastating consequences.

Other injuries may occur during the event: for example, the child may fall or be thrown from the source. As with all injuries, a systematic approach is required.

Pathophysiology

Alternating current (AC) produces cardiac arrest at lower voltages than does direct current (DC). Regardless of whether the electrocution is caused by AC or DC, the risk of cardiac arrest is related to the size of the current and the duration of exposure. The current is highest when the resistance is low and the voltage is high.

Current

A lightning strike is a massive direct current of very short duration which can depolarise the myocardium and cause an immediate asystole. On average two people are killed by lightning in the UK per year, and in May 2021 a 9-year-old boy lost his life after being struck by lightning while playing football in an open field in the UK.

Advanced Paediatric Life Support: A Practical Approach to Emergencies, Seventh Edition. Edited by Stephanie Smith.
© 2023 John Wiley & Sons Ltd. Published 2023 by John Wiley & Sons Ltd.

The typical effects of an increase in current are given in the following list:

- Above 10 mA: tetanic contractions of muscles may make it impossible for the child to let go of the electrical source
- 50 mA: tetanic contraction of the diaphragm and intercostal muscles leads to respiratory arrest, which continues until the current is disconnected. If hypoxia is prolonged, secondary cardiac arrest will occur
- Over 100 mA to 50 A: primary cardiac arrest may be induced (defibrillators used in resuscitation deliver around 10 A)
- 50 A to several hundreds of amps: massive shocks cause prolonged respiratory and cardiac arrest and more severe burns

Resistance

The resistance of the tissues determines the path that the current will follow. Generally, the current will follow the path of least resistance from the point of contact to the earth. The relative resistance of the body tissues, in increasing order, is: tissue fluid, blood, muscle, nerve, fat, skin and bone. Electrocution generates heat, which causes a variable degree of tissue damage. Nerves, blood vessels, the skin and muscles are damaged the most. Swelling of damaged tissues, particularly muscle, can lead to a crush or compartment syndrome requiring fasciotomy. Water decreases the resistance of the skin and will increase the amount of current that flows through the body. Because of the variability of tissue resistance, surface area and volume of tissue exposed, it is extremely difficult to predict the actual course of current flow and to infer the type and extent of injuries to internal organs.

Voltage

High-voltage sources such as lightning or high-tension cables cause extremely high currents and severe tissue damage. However, very high voltages can cause severe superficial burns without damage to deeper structures (flash burns and arcing).

14.2 Injury pattern

The classic injury pattern develops when the body becomes part of a circuit and is usually associated with entrance and exit wounds. These wounds generally do not help predict the path of the current, and the skin findings can significantly underestimate the degree of internal thermal injury.

Flash burns occur when the current arc strikes the skin but does not enter the body.

Flame injuries result from clothing catching fire in the presence of an electrical source.

Lightning injury is caused by DC exposure that lasts from 1/10 to 1/1000 of a second, but often has voltages that exceed 10 million volts. Peak temperature within a bolt of lightning rises within milliseconds to 30 000 Kelvin (five times hotter than the sun), generating a shock wave of up to 20 atm induced by the rapid heating of the surrounding air. This shock wave then can be transmitted through the body and result in mechanical trauma.

14.3   Initial treatment

The priority is to disconnect the current. Be aware that high-voltage sources can discharge through several centimetres of air.

Primary survey and resuscitation

Following severe electrical exposures, some injuries may not be apparent initially and frequent reassessment is essential.

- Airway, breathing and circulation
- Cardiovascular function: assess cardiac rhythm; examine pulses
- Skin: inspect for burns; look for blisters, charred skin and other lesions; pay attention to skin creases, areas around joints and the mouth
- Neurological function: assess mental status, pupillary function, strength and motor function and sensation
- Ophthalmological function: assess visual acuity; inspect the eyes, including a funduscopic examination
- Ear, nose and throat: inspect the tympanic membranes; assess hearing
- Musculoskeletal: inspect and palpate for signs of injury (e.g. fracture, acute compartment syndrome), and be certain to examine the spine

14.4   Secondary survey and looking for key features

Associated injuries are common in electrocution. Almost all possible injuries can occur as a result of falls or being thrown from the source. Burns are particularly common and are caused either by the current itself or by burning clothing. Tetanic contraction of muscles can cause fractures, luxations or muscle tearing.

Associated problems

Burns cause oedema and fluid loss. Myoglobinuria occurs after significant muscle damage. In this case it is important to maintain a urine production of more than 2 ml/kg/h with the judicious use of diuretics such as mannitol and appropriate fluid loading. Alkalisation of the urine with sodium bicarbonate increases the excretion of myoglobin. Children with significant internal injuries have a greater fluid requirement than one would suspect on the basis of the area of the burn.

14.5   Stabilisation and transfer to definitive care

A significant electrical burn is an indication for transfer to a burns centre.

14.6   Summary

This chapter has covered the important strategies for managing electrical injuries in addition to the ABCDE approach: switch off the current, and check all systems for possible injury.

CHAPTER 15

Special considerations

Learning outcomes

After reading this chapter, you will be able to:

- Describe how to manage different presentations of complex traumatic injuries which include:
  - Penetrating injury
  - Blast injury
  - Paediatric traumatic cardiac arrest
  - Bariatric trauma
  - Trauma in pregnancy

15.1   Introduction

This chapter highlights the conditions for which the trauma team may be required to modify their approach to manage the needs of the individual child's care and their specific circumstances. Although most of these exceptional circumstances are rarely seen within the child and young person population, they involve a high risk of complex, multiple region trauma, which requires a great deal of organised thought and preparation. These presentations can be exceptionally challenging, especially when managed outside specialist trauma centres. The structured system-based approach as discussed in previous chapters must be adhered to in order to ensure optimal care and assessment.

15.2   Penetrating injury

Whilst penetrating injury is less common than blunt injury, with a ratio of approximately 1:12 cases, it is associated with an increased rate of mortality and morbidity. The mechanisms of injury for penetrating trauma are broadly gun shot wounds and stab wounds which include impalement.

Violent crime amongst young people is rising in the UK. The most common method of murder in the UK is stabbing, although homicide rates in children under 16 years remain low. Non-fatal stabbing can occur as a result of assault or accident in children as young as 2 years of age. The majority of stab injuries are non-fatal and superficial but almost a fifth of cases presenting to hospital have injury of multiple organs; 25% of those with an abdominal injury have an associated chest injury, highlighting the need to be vigilant for injury of more than one body area. The limbs are the most commonly injured area due to stabbing, accounting for over 60% of cases; 90% of these are superficial injuries. One in 10 may have damage to the neurovascular bundle, necessitating vascular and plastic surgery input.

Advanced Paediatric Life Support: A Practical Approach to Emergencies, Seventh Edition. Edited by Stephanie Smith.
© 2023 John Wiley & Sons Ltd. Published 2023 by John Wiley & Sons Ltd.

Impalement injuries can occur in isolation, or in conjunction with blunt injury (e.g. after a fall from a height). Impalement injuries affect the oral cavity of children most commonly, but significant injury is most often seen after perineal impalement, the second most common site of injury.

The approach to penetrating injury follows that of the approach to blunt injury, with a focus on the <c>ABCDE approach, resuscitation and imaging as appropriate. In addition, it is imperative that if the penetrating object remains in situ then it should not be removed until the appropriate surgical teams are in attendance, preferably in theatre. The child should be given antibiotics as the wound is inherently dirty and the wound should be cleaned and dressed. The management of specific injuries has been detailed in their relevant chapters previously.

An important non-clinical note is that injuries of this nature will often be part of a forensic/police investigation and as such the trauma team should be aware of forensic considerations and the handling of evidence. Photos should be taken as soon as possible and stored securely, and no foreign bodies or items of apparel should be disposed of.

Ballistics

When a child presents after being shot, it is important to understand that bullets do not necessarily create a linear wound as would a knife. There may be two wounds (possibly an entry and an exit site). The bullet may not, however, have taken a linear path through the tissues. It is also possible that a great deal of tissue damage, with contamination, has occurred due to the way a bullet works and this may not be externally obvious. A description of 'entry' and 'exit' should also not be made as this is a forensic matter, and is irrelevant for immediate management. Any evidence retrieved as part of management should be handled with care (gloves) and bagged for the police.

Below is a brief description of some of the variables affecting injuries sustained during gun shot wounds.

There are several key elements to consider when understanding ballistics. Kinetic energy (KE) in this context will represent the transfer of energy from the bullet to the structures as it enters and decelerates. The equation for KE is:

$$KE = \tfrac{1}{2}\,mv^2$$

What this means is the energy of the bullet is derived from both the mass (*m*) and velocity (*v*) (speed). A doubling of mass results in a doubling of the energy, however a doubling of velocity quadruples the energy.

We then need to consider the amount of energy transferred into the tissues. This is solely dependent upon the change in velocity. If the bullet enters but does not exit, all of the energy is dumped. If there is also an exit site then not all of the energy has been dumped within the tissues, however this may be due to the bullet having more energy at entry. The magnitude of energy dumped depends upon the type of tissue and therefore the drag or retardation that tissue type offers, for example the lung would offer little resistance whereas liver or bone would offer a greater resistance.

The energy dump is also affected by the type of bullet, of which there are many, such as the full metal jacket, partial metal jacket or shot gun cartridges. The full metal jacket bullet retains its shape, producing a smaller tract through the tissue, whereas unjacketed or partially jacketed bullets deform more on impact causing greater dumping of energy. The Hague convention in 1899 prohibited the use of partial metal jacketed bullets in warfare situations. They are, however, still in use for hunting and law enforcement.

Tissue injury occurs directly from the trajectory of the bullet. This is called the permanent tract. Severe stretching of the tissues can also occur by the energy transferred to the tissues in what is a temporary tract. The temporary tract is perpendicular to the permanent tract and represents the width of damaged tissue. The path of the bullet through the body may be affected by tissue, angle of entry and possible tumbling of the bullet – do not assume a direct passage from A to B. Due to cavitation, contamination may be sucked into the wound. This poses an increased infection risk in already damaged tissue from bacteria or foreign bodies.

Stab wounds

Stab wounds are caused by penetration of the skin and tissues by a sharp object. These wounds are generally more predictable than those inflicted by bullets and will only have direct injury. However, it is important to follow the structured approach when assessing these patients, fully exposing them and thoroughly examining their back and torso.

Assessment of penetrating trauma

Important history

Important things to consider are the method of injury, type and number of injuries and anatomy of the patient. Blood loss at the scene and character of bleeding should be ascertained if possible, and the level of consciousness and ongoing resuscitative measures documented.

Primary survey and resuscitation of penetrating trauma

If exsanguinating, immediate resuscitative measures should occur alongside surgical exploration.

If haemodynamically stable, the primary and secondary surveys should be completed along with an inspection of the wounds.

15.3   Blast injury

Although infrequently seen in many countries, on a global scale blast injury is a common mechanism of injury in children and a persistent threat. In 2019, 426 million children lived in conflict zones, 160 million of them in high-intensity areas. A high proportion of children injured in conflict are exposed to blast injury mechanisms and these children have a higher mortality than adults in an equivalent healthcare system.

In recent years there have been several attacks using explosive devices outside conflict zones, including Manchester 2017, Brussels 2016 and Boston 2013. These attacks often result in a mass casualty event, and they are something a trauma centre should be prepared for.

Mechanism

The key to blast injury, as for all trauma, is to understand the mechanism of injury the child is exposed to and therefore be able to predict, prepare and respond when faced with a paediatric blast victim. Blast does not present a single mechanism of injury and can be complex. However, it is important not to view it as an entirely different situation as much of it will be familiar to the trauma team and entirely manageable with the team's skill set. Children exposed to blast events will be injured via a number of mechanisms.

A blast wave is produced when the chemical energy of an explosive substance is near-instantaneously converted to heat, light and kinetic energy. This produces a high-pressure wave that travels from the centre of the explosion (Figure 15.1).

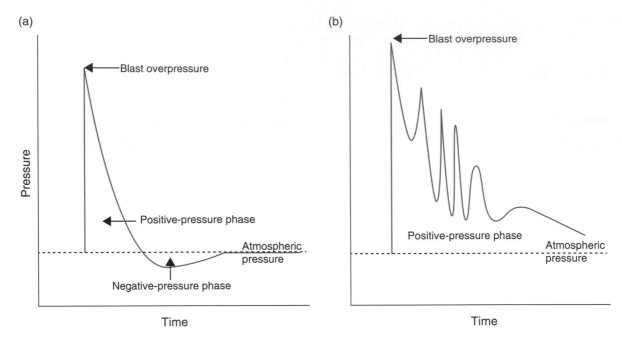

Figure 15.1 (a) Open air explosion pressure–time curve, and (b) closed space explosion pressure–time curve
Reproduced from Wolf et al. (2009) with permission of Elsevier

Blast injury can be classified as follows.

Primary injury

Injuries result from the effect of the blast pressure wave as it passes through tissues, depositing energy and causing tissue damage. Close to the blast, this will cause death and dismemberment. All tissues are affected, in particular where there is a gas–liquid interface or a change in density. Acutely, clinical effects are most pronounced in the lungs and gastrointestinal tract. The degree of primary injury is determined by a number of factors including the size of the explosive blast, proximity and, if in an enclosed space, the amplification and reflection of the wave as it 'bounces' back and forth causing multiple exposures.

Secondary injury

The blast will carry fragments from the explosive casing, any objects placed in the device (e.g. ball bearings, nuts and bolts) and surrounding debris. These will become missiles that cause either penetrating or blunt trauma to the child depending on the shape, energy and where they strike the victim. This trauma can be viewed in the same way as isolated blunt or penetrating injuries.

Tertiary injury

These injuries are a result of the blast wave causing bodily displacement or crush injuries when structures collapse onto the victim. A child is more vulnerable to both of these. They will be predominantly blunt injuries and again can be viewed in the same way as all other blunt injuries.

Quaternary injury

This includes all other injuries sustained in the blast not described above such as burns, inhalation injuries, toxic exposure, psychological impact and exacerbation of underlying health conditions.

Blast injury characteristics

Paediatric blast injury characteristics

- **Blast injuries cause an in-hospital mortality of 8%**
- **Children are at higher risk for all the reasons previously highlighted in this manual**
- Multiple body region involvement in 65%
- Burns in 70%
- Penetrating injury in 80%
- Double (56%) the requirement for surgery vs non-blast paediatric trauma
- Principle cause of death is total body surface area burns exceeding 30%
- 30% with severe injury and 18% critically injured
- Higher risk of coagulopathy in blast injury compared with isolated penetrating and blunt mechanisms
- A 100 kg projectile with a few kilos of explosive charge can cause injury up to 550 metres from the centre of the explosion

---

Table 15.1 shows typical blast injuries by system condition.

Table 15.1 Typical blast injuries by system condition	
Auditory	Tympanic membrane rupture,* ossicle disruption, cochlear injuries, foreign body
Eye, orbit, face	Globe perforation, foreign body penetration, air embolism, fractures
Respiratory	Blast lung, haemothorax, pneumothorax, pulmonary contusion and haemorrhage, A-V fistulae, thermal inhalation injury
Gastrointestinal	Ischaemia, bowel perforation and haemorrhage, ruptured liver or spleen
Circulatory	Cardiac contusion, air embolism, shock, vasovagal hypotension, peripheral vascular injury
CNS injury	Concussion, intracranial haemorrhage, closed and open brain injury, stroke, spinal cord injury
Renal Injury	Renal contusion, laceration, acute renal failure
Extremity injury	Traumatic amputation, fractures, crush injuries, compartment syndrome, burns, lacerations, acute arterial occlusion

* Whilst the presence of tympanic membrane rupture confirms significant exposure, absence **does not** exclude it.
A-V, arteriovenous; CNS, central nervous system.

Assessment and intervention

The assessment and management of a blast-injured child should be performed by a fully trained trauma team using the paradigm <c>ABCDE.

There is no blast-specific deviation required. Life-threatening injuries should be dealt with as found using the standard interventions, and subsequent injuries should be treated as they are in non-blast trauma.

Primary injury

The main primary injuries that threaten life are traumatic amputation and blast wave injury to the lungs and gastrointestinal tract. It is possible to have isolated primary injury so it is vital to assess any child exposed to a blast event carefully. The degree of primary injury will have been determined at the time of exposure by the 'dose' of energy the child was exposed to. Any signs or symptoms of injury will necessitate a period of observation and review as primary injuries evolve over time. The capacity to observe asymptomatic children with abnormal physiology will be affected by the number and severity of casualties a team is dealing with.

Blast lung injury

Blast lung injury is the commonest fatal primary injury. Pressure and volume trauma to the lung causes alveolar haemorrhage, pulmonary contusions, oedema and pneumothorax. Signs and symptoms may take several hours to present, with a clinical appearance similar to acute respiratory distress syndrome (ARDS) usually appearing within hours but this can take up to 48 hours to appear. Be suspicious of primary blast lung injury in children with any of the signs and features in Box 15.1.

Box 15.1 Common symptoms and signs that should be sought in primary blast lung injury

Signs and symptoms
- Cough
- Dyspnoea
- Haemoptysis
- Tachypnoea
- Tachycardia
- Hypoxia
- Cyanosis

Associated features
- Pneumothorax
- Haemothorax
- Pneumomediastinum
- Air embolus

Tachycardia may be a physiological response to a blast wave and may not represent lung injury, hence observation is important. Imaging will be consistent with ARDS or injuries listed in Box 15.1. Imaging is recommended in children who develop respiratory signs or symptoms. Treatment is supportive, and up to 80% require respiratory support. If ventilation is required, use a lung protective strategy to reduce lung injury (Paediatric Acute Lung Injury Consensus Conference (PALLIC) guidelines). Excessive fluids should be avoided.

Primary blast gastrointestinal tract injury

Compression–decompression injury to the bowel results in mucosal separation, haemorrhage and ischaemia. Again, presentation may take hours or days. Serial examination is required to identify ischaemia, perforation and peritonism. Reimaging and early surgical review is recommended in any child who develops abdominal signs or symptoms.

Imaging

Children exposed to blast often have multiple body region and organ involvement. It can be very difficult to exclude injury on the basis of clinical examination. It is recommended that there is a low threshold for computed tomography (CT) trauma scanning in any child with evidence of significant injury. There is a high chance of significant occult injury in blast victims, and whilst amputations, blunt and penetrating trauma may be obvious, other primary injuries are far less so. In a mass casualty situation where the capacity to serially review children is reduced and capacity demand is vital, CT scanning will aid the identification of life-threatened children early.

It is important to note that children injured by blast have a high risk of complex, multiple region trauma and primary injuries that evolve over time and so require serial assessment. Use the <c>ABCDE for assessment and intervention and have a low threshold for imaging.

15.4   Paediatric traumatic cardiac arrest

Survival from cardiac arrest following trauma was traditionally described as being extremely poor, but more recent studies have demonstrated that this is not the case, with survival rates comparable to that of out-of-hospital cardiac arrest from medical causes. Key to survival is the aggressive and early management of these children to target the possible reversible causes of traumatic cardiac arrest (TCA).

Paediatric TCA is a low-frequency but high-acuity event that is associated with high mortality. The majority of patients are male and have sustained blunt injuries following a road traffic collision. With a large proportion of paediatric TCA patients managed outside major trauma centres, it is imperative that clinicians have an appropriate framework with which to manage these children.

The algorithm shown in Figure 15.2 was derived from available evidence and as a result of a consensus-based process to determine the optimum management of the child in TCA.

The management of the child in TCA is different to the management of cardiac arrest secondary to illness. The initial step is to ascertain cardiac arrest and to determine that it is indeed as a result of trauma, that is, with a mechanism associated with a direct transfer of energy.

1. **Bundle of life-saving interventions.** Key to the management of TCA is the rapid and aggressive correction of potential reversible causes – hypoxia, hypovolaemia, tension pneumothorax and cardiac tamponade. The bundle of life-saving interventions addresses these, and should be performed concurrently and should be **prioritised over chest compressions and defibrillation**.

2. **Thoracotomy:**
   - Thoracotomy is advocated in TCA following penetrating trauma to relieve possible cardiac tamponade. Additionally, it may allow the clinician to gain control of pulmonary haemorrhage or enable proximal occlusion of the descending aorta. The role of thoracotomy in TCA following blunt trauma is unclear, but is included within the algorithm for providers to consider if deemed appropriate
   - Thoracotomy should only be undertaken if there has been a witnessed loss of cardiac output within the preceding 10 minutes
   - A clamshell approach is advocated and should be undertaken by clinicians trained in the procedure

3. **Cardiac compressions.** External cardiac compressions are unlikely to be effective in TCA and should not be performed especially if they inhibit or divert attention from carrying out the bundle of life-saving interventions. Once these interventions have been completed then compressions can be performed, particularly if correction of hypovolaemia has been achieved.

4. **Adrenaline.** The use of adrenaline (or other inotropes) is not recommended during TCA. Once return of spontaneous circulation (ROSC) has been achieved, a vasopressor should be considered in those children who have sustained an isolated traumatic brain injury or high spinal injury.

5. **Terminating resuscitation.** The decision to terminate a paediatric resuscitation attempt is challenging and the ability to recognise features suggesting futility are important in this decision-making process. Reaching the end of the treatment algorithm without achieving ROSC, having a persistently low end-tidal carbon dioxide and the presence of cardiac standstill on ultrasound are all features associated with futility of continued resuscitation and may guide the decision to stop resuscitation.

Paediatric traumatic cardiac arrest

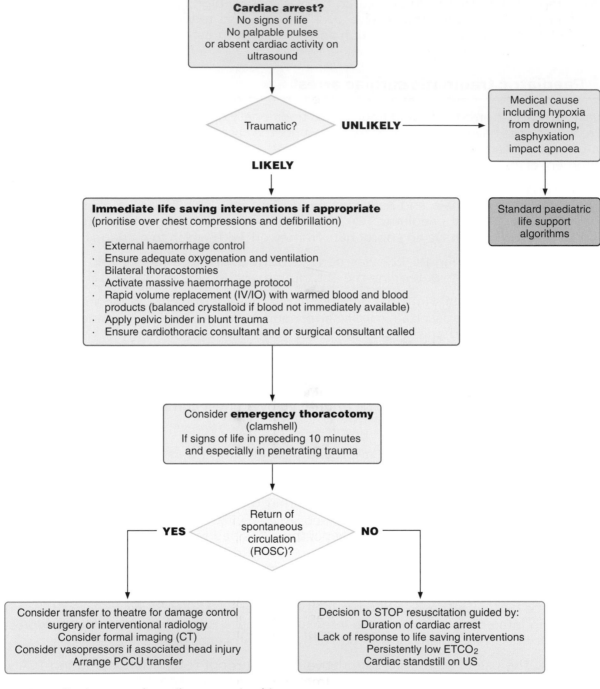

Figure 15.2 Paediatric traumatic cardiac arrest algorithm
Reproduced from Vassallo et al. (2018) by kind permission of the PTCA Research Group on behalf of PERUKI
CT, computed tomography; $ETCO_2$, end-tidal carbon dioxide; PCCU, paediatric critical care unit; US, ultrasound

15.5   Bariatric trauma

Obesity is increasing in prevalence in children and young people. Co-morbidities such as diabetes and hypertension may contribute to increased mortality and morbidity as well. There are several additional considerations when managing a severely injured obese child:

- **Catastrophic haemorrhage.** It can be difficult to apply sufficient pressure to stop bleeding in deeper structures such as arteries in children with large amounts of soft tissue. Considerable force may be required and the use of tourniquets may be helpful
- **Airway.** Large necks and tongues can make mask ventilation difficult. An appropriately fitting mask must be found and a two-person technique may need to be used. The anatomy can make intubation more difficult. Pillows or blankets may be used to raise up the head to bring the ear into horizontal alignment with the sternal notch; this may be required to achieve correct airway positioning (Figure 15.3)

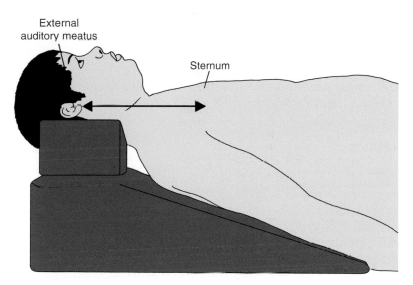

Figure 15.3 Airway positioning for a bariatric patient

- **Breathing.** There may be reduced chest wall compliance, increased abdominal contents, reduced functional residual capacity and increased oxygenation, meaning the patient is more prone to hypoxia and acidosis. Chest compressions if required are more difficult
- **Circulation.** Obese children have relatively larger circulating volume. Consequently, shock can be difficult to assess in obese patients who risk being under-resuscitated. Larger abdominal contents can obstruct the inferior vena cava when lying on their back. Placing a patient in a lateral tilt may help to improve blood flow and perfusion. A head-up position (20°) may reduce pressure on the lungs and abdomen and improve breathing or circulation. A left lateral position will also help in this regard
- **Types of injury.** Abdominal fat is protective to a degree, with fewer severe intra-abdominal injuries and head injuries. Rib fractures, pulmonary contusions, limb and pelvic injuries are more likely. Overall, mortality is greater in obese children, especially in burns patients when body surface area (BSA) can be hard to estimate, again risking inadequate fluid resuscitation
- **Radiology.** Imaging an obese child can be challenging, including physically fitting them in a CT scanner. It may only be possible to scan part of the patient (such as the head or chest). Radiation doses may need to be adjusted
- **Resources to be considered.** Is there an appropriately sized trolley or bed? If the child is on a bariatric ambulance stretcher, should they remain on this for resuscitation and transfer to definitive care to reduce risky transfers? Are there sufficient staff to safely transfer the patient from the trolley to the scanner or theatre bed? Can the child slide across or should a hoist be used for transfer if spinal mobilisation can be maintained?

15.6   Trauma in pregnancy

Although pregnancy in trauma is rare it remains the highest non-obstetric cause of death during pregnancy. Management of the pregnant trauma victim requires an urgent but considered approach as there are two patients requiring stabilisation. Coupled with the associated anatomical and physiological changes, the management approach can be very challenging. Pre-alert is essential so that the right team can be assembled including the obstetric and neonatal resuscitation team. This is not always possible in the cases of unrecognised or undisclosed pregnancy. It is essential that local protocols are established to provide guidance in such an event.

Anatomical and physiological changes of pregnancy influence the assessment and management of major trauma and must be considered, especially if the patient appears shocked and needing resuscitation.

Physiological changes

These include:

- A 30–50% increase in blood volume which contributes to dilutional 'anaemia of pregnancy' and ability to compensate. Signs of shock may appear later
- A 40–50% increase in respiratory rate which reduces ability to compensate for acidosis
- A reduction in functional respiratory capacity which makes hypoxia more likely

Anatomical considerations

Anatomical considerations in the management of trauma in pregnancy include:

- Delayed gastric emptying – there is an increasing risk of aspiration, therefore early intubation with a cuffed tracheal tube must be considered. This should be carried out by an experienced team as the anatomical changes such as breast hypertrophy, glottic oedema and neck obesity and diaphragmatic splinting can make intubation more difficult and thus appropriately experienced and trained anaesthetic support is essential
- Progressive uterine growth – the weight of the uterus and fetus, especially in third trimester may compress the abdominal aorta or vena cava, contributing to shock. An essential manoeuvre is to relieve this pressure by manual displacement of the uterus or tilting the patient 15° to the left (Figures 15.4 and 15.5). This may improve blood flow

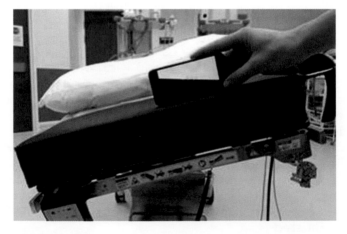

Figure 15.4 Fifteen degrees of left lateral tilt
Courtesy of Rosamunde Burns

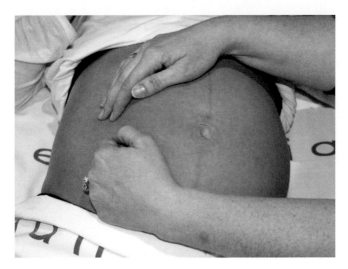

Figure 15.5 Manual uterine displacement
Victorian Department of Health / http://trauma.reach.vic.gov.au/ (last accessed November 2022)

- It is important to recognise that hypovolaemia may be difficult to detect. Initial haemodynamic parameters may be normal even with significant blood loss. Any altered physiology such as tachycardia or hypotension must be managed vigorously. Falls in blood pressure will trigger placental vasoconstriction and therefore result in a fall in fetal oxygenation. Any hypovolaemia in the mother will gravely compromise the fetus
- During the first trimester, the thick-walled uterus is well protected from trauma by the pelvic girdle. In the second trimester, relatively abundant amniotic fluid volume protects the fetus. By the third trimester, however, the now thin-walled and prominent uterus is exposed to blunt and penetrating abdominal trauma and is the most vulnerable of intra-abdominal structures. The placenta is an inelastic organ attached to an elastic organ (the uterus). Placental abruption may occur when trauma involving acceleration and deceleration deforms the uterus and shears the placenta off its implantation site, causing placental abruption and significant bleeding. Abdominal tenderness, guarding, rigidity, easy palpation of the fetal part are all signs of placental abruption
- In any visibly pregnant woman, aortocaval compression will occur. This will case a reduction in venous return to the mother compromising her cardia output and consequently reduce the blood flow to the fetus. Manual displacement is therefore essential
- In rhesus-negative women with uterine bleeding, an early prophylactic dose of anti-D immunoglobulin should be given

Traumatic perimortem caesarean section

This may be required as part of resuscitation primarily to improve maternal survival but may also achieve neonatal survival. It is undertaken if cardiac arrest has occurred or is impending in the pregnant women over 20 weeks' gestation and must be undertaken within a few minutes (no more than 5 minutes of cardiopulmonary resuscitation (CPR)). The aim is to deliver the fetus to reduce pressure on the aorta and vena cava, reduce blood demand from the uterus and increase the overall effectiveness of CPR, which may be hampered by a large fetus and uterus. It may also allow access to and damage control of intra-abdominal injuries.

15.7   Summary

This chapter has described how specific circumstances can be exceptionally challenging especially when managed outside specialist trauma facilities. The system based approach as discussed in previous chapters should be adhered to, to ensure optimal care and assessment.

PART 4
Life support

CHAPTER **16**

Basic life support

Learning outcomes

After reading this chapter, you will be able to:

• Assess the collapsed child and perform basic life support

16.1   Introduction

Paediatric basic life support (BLS) is not simply a scaled-down version of the adult algorithm. The epidemiology, pathophysiology and common aetiologies of paediatric cardiorespiratory arrest are different from those in adults. Cardiorespiratory arrest in infants and children is not usually the result of a primary cardiac cause, but instead is the end result of progressive respiratory failure or shock. To reflect these differences, the ideal sequence of BLS is different in the paediatric, newborn and adult populations. This must be balanced against the educational advantages of training using a general BLS algorithm so, where possible, guidelines are standardised for all ages to aid teaching and retention.

For the purposes of paediatric life support guidelines, some of the techniques employed need to be varied according to the size of the child. Paediatric patients include *infants* (under 1 year) and *children* (from 1 year to puberty), excluding newborns. The guidelines for newborn babies (transition at birth) are described separately. From a practical perspective, if the rescuer believes that the patient is a child, then they should follow paediatric guidelines, and adult guidelines should be used for anyone who appears to be an adult. If paediatric guidelines are followed but the victim is, in fact, a young adult, no harm will be caused as the aetiology of cardiac arrest is, in general, similar in this age group to that in childhood.

By applying the basic techniques described, a single rescuer can support the vital respiratory and circulatory functions of a collapsed child with no equipment. However, suitably trained health professionals should use bag–mask ventilation with oxygen, if available, to deliver rescue breaths.

Basic life support is the foundation on which advanced life support is built. Therefore, it is essential that all advanced life support providers are proficient at basic techniques, and that they are capable of ensuring that basic support is provided continuously and effectively during resuscitation.

Advanced Paediatric Life Support: A Practical Approach to Emergencies, Seventh Edition. Edited by Stephanie Smith.
© 2023 John Wiley & Sons Ltd. Published 2023 by John Wiley & Sons Ltd.

16.2   Primary assessment and resuscitation

Once the child has been approached safely, checked for responsiveness (signs of life) and help has been summoned, assessment and treatment follow the familiar ABCDE pattern. The overall sequence of BLS in paediatric cardiorespiratory arrest is summarised in Figure 16.1. Note that this guidance is for one or more health professionals trained in paediatric BLS.

Paediatric basic life support

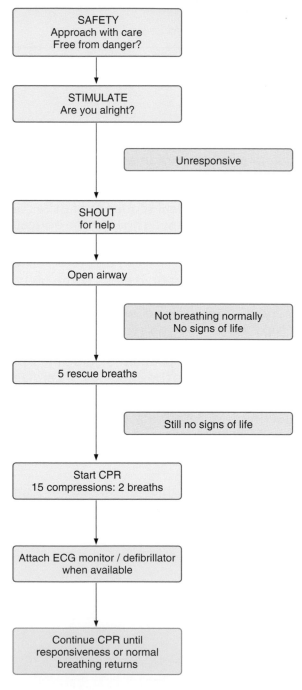

Figure 16.1 Basic life support algorithm
CPR, cardiopulmonary resuscitation; ECG, electrocardiogram

General BLS guidance for lay people (or health professionals unfamiliar with paediatric techniques) can be found later in this section.

The initial SSS approach – safety, stimulate, shout – is summarised in Figure 16.2.

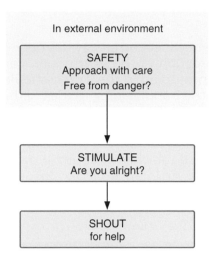

Figure 16.2 The initial SSS approach: safety, stimulate, shout

S – Safety

In the external environment, it is essential that the rescuer does not become a second victim, and that the child is removed from continuing danger as quickly as possible. These considerations should precede the initial airway assessment. Within a healthcare setting, the likelihood of risk is minimal and help should be summoned as soon as the victim is found to be unresponsive.

S – Stimulate

The initial simple assessment of responsiveness consists of asking the child loudly 'Are you alright?' and gently applying a stimulus, such as holding the head and shaking the arm. This will avoid exacerbating a possible neck injury whilst still waking a sleeping child. Infants and very small children who cannot talk yet, and older children who are very scared, are unlikely to reply meaningfully, but may make some sound or open their eyes to the rescuer's voice or touch.

S – Shout for help

When more than one rescuer is present, one should commence BLS while others activate the emergency medical services (EMS) system, collect the emergency equipment (e.g. manual defibrillator or automated external defibrillator (AED)) and then return to assist in the BLS effort (including application of defibrillator pads). Bystanders may be asked to help.

If there is only one rescuer, they should call for help immediately (preferably using a mobile phone with speaker function) and then commence cardiopulmonary resuscitation (CPR). If no phone is available, the single rescuer should perform 1 minute of CPR before leaving the child to activate the EMS system. If the patient is a baby or small child, the rescuer may be able to take the patient with them to a telephone whilst performing CPR on the way.

A single rescuer witnessing a sudden collapse or collapse in a child with a known cardiac condition (i.e. there is a higher risk that the cardiac arrest is caused by arrhythmia) should prioritise obtaining help and then start CPR, as urgent defibrillation may be life saving.

The increasingly wide availability of public access defibrillation programmes with AEDs may result in a better outcome for this small group (see the section on AEDs in children in this chapter).

[A] Airway

If a child is having difficulty breathing, but is conscious, transport to hospital should be arranged as quickly as possible. A child will often find the best position to maintain their own airway and should not be forced to adopt a position that may be less comfortable. In environments where immediate advanced support is not available, attempts to improve a partially maintained airway in a conscious child can be dangerous as total obstruction may occur.

If a child is not breathing, it may be because the airway has been blocked by the tongue falling back and obstructing the pharynx. Correction of the obstruction can result in rapid recovery without further intervention. An initial attempt to open the airway should be made using the head tilt/chin lift manoeuvre. The rescuer places the hand nearest to the child's head on the forehead and applies pressure to tilt the head back gently. The fingers of the other hand should be placed under the chin and the chin should be lifted upwards in an attempt to lift the tongue base away from the posterior pharynx, thus improving airway patency. Care should be taken not to injure the soft tissue by gripping too hard. As this action can close the child's mouth, it may be necessary to use the thumb of the same hand to part the lips slightly. An infant's airway is usually optimised by tilting the head into a neutral position, while the older child's airway is better placed with the neck more extended in the 'sniffing' position. These are shown in Figures 16.3 and 16.4.

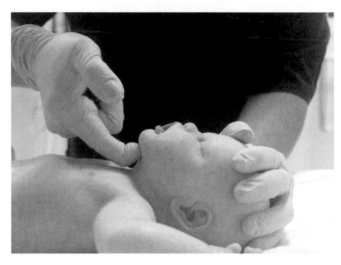

Figure 16.3 Head tilt and chin lift in infants: neutral position in an infant
Children's Health Queensland/CC BY 4.0

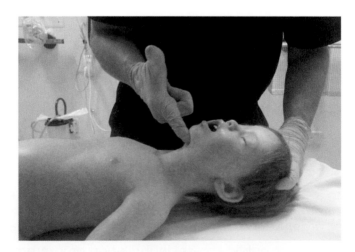

Figure 16.4 Head tilt and chin lift: 'sniffing' position in a child
Children's Health Queensland/CC BY 4.0

The patency of the airway should then be assessed.

LOOK	for chest and/or abdominal movement
LISTEN	for breath sounds
FEEL	for breath

This is best achieved by the rescuer placing their face above the child's, with the ear over the nose, the cheek over the mouth and the eyes looking along the line of the chest (for a maximum of 10 seconds), as shown in Figure 16.5.

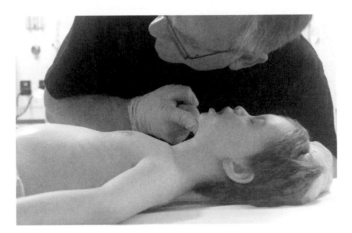

Figure 16.5 Looking, listening and feeling
Children's Health Queensland/CC BY 4.0

If there is a risk of disease transmission by aerosol, avoid approaching the nose and mouth of the child. Instead, assess breathing visually and by feeling for respiratory movement (e.g. placing a hand on the abdomen).

If the head tilt/chin lift manoeuvre is not possible or is contraindicated (e.g. suspected neck injury) then the jaw thrust manoeuvre can be performed. This is achieved by placing one or two fingers under the angle of the mandible bilaterally and lifting the jaw upwards (towards the sky). This technique may be easier if the rescuer's elbows are resting on the same surface as the child is lying on. A small degree of head tilt may also be applied if there is no concern about neck injury. This is shown in Figure 16.6.

(a)

(b)

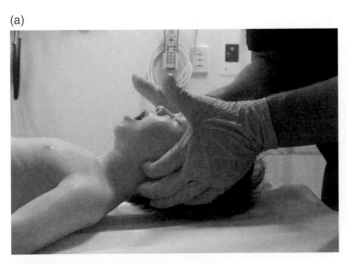
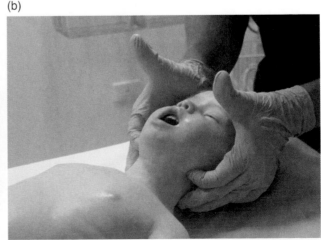

Figure 16.6 (a, b) Jaw thrust
Children's Health Queensland/CC BY 4.0

As before, the success or failure of the intervention is assessed using the technique described above:

- LOOK
- LISTEN
- FEEL

It should be noted that, if there is a history of trauma, then the head tilt/chin lift manoeuvre may exacerbate cervical spine injury. In general, the safest airway intervention in these circumstances is the jaw thrust without head tilt. However, on rare occasions in trauma, it may not be possible to control the airway with a jaw thrust alone. In these circumstances, an open airway takes priority over cervical spine risk and a gradually increased degree of head tilt may be tried. Cervical spine control should be achieved by a second rescuer maintaining manual in-line cervical stabilisation throughout.

The blind finger sweep technique for removal of a foreign body (see Section 16.4) should not be used in children. The child's soft palate is easily damaged and bleeding from within the mouth can worsen the situation. Furthermore, foreign bodies may be forced further down the airway, becoming lodged below the vocal cords (vocal folds) making removal even more difficult. In the child with a tracheostomy, additional airway opening procedures may be necessary (see Chapter 19).

[B] Breathing

If normal breathing recommences after the airway is open, the child should be turned onto their side in the recovery position, maintaining the open airway. Someone should continue to monitor the child for normal breathing while help is sought.

If the airway-opening techniques described earlier do not result in the resumption of adequate breathing within 10 seconds, **five initial rescue breaths should be given**. The rescuer should distinguish between adequate breathing and ineffective, gasping or obstructed breathing. Agonal gasps are characterised by irregular, infrequent, deep breaths. If in doubt, attempt rescue breathing.

While the airway is kept open as described, the rescuer breathes in and seals their mouth around the victim's mouth (for a child), or mouth and nose (for an infant, as shown in Figure 16.7). If the mouth alone is used, then the nose may be pinched closed using the thumb and index fingers of the hand that is maintaining the head tilt. Slow exhalation (1 second) by the rescuer should cause the patient's chest to visibly rise. Too vigorous a breath will cause gastric inflation and increase the chance of regurgitation of stomach contents into the lungs. The rescuer should take a breath between rescue breaths to maximise oxygenation of the victim.

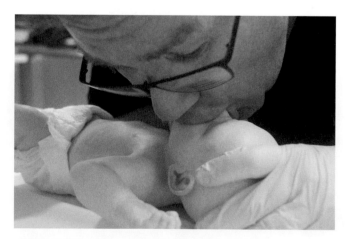

Figure 16.7 Mouth to mouth and nose in an infant
Children's Health Queensland/CC BY 4.0

General guidance for exhaled air resuscitation

- The chest should be seen to rise
- Inflation pressure may be higher because the airway is small
- Slow breaths at the lowest pressure reduce gastric distension
- As soon as possible, change to a self-inflating bag

Competent providers should use bag–mask ventilation (BMV) with oxygen, when available, instead of expired air ventilation. In larger children when BMV is not available, equipped providers can also use a pocket mask for rescue breaths.

If the chest does not rise, then the airway is not clear. The usual cause is failure to correctly apply the airway-opening techniques discussed. Therefore, the first thing to do is to readjust the head tilt/chin lift position and try again. If this does not work, a jaw thrust should be tried. It is not always feasible for a single rescuer to open the airway using this technique and perform exhaled air resuscitation; if two rescuers are present, one should maintain the airway whilst the other breathes for the child. Up to five attempts should be attempted to achieve effective breaths. If still unsuccessful, the rescuer should move on to chest compressions.

Failure of both head tilt/chin lift and jaw thrust should lead to the suspicion that a foreign body is causing the obstruction and appropriate action should be taken (see Section 16.4).

While performing rescue breaths, any gagging or coughing in response to these actions should be noted. These responses, or their absence, will form part of the assessment of 'signs of life' described in the next section.

[C] Circulation

Once the rescue breaths have been given, attention should turn to the circulation. Fifteen chest compressions should be given unless there are clear 'signs of life' (e.g. spontaneous movement, coughing, gagging, normal breathing). Agonal gasps (irregular, infrequent breaths) may be present in a cardiac arrest but are not a sign of life. Compressions should also be provided in patients with a very low heart rate (less than 60 beats/min) accompanied by signs of circulatory inadequacy (e.g. absence of signs of life).

Early institution of CPR maximises the chance of intact neurological survival. 'Unnecessary' chest compressions are almost never harmful and it is important not to delay starting CPR because of fear of causing harm to the patient. If signs of life are present but apnoea persists, ventilation (via expired air resuscitation or using resuscitation equipment, e.g. bag–valve device) must be continued until spontaneous breathing resumes.

Chest compressions

To best provide effective compressions, the child should be placed lying flat on their back, on a hard surface. A backboard may be useful when available. Clothing should be removed only if it severely hinders chest compressions. (Clothing should be removed with minimal delay of starting chest compressions.)

Children vary in size, and the exact nature of the compressions given should reflect this. Compressions should be at least one-third of the depth (anteroposterior) of the patient's chest – at least 5 cm for a child and at least 4 cm in an infant.

Position for chest compressions

Chest compressions should compress the lower half of the sternum. The rescuer should avoid placing the hand/fingers too low so as to avoid pressing the xiphisternum into the abdomen. It is important to allow the chest wall to recoil fully before the next compression starts – this will ensure that the coronary arteries fill adequately.

Infants. Infant chest compression is most effectively performed using the two-thumb technique: the infant is held with both the rescuer's hands encircling or partially encircling the chest. The thumbs are placed over the lower half of the sternum and compression performed (Figure 16.8). The single rescuer may alternatively use the two-finger method, placing two fingers on the lower half of the sternum and employing the other hand to maintain the airway position (Figure 16.9).

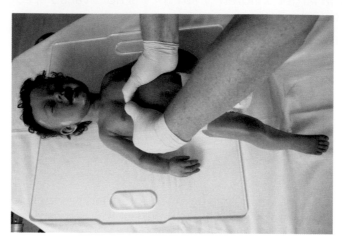

Figure 16.8 Chest compressions: two-thumb technique in an infant
Children's Health Queensland/CC BY 4.0

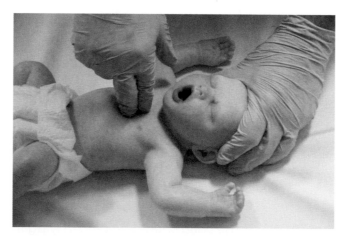

Figure 16.9 Chest compressions: two-finger technique in an infant
Children's Health Queensland/CC BY 4.0

Children. The rescuer should place the heel of one hand over the lower half of the sternum. The fingers should be lifted to ensure that pressure is not applied over the child's ribs. The rescuer is best positioned vertically above the child's chest and, with a straight arm (elbow extended), the sternum is compressed to depress it by at least one-third of the depth of the chest (at least 5 cm) as shown in Figure 16.10. For larger children, or for small rescuers, this may be achieved more reliably by using both hands with the fingers interlocked (Figure 16.11). The rescuer should choose one or two hands to achieve the desired compression of at least one-third of the depth of the chest. It is important to avoid leaning and to allow for complete chest recoil in between.

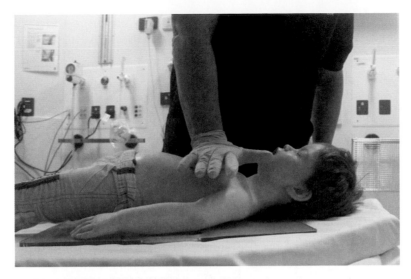

Figure 16.10 Chest compressions: one-handed technique in a child
Children's Health Queensland/CC BY 4.0

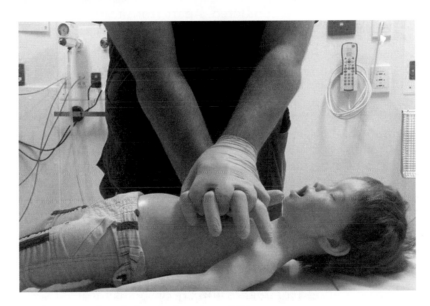

Figure 16.11 Chest compressions: two-handed technique in a child
Children's Health Queensland/CC BY 4.0

Once the correct technique has been chosen and the area for compression identified, 15 compressions should be given to two ventilations (in each duty cycle).

Compression : ventilation ratios

Experimental work has shown that coronary perfusion pressure in resuscitation increases if sequences of compressions are prolonged rather than curtailed. In infants and children, early ventilations are also a vital part of all resuscitation, especially in the hypoxic/ischaemic arrests characteristic of childhood. Once CPR has started, interruptions to chest compressions should be minimised (e.g. only for ventilations). Pausing compressions decreases coronary perfusion pressure to zero and several compressions will be required before adequate coronary perfusion restarts. There is no experimental evidence to support any particular compression : ventilation ratio in childhood but a 15:2 ratio has been validated by experimental and mathematical studies and is the recommended ratio for healthcare professionals performing paediatric basic or advanced life support.

Where possible, once the child has been intubated during advanced life support, compressions may be continued without pauses for ventilation. The ventilation rate should approximate the lower limit of normal for age:

- Infants: 25 breaths per minute
- Children 1–8 years: 20 breaths per minute
- Children 8–12 years: 15 breaths per minute
- Children over 12 years: 10–12 breaths per minute

Continuing cardiopulmonary resuscitation

The compression rate at all ages is 100–120 per minute. A ratio of 15 compressions to 2 ventilations is maintained whatever the number of rescuers. Ideally, rescuers performing compressions should change every 2 minutes to avoid fatigue and maintain optimal performance. With pauses for ventilation, there will effectively be fewer than 100–120 compressions per minute although the **rate is 100–120 per minute**. Compressions should be recommenced immediately after the second ventilation in each duty cycle and may augment exhalation. If no help has arrived after 1 minute of CPR, the emergency services must be contacted. Apart from this interruption to summon help, CPR should not be interrupted unless the child moves or takes a breath.

Research on the delivery of CPR has shown that many rescuers tend to perform compressions too slowly and/or too gently. Consequently, the current focus in CPR quality improvement initiatives is on the delivery of effective CPR, with adequate compression depth (at least one-third of the patient's anteroposterior chest diameter), a rate of between 100 and 120 compressions a minute, allowing full chest recoil after each compression, and with minimal interruptions to compressions. Any time spent readjusting the airway or re-establishing the correct position for compressions will negatively impact on the number of compressions given per minute. This can be particularly difficult for the solo rescuer. In the infant and small child, the free hand may be used to maintain the head position during two-finger or one-handed chest compressions to prevent the need for repositioning. The correct position for compressions does not need to be remeasured after each ventilation.

Biometric devices may be used to provide feedback on the quality and speed of chest compressions. These are best employed as part of a quality improvement process and their use should not result in delay in starting chest compressions.

The CPR manoeuvres recommended for infants and children are summarised in Table 16.1.

Table 16.1 Summary of basic life support techniques in infants and children

	Infant (under 1 year)	Child (1 year to puberty)
Airway		
Head tilt position	Neutral	Sniffing
Breathing		
Initial slow breaths	Five	Five
Chest compressions		
Landmark	Lower half of sternum	Lower half of sternum
Technique	Two-thumb or two-finger	One-hand or two-hand
CPR ratio	15:2	15:2

Lay rescuers

Bystander CPR is associated with better neurological outcome in adults and children. However, it has become clear that bystanders often are unwilling to perform BLS either because they are afraid of doing it wrongly or because of anxiety about performing mouth-to-mouth resuscitation on strangers. For lay rescuers, therefore, the adult compression : ventilation ratio of 30 compressions to 2 ventilations is also recommended for children to simplify the guidance. It may also be appropriate for healthcare providers trained in adult resuscitation (but with limited paediatric training) to apply adult BLS techniques if this creates less confusion for them and their team.

To increase the appropriateness for children, lay rescuers should be advised to precede their efforts by five rescue breaths if the victim is a child. If lay rescuers are unable or unwilling to perform mouth-to-mouth resuscitation, they may perform compression-only CPR.

Single healthcare professional rescuers can also perform five rescue breaths followed by a ratio of 30 compressions to 2 ventilations for children if they find difficulty in the transition from compressions to ventilations.

Automatic external defibrillators in children

The use of the AED is now included in BLS teaching for adults because early defibrillation is the most effective intervention for the large majority of unpredicted cardiac arrests in adults. As has been stated, in children and young people, circulatory or respiratory causes of cardiac arrest predominate. However, in circumstances where the likelihood of a primary shockable rhythm is very high, the use of an AED may be life saving. Recently there has been a large increase in the number of AEDs, together with trained operators, made available in public places such as airports, entertainment venues and retail precincts. The use of AEDs in children is discussed in Chapter 18.

Paediatric basic life support in the setting of traumatic cardiac arrest

Paediatric BLS in the setting of traumatic cardiac arrest (TCA) requires some additional considerations. Bystander CPR should be commenced immediately provided it is safe to do so.

Spinal movement should be minimised as far as possible during CPR without hampering the process of resuscitation (which is the priority). An AED should not be routinely applied in the setting of paediatric TCA unless there is a high likelihood of shockable underlying rhythm (e.g. after electrocution) or in the event of a sudden collapse during exertion in sport where there is no immediate clarity of the cause (e.g. in a rugby scrum or collision of players).

If massive external haemorrhage is present, direct pressure should be applied, if possible, using haemostatic dressings. If direct pressure is not effective, a tourniquet (preferably manufactured but otherwise improvised) may be used to manage uncontrolled, life-threatening external bleeding.

Recovery position

No specific recovery position has been identified for children. An example of one recovery position is shown in Figure 16.12. The child should be placed in a stable, lateral position that ensures maintenance of an open airway with free drainage of fluid from the mouth; the ability to monitor and gain access to the patient; security of the cervical spine; and attention to pressure points.

The following is a description of the technique for adults and is suitable for use in children:

- Kneel beside the victim and make sure that both their legs are extended
- Place the arm nearest to you out at right angles to the child's body, elbow flexed with the hand palm up
- Bring the far arm across the chest, and hold the back of the hand against the child's cheek nearest to you

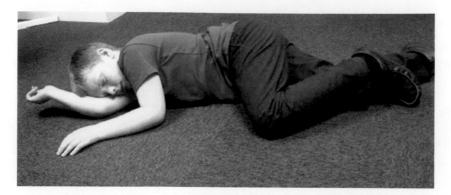

Figure 16.12 Example recovery position

- With your other hand, grasp the far leg just above the knee and pull it up, keeping the foot on the ground
- Keeping the child's hand pressed against their cheek, pull on the far leg to roll the child towards you onto their side
- Adjust the upper leg so that both the hip and knee are bent at right angles
- Tilt the head back to make sure that the airway remains open
- If necessary, adjust the hand under the cheek to keep the head tilted and facing downwards to allow liquid material to drain from the mouth
- Check breathing regularly, for example every minute
- If the victim has to be kept in the recovery position for more than 30 minutes, turn them to the opposite side to relieve the pressure on the lower arm

16.3   Basic life support and infection risk

Before the COVID-19 pandemic, there were only a few reports of transmission of infectious diseases from casualties to rescuers during mouth-to-mouth resuscitation. The most serious concern was meningococcus, and rescuers involved in the resuscitation of the airway in such patients took standard prophylactic antibiotics (rifampicin or ciprofloxacin). Tuberculosis can be transmitted during CPR and appropriate precautions should be taken when this is suspected. There have been no reported cases of transmission of human immunodeficiency virus (HIV) through mouth-to-mouth ventilation. Blood-to-blood contact is the single most important route of the transmission of such viruses and, in non-trauma resuscitations, the risks are negligible. Sputum, saliva, sweat, tears, urine and vomit are low-risk fluids. Precautions should be taken, if possible, in cases where there might be contact with blood, semen, vaginal secretions, cerebrospinal fluid, pleural and peritoneal fluids or amniotic fluid. Precautions are also recommended if any bodily secretion contains visible blood.

The COVID-19 pandemic has now drawn much attention to the safety of healthcare workers during BLS and has led to modifications in treatment approaches. Although children are less susceptible to COVID-19, they may be infectious even when they are asymptomatic. Although there are no reports of transmission of SARS-CoV-2 during paediatric BLS, bystanders should protect themselves as far as feasible and healthcare professionals should use proper personal protective equipment (PPE) as per local guidelines in any cases where aerosol contamination can occur. In most paediatric out-of-hospital cardiac arrests, rescuers are likely to be family members and therefore to have had previous exposure to SARS-CoV-2 (if the child was infected). It may be expected that rescuers will consider their personal risk far less important than the potential benefit for the child. This is less likely to be true for random bystanders. Healthcare providers may also value the benefit for the child higher than their personal risk, but they should also consider their responsibility towards their relatives, colleagues and the wider community as well.

There are specific modifications in the potentially infectious child by aerosol:

- Proper airway maintenance remains a crucial part of the respiratory management of any critically ill or injured child
- Breathing should be assessed visually (chest rise) and optionally by placing a hand on the child's abdomen
- If cardiac arrest is identified, rescuers should provide at least compression-only CPR. Those rescuers willing and able should also provide rescue breaths, knowing that this is likely to increase the risk of infection (if the child has COVID-19) but can significantly improve the outcome. If available, a face mask can be provided for the child. Whenever possible, healthcare workers should use BMV with an adequate filter between the mask and bag. Rescuers should aim for a good seal with no leak, preferably by a two-person technique. Intubation should be considered early but should only be attempted by an experienced provider with air-borne precaution PPE including face shields. Cuffed tubes should be used to avoid leakage afterwards. Cuffs should be inflated before the first insufflation

16.4   The choking child

The vast majority of deaths from foreign body airway obstruction (FBAO) occur in pre-school-age children. Virtually anything may be inhaled, with foodstuffs predominating. The diagnosis may not be clear-cut but should be suspected if the onset of respiratory compromise is sudden and is associated with coughing, gagging and/or stridor.

Airway obstruction may also occur with infectious conditions such as acute epiglottitis and croup. In these cases, attempts to relieve the obstruction using the methods described here are danger-ous. Children with known or suspected infectious causes of obstruction, and those who are still breathing and in whom the cause of obstruction is unclear, should be taken to hospital urgently. The treatment of these children is dealt with in Chapter 4.

If a foreign body is easily visible and accessible in the mouth, an attempt may be made to remove it, but great care should be taken to not push it further into the airway. **Blind finger sweeps of the mouth or upper airway should not be performed** as these may further impact a foreign body and damage tissues without removing the object.

The physical methods of clearing the airway, described here, should therefore only be performed if:

1. The risk of FBAO is identified (either directly witnessed or strongly suspected on history) and ineffective coughing and increasing dyspnoea, loss of consciousness or apnoea have occurred.
2. Head tilt/chin lift and jaw thrust have failed to open the airway of an apnoeic child. (The sequence of instructions is shown in Figure 16.13.)

Infant or child with foreign body airway obstruction coughing effectively

If the child is coughing effectively, they should be encouraged to cough. A spontaneous cough is more effective at relieving an obstruction than any externally imposed manoeuvre. An effective cough is recognised by the victim's ability to speak or cry and to take a breath between coughs. The child should be continually assessed and not left alone at this stage. No intervention should be made unless the cough becomes ineffective (i.e. quieter or silent) and the victim cannot cry, speak or take a breath or if they becomes cyanosed or start to lose consciousness. If this happens, then call for help and start the intervention.

Conscious infant or child with foreign body airway obstruction coughing ineffectively

If the child or infant is still conscious but coughing ineffectively, the following manoeuvres should be attempted in sequence followed by re-examination of the mouth and attempted breaths as shown in Figure 16.13.

Paediatric foreign body airway obstruction

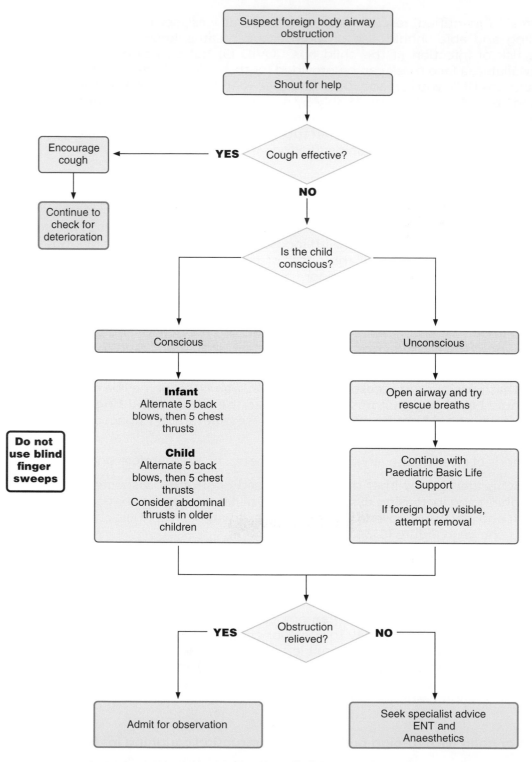

Figure 16.13 Paediatric foreign body airway obstruction algorithm

Infants

Abdominal thrusts may cause intra-abdominal injury in infants. A combination of back blows and chest thrusts is recommended for the relief of FBAO in this age group.

The baby is placed along one of the rescuer's arms in a head-down position, with the rescuer's hand supporting the infant's jaw in such a way as to keep it open, in the neutral position. The rescuer then rests their arm along their own thigh and delivers five back blows between the infant's shoulder blades with the heel of the free hand.

If the obstruction is not relieved the baby is turned over and laid along the rescuer's thigh, still in a head-down position. Five chest thrusts are given – using the same landmarks as for cardiac compression but at a slower rate of 1 per second and sharper than chest compressions. If an infant is too large to allow use of the single-arm technique described, then the same manoeuvres can be performed by laying the baby across the rescuer's lap. These techniques are shown in Figures 16.14 and 16.15. In a large infant the heel of the hand can be used if the two-finger technique is not effective or deemed too difficult to do.

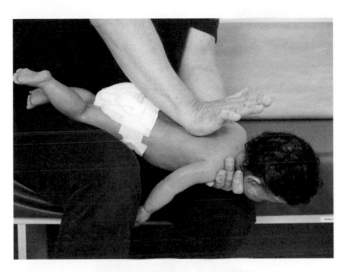

Figure 16.14 Back blows in an infant
Children's Health Queensland/CC BY 4.0

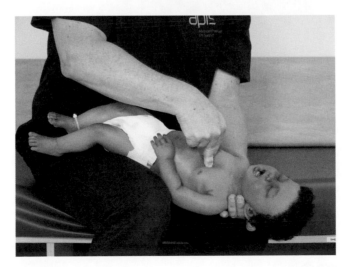

Figure 16.15 Chest thrusts in an infant
Children's Health Queensland/CC BY 4.0

Children

Back blows can be used as in infants or, in the case of a larger child, with the child supported in a forward-leaning position (Figure 16.16).

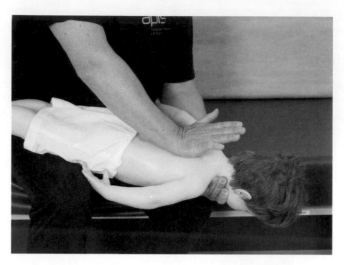

Figure 16.16 Back blows in a child
Children's Health Queensland/CC BY 4.0

In the child, the abdominal thrust (Heimlich manoeuvre) is recommended instead of chest thrusts. This can be performed with the victim either standing (Figure 16.17) or lying on the ground (Figure 16.18), but the former is usually more appropriate.

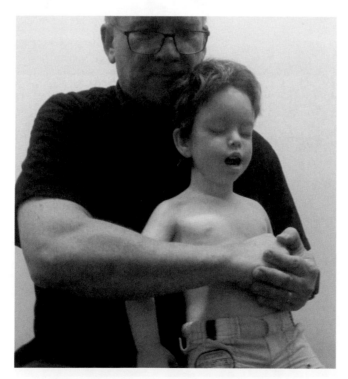

Figure 16.17 Abdominal thrust in a child
Children's Health Queensland/CC BY 4.0

If abdominal thrusts are to be attempted with the child standing, the rescuer moves behind the victim and passes their arms around the victim's body. Owing to the smaller stature of children, it may be necessary for an adult to raise the child or kneel behind them to carry out the standing manoeuvre effectively. One hand is formed into a fist and placed against the child's abdomen above the umbilicus and below the xiphisternum. The other hand is placed over the fist, and both hands are thrust sharply upwards into the abdomen. This is repeated five times unless the object causing the obstruction is expelled before then.

To carry out the abdominal thrust in a supine child, the rescuer kneels at the child's feet. If the child is large, it may be necessary to kneel astride the child. The heel of one hand is placed against the child's abdomen above the umbilicus and below the xiphisternum. The other hand is placed on top of the first, and both hands are thrust sharply upwards into the abdomen, with care being taken to direct the thrust in the midline. This is repeated five times unless the object causing the obstruction is expelled before that. This technique is shown in Figure 16.18. When performing the abdominal thrust make sure that the pressure is not applied to the xiphisternum or the lower rib cage to avoid abdominal trauma.

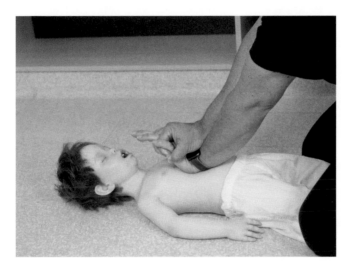

Figure 16.18 Abdominal thrust with the child in a supine position
Children's Health Queensland/CC BY 4.0

If the foreign body has not been expelled and the child or infant is still conscious, continue the sequence of back blows and chest (for infants) or abdominal (for children) thrusts. Do not leave the child unattended.

Following successful relief of the obstructed airway, assess the child or infant clinically. There may still be some part of the foreign material in the respiratory tract. If abdominal thrusts have been performed, the child should be assessed for possible abdominal injuries.

Unconscious infant or child with foreign body airway obstruction

If the child or infant is unconscious, or loses consciousness during the performance of manoeuvres, the following should be attempted in sequence:

- Call for help
- Place the child supine on a flat surface
- Open the mouth and attempt to remove any visible object
- Open the airway and attempt five rescue breaths, repositioning the airway with each breath if the chest does not rise
- Start chest compressions even if the rescue breaths were ineffective
- Continue the sequence for single-rescuer CPR for 1 minute then summon help again if none is forthcoming

Each time breaths are attempted, the rescuer should look in the mouth for the foreign body and remove it if visible. Care should be taken not to push the object further down and to avoid damaging the tissues.

If the obstruction is relieved, the patient may still require either continued ventilations (if not breathing but is moving or gagging), or both ventilations and chest compressions if there are no signs of life. Advanced life support may also be needed. If the child breathes effectively then they should be placed in the recovery position and should be monitored regularly.

16.5 Summary

This chapter is consistent with the International Liaison Committee on Resuscitation (ILCOR) 2021 resuscitation guidelines – the references used in this process are available on the ALSG website (see details in the prelims).

Paediatric basic life support

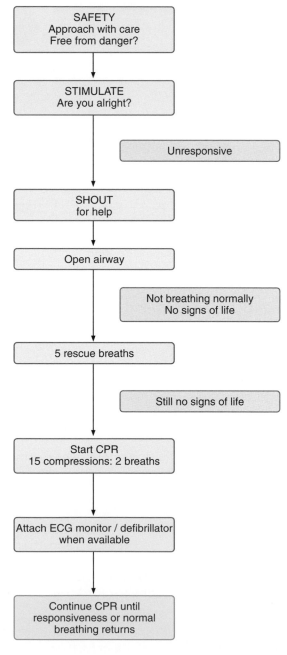

Figure 16.19 Basic life support algorithm
CPR, cardiopulmonary resuscitation; ECG, electrocardiogram

CHAPTER **17**

Support of the airway and ventilation

Learning outcomes

After reading this chapter, you will be able to:
- Describe how to respond to airway and breathing problems with a structured approach
- Recognise equipment that may be used to assess and support airway and breathing

---

17.1 Introduction

Along with control of catastrophic haemorrhage, assessment and management of airway and breathing has priority in the resuscitation of patients of all ages. Respiratory function can deteriorate rapidly in children. Effective resuscitation techniques aimed at resolving problems identified in the primary survey should be applied quickly and in order of priority.

It is important to recognise differences between adults and children and be familiar with appropriate paediatric equipment. Techniques for obtaining a patent and protected airway, and for achieving adequate ventilation and oxygenation, should be learned and practised frequently to best maintain competence.

> It should be stressed that basic, simple techniques are often effective and therefore life saving. When this is the case, prolonged or repeated attempts at advanced airway techniques (that interrupt ventilation or other ongoing resuscitation) may be detrimental

17.2 Airway and breathing management: principles

A systematic, prioritised approach to emergency airway management allows a rapid response while maintaining thoroughness. As with other aspects of resuscitation, care can be structured into the standard ABCDE phases.

Advanced Paediatric Life Support: A Practical Approach to Emergencies, Seventh Edition. Edited by Stephanie Smith.
© 2023 John Wiley & Sons Ltd. Published 2023 by John Wiley & Sons Ltd.

17.3   Primary survey and resuscitation

This consists of a rapid 'physiological' examination to identify immediately life-threatening emergencies. From the respiratory viewpoint, the following assessments should be performed as part of the primary survey:

- Look, listen and feel for airway obstruction, respiratory arrest, depression or distress (NB: should the patient have undergone prior intubation, the correct placement and functioning of the endotracheal tube should be checked by the receiving team at this stage)
- Assess the effort of breathing
- Auscultate for breath sounds, including any stridor
- Assess skin colour

If a significant problem is identified, management of that problem should be started immediately. After appropriate interventions have been performed and their effect assessed, primary assessment may be resumed or repeated.

Life-saving interventions should be performed during this phase. In the critically unwell or injured child, the resuscitation phase and primary assessment occur together and problems should be dealt with as they are found. This may include emergency procedures such as intubation, ventilation, cannulation and fluid resuscitation. At the same time, oxygen should be provided, vital signs recorded and essential monitoring established.

From the respiratory viewpoint, the following management should be performed.

Airway

- Perform basic airway-opening manoeuvres
- Give high-concentration oxygen
- Provide suction if necessary
- Place airway adjuncts if necessary
- Proceed to advanced airway management if required

Breathing

- Establish adequate ventilation via a bag–valve–mask ventilation
- Intubate if necessary
- Decompress the stomach with a large-bore orogastric or nasogastric tube if necessary
- Perform chest decompressions if necessary
- Consider alternative advanced airway management techniques or (very rarely) surgical airway if it is not possible to intubate or ventilate
- Apply monitoring including oxygen saturation and capnography (in intubated patients) (Cook et al., 2011a, 2011b; AAGBI, 2016)

17.4   Secondary survey

This consists of a thorough physical examination with appropriate investigations. Before embarking on this phase, it is important that any required resuscitative measures are already underway.

From the respiratory viewpoint, the following should be done as part of the secondary assessment:

- Perform a detailed examination of the airway, neck and chest
- Identify any swelling, bruising or wounds
- Re-examine for symmetry of chest movement and air entry
- Do not forget to inspect and listen to the whole of the chest, including the back

17.5   Emergency treatment

All other urgent interventions are included in this phase. If at any time the child deteriorates, the team should return to the primary assessment and recycle through the system.

Box 17.1 Airway and breathing management protocol

Assess airway and give oxygen
- If dealing with a trauma case:
  - control of major haemorrhage occurs simultaneously
  - consider cervical spine (see Chapters 8 and 12)
- If evidence of obstruction or altered consciousness:
  - perform airway-opening manoeuvres (**common**)
  - consider suction and foreign body removal (**common**)
- If obstruction persists:
  - consider oro- or nasopharyngeal airway or supraglottic airway device (laryngeal mask airway/i-gel®) (**common**)
- If obstruction still persists:
  - consider intubation (**uncommon**)
- If performed, immediately check position of tracheal tube (auscultation and capnography)
- If intubation is difficult or impossible:
  - see failed intubation algorithm (see Figure 19.8)
  - consider surgical airway (**very uncommon**)
- If stridor but relatively alert:
  - allow self-ventilation whenever possible
  - encourage oxygen but do not force to wear mask
  - do not force to lie down; sitting on parent's knee may be preferred
  - do not inspect the airway (except as a definitive procedure under controlled conditions)
  - assemble expert team and equipment

Assess breathing
- If respiratory arrest or depression:
  - administer oxygen by bag–valve–mask
  - SpO_2 monitoring
  - consider supraglottic airway device
  - consider intubation
  - check the position of tube if inserted (capnography and auscultation)
- If sedative or paralysing drugs are possible:
  - administer reversal agent
- If respiratory distress or tachypnoea:
  - administer oxygen
- If lateralised ventilatory deficit:
  - consider haemo- or pneumothorax, or inhaled foreign body
  - consider lung consolidation, collapse or effusion
- If chest injury:
  - consider tension haemo- or pneumothorax, flail segment and open pneumothorax
- If evidence of tension pneumothorax:
  - perform immediate thoracotomy or needle decompression
  - follow with chest drain
- If evidence of massive haemothorax:
  - insert chest drain
  - commence blood volume replacement, simultaneously if possible
- If wheeze or crackles:
  - consider asthma, bronchiolitis, pneumonia and heart failure
  - consider inhaled foreign body
- If evidence of acute severe asthma:
  - give inhaled or intravenous β-agonists
  - give steroids and consider aminophylline or magnesium
- Continue primary assessment:
  - proceed to assess the circulation and nervous system
- **If there is deterioration from any cause: reassess airway and breathing**

17.6   Team aspects of airway management

Resuscitation team members will generally have designated roles, with a team leader having a coordinating role. In many paediatric resuscitation teams, an anaesthetist or paediatric intensivist will take charge of airway management. As this role involves taking a position at the head of the trolley, the person in this 'airway' role should also be responsible for protecting and managing the cervical spine if this is necessary. The airway doctor/nurse will have a key role in the coordination of log-rolling manoeuvres during the secondary assessment and in any subsequent transfer of the child for medical imaging or to intensive care. Being at the child's head, they will be in a position to see (and bring to the team leader's attention to) any significant untreated scalp lacerations, which can be a cause of significant blood loss in children. The person managing the airway will need at least one skilled assistant to help with drugs and equipment if advanced airway techniques become necessary.

The decision to embark on endotracheal intubation or other advanced airway techniques should be made by the team leader, after discussion with the team member/s managing the airway and other team members. Members of the airway team should prepare for intubation while other members of the team complete their part of the secondary assessment. Should a person skilled in paediatric airway management not be present, every effort should be made by the team to contact an appropriate expert (anaesthetist, intensivist or emergency physician) to discuss the situation and plan. Except in life-threatening situations, the team should wait for senior help to arrive before embarking on advanced airway management.

In the setting of severe trauma, children may require early intubation even if the airway is not compromised by the injury. However, the process of intubation may itself cause coughing, vomiting and 'bucking', associated with potentially harmful increases in intracranial pressure. In these situations, general anaesthesia will be required to best achieve a smooth intubation. As induction of anaesthesia makes neurological assessment impossible, an initial neurological assessment should be performed prior to induction (Box 17.1).

17.7   Equipment for providing oxygen and ventilation

Oxygen source

A wall oxygen supply (at a pressure of 4 bar, 400 kPa) is provided in most resuscitation rooms. A flow meter capable of delivering at least 15 l/min should be fitted. Air outlets may also be available but these should remain capped unless specifically needed for a particular patient or for use with a ventilator.

Masks for spontaneous breathing

A mask with a reservoir bag (Figure 17.1) should be used in the first instance so that a high concentration of oxygen is delivered. A simple mask or other device such as a head box may be used later if a high oxygen concentration is no longer required. Nasal prongs are often well tolerated, but they may cause drying of the airway, hence flow rates are limited. Younger children are more susceptible to the drying effect of a non-humidified oxygen supply. Devices providing high-flow, high-humidity inspired gases with air/oxygen blenders permit titration of inspired oxygen levels whilst maintaining high flow rates. These may also provide additional non-invasive respiratory support.

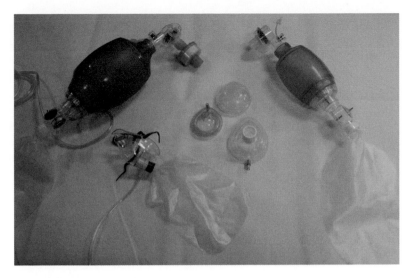

Figure 17.1 Equipment for providing oxygen and ventilation
Children's Health Queensland/CC BY 4.0

Face masks (for artificial ventilation)

Face masks for mouth-to-mouth or bag–valve–mask ventilation in infants are of two main designs (Figure 17.2). Some masks are shaped to conform to the anatomy of the child's face and have a low dead space. Circular, soft plastic masks give a good seal and are preferred by many. Clear masks allow the presence of vomit to be seen, and also misting during effective ventilation.

The standard position of the 'tear-drop' shaped mask has the narrow top end over the nose; however by using it upside down, it may be used to help ventilate an infant.

(a)

(b)

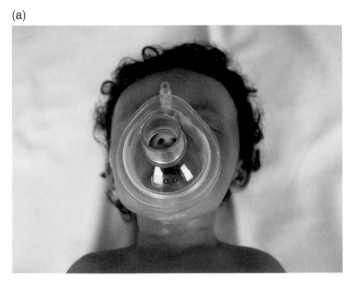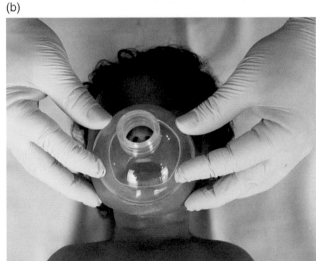

Figure 17.2 (a, b) Face masks
Children's Health Queensland/CC BY 4.0

Self-inflating bags

Self-inflating bags come in three sizes: 250, 500 and 1500 ml. The smallest bag is ineffective except in very small babies. The two smaller sizes usually have a pressure-limiting valve set at 4.5 kPa (45 cmH$_2$O), which may occasionally need to be over-ridden for high-resistance/low-compliance lungs, but which protects normal lungs from inadvertent barotrauma. The patient end of the bag connects to a one-way valve of a fish-mouth or leaf-flap design. The opposite end has a connection to the oxygen supply and to a reservoir attachment. The reservoir enables high oxygen concentrations to be delivered. Without a reservoir bag, it is difficult to supply more than 50% oxygen to the patient whatever the fresh gas flow, whereas with a reservoir bag and high-flow oxygen, an inspired oxygen concentration of 98% can be achieved. Should the oxygen supply fail, ventilation continues with air.

Anaesthetic breathing systems (e.g. T-piece with open-ended bag)

This equipment may be chosen by those experienced in its use. The T-piece provides useful tactile feedback, and also allows positive end-expiratory pressure (PEEP) to be delivered either by means of an adjustable valve or by the operator varying the degree of occlusion of the bag outlet, often with the little finger. T-pieces are difficult to use by inexperienced operators, particularly if one-handed when the other hand is holding a face mask. High gas flows are necessary to prevent re-breathing of expired CO$_2$, and although T-pieces could be used for patients of any size, in practice they are usually used for infants and sometimes for younger children. The open-ended bag on T-piece systems is usually a small size (0.5 or 1 litre) suitable for these smaller patients (typically weight less than 15–20 kg). Unlike self-inflating bags, they are totally dependent on a pressurised supply of fresh gas. When in use, particularly during transportation, a back-up self-inflating bag should be available in case of gas supply failure.

Mechanical ventilators

A detailed discussion of individual mechanical ventilators is beyond the scope of this book. If a ventilator is used, frequent re-evaluation is necessary, with mandatory monitoring of expired carbon dioxide (CO$_2$) and pulse oximetry (Cook et al., 2011a, 2011b; AAGBI, 2016).

Chest tubes

These are included because haemothorax or pneumothorax may severely limit ventilation. They are described elsewhere (see Chapter 21).

Gastric tubes

Children are prone to air swallowing and vomiting. Air may also be forced into the stomach during bag–mask ventilation. This may cause vomiting, vagal stimulation and diaphragmatic splinting. A gastric tube will decompress the stomach and significantly improve both breathing and general well-being. Withholding the procedure 'to be kind to the child' may cause more distress than performing it.

17.8   Equipment for managing the airway

Equipment for managing the airway should be available in a variety of sizes and should be present in all resuscitation areas. Complete familiarity with airway equipment should be gained before an emergency occurs.

Airway equipment

- Face masks
- Oropharyngeal and nasopharyngeal airways
- Supraglottic airways (pharyngeal airway, laryngeal mask airway (LMA)/i-gel®))
- Laryngoscopes with a selection of blades
- Tracheal tubes, introducers and connectors
- Magill forceps
- Suction devices

Assessment and continued monitoring is a vital part of the safe use of an airway device, and appropriate equipment for this should also be available.

Pharyngeal airways

There are two main types of pharyngeal airway:

- Oropharyngeal airway
- Nasopharyngeal airway

Oropharyngeal airway

An oropharyngeal airway, otherwise referred to as an oral airway or Guedel® airway, may be used in the unconscious or obtunded patient for short-term airway management. It is frequently used as the first intervention when a patent airway cannot be achieved by manual methods. It provides a patent airway channel between the tongue and the posterior pharyngeal wall. It may also be used to stabilise the position of an oral endotracheal tube (ETT) following intubation. In a patient with an intact gag reflex it may not be tolerated; in this situation attempted forced insertion may cause vomiting. During use, if the patient begins to gag as the level of consciousness improves, the airway should be removed.

A correctly sized airway when placed with its flange at the centre of the incisors, then curved around the face, will reach the angle of the mandible (Figure 17.3). This method of sizing is an estimate only, and a larger or smaller airway should be tried if no immediate improvement is seen. Too small an airway may be ineffective, too large an airway may cause laryngospasm. Either may cause oral trauma or may worsen airway obstruction.

Nasopharyngeal airway

A nasopharyngeal airway is often better tolerated than a Guedel® airway. It is contraindicated in fractures of the anterior base of the skull. Insertion may cause haemorrhage from the vascular nasal mucosa, especially if it is not well lubricated. A suitable length can be estimated by measuring from the lateral edge of the nostril to the tragus of the ear (Figure 17.4). An appropriate diameter is one that just fits into the nostril without causing blanching. As small-sized nasopharyngeal airways may not be available, shortened ETTs may be used with a large safety pin to prevent loss into the nose.

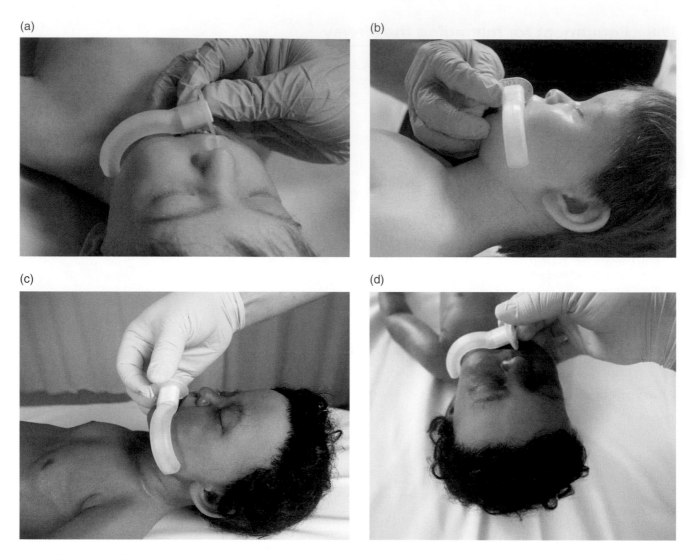

Figure 17.3 (a, b) Sizing an oropharyngeal airway in a child, and (c, d) sizing an oropharyngeal airway in an infant
Children's Health Queensland/CC BY 4.0

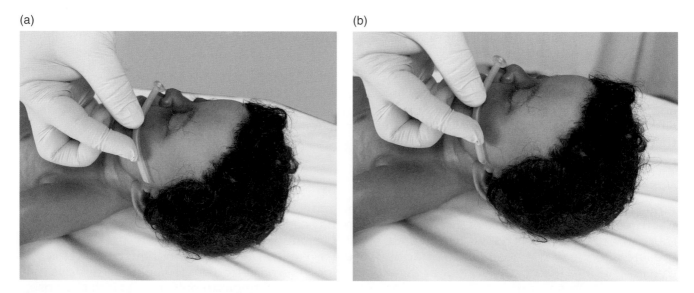

Figure 17.4 (a, b) Sizing a nasopharyngeal airway
Children's Health Queensland/CC BY 4.0

Supraglottic airways and related devices

The laryngeal mask airway (LMA) was originally designed for use in elective anaesthesia, but is increasingly used for the management of the airway in emergencies. The LMA has an inflatable elliptical mask that sits around the laryngeal inlet. At the proximal end is a tube similar to a large ETT, with a pilot tube to inflate the cuff. The original LMAs were reusable, but disposable LMAs and other designs such as the intubating LMA are now available, some designs incorporating a channel for the suctioning of gastric contents.

The i-gel® is based on similar design principles to the LMA, but has a soft, gel-like cuff that does not require inflation and a more rigid, flatter tube that may be less prone to rotation after insertion than the round tube of the LMA. It also incorporates a suction channel. Both the LMA and i-gel® are available in paediatric sizes (Tables 17.1 and 17.2).

Table 17.1 Laryngeal mask airway (LMA) sizes

Patient weight (kg)	LMA size (standard disposable LMA)	Maximum cuff volume (ml)
Less than 5	1	5
5–10	1.5	7
10–20	2	10
20–30	2.5	15
30–50	3	20
50–70	4	30
More than 70	5	40

Recommended maximum inflation volumes vary slightly between manufacturers and different models of LMA. Check packaging.

Table 17.2 I-gel® sizes

Patient weight (kg)	I-gel® size
Less than 5 (neonate)	1
5–12 (infant)	1.5
10–25 (small paediatric)	2.0
25–35 (large paediatric)	2.5
30–60 (small adult)	3
50–90 (medium adult)	4

The LMA and i-gel® have an established role in many areas, including the emergency department and in pre-hospital care, as they are relatively easy and quick to insert even for non-expert users, particularly the i-gel®. Training in their use is still advisable, as in the hands of inexperienced users it is possible for them to be misplaced. Success rates are high in those experienced in their use, and reach near 100% when used electively by anaesthetists. Success rates are lower in infants.

Use of these devices may result in less gastric distension than with bag–valve–mask ventilation. This reduces, but does not eliminate, the risk of aspiration: the seal is less effective than the cuff of an ETT in protecting the trachea against contamination.

Note that the manufacturers' recommended sizes for different patient weights differ slightly between LMAs and i-gels®.

Laryngoscopes

Intubation should take no longer than approximately 30 seconds, or, as a very rough guide, for how long the operator can hold their breath easily. If intubation has not been achieved within this timescale, or the child is desaturating, the child should be re-ventilated/re-oxygenated with the bag–valve–mask device before any further intubation attempt is made. Oxygen saturations should not normally fall during intubation.

There are many designs of laryngoscope available for paediatric use, and choice is to some degree a matter of the personal preference of the user. There are two principal design categories: straight bladed and curved bladed. Most blade designs are available in varying sizes. The appropriate size of laryngoscope blade should be chosen for the age of the child. It is possible to intubate with a blade that is too long but not one that is too short.

The straight-bladed laryngoscope (e.g. Miller, Robertshaw) may be used to directly lift the epiglottis, thereby uncovering the vocal folds. The advantage of this approach is that the epiglottis is moved sufficiently so that it does not obscure the cords.

The curved-bladed laryngoscope (e.g. Macintosh) is designed to move the epiglottis forward by lifting it from in front. The tip of the blade is inserted into the mucosal pocket, known as the vallecula (Figure 17.5), anterior to the epiglottis and the epiglottis is then moved forward by anterior

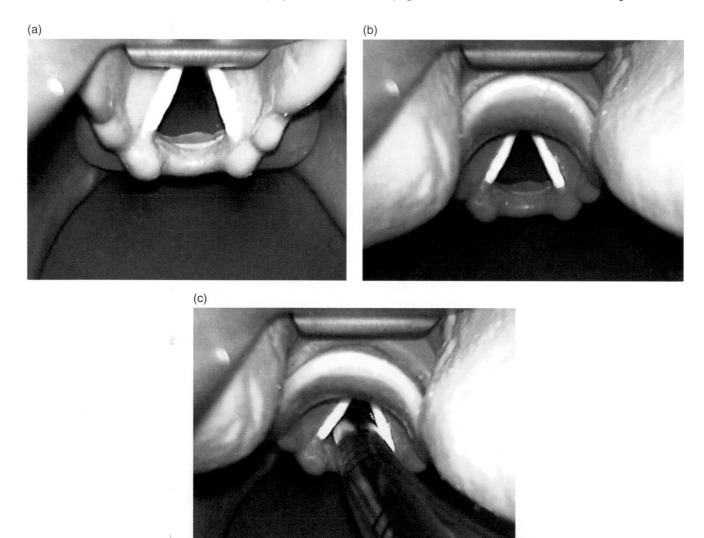

(a)

(b)

(c)

Figure 17.5 Curved-blade laryngoscope. **(a)** Tip of Macintosh blade directly lifting the epiglottis to reveal the vocal cords. **(b)** Tip of Macintosh blade in the vallecular above the epiglottis to reveal the vocal cords beneath the epiglottis. **(c)** Endotracheal tube inserted through vocal cords

pressure in the vallecula. (This has the possible advantage that less vagal stimulation ensues, as the mucosa of the vallecula is innervated by the glossopharyngeal nerve; however children should be anaesthetised before intubation, so this should not be a major issue.)

Either technique can be equally effective at obtaining a view of the cords. In practice, either technique may be used with either type of blade according to user preference. Users should simply choose whichever combination of blade design and intubation technique gives the best view of the cords in their hands.

Modern laryngoscopes have a fibreoptic light guide carrying light to the blade from a light source in the handle. This design is replacing the former arrangement whereby small, unreliable and possibly loose light bulbs in the blade were powered by a battery in the handle. As fibreoptic laryngoscopes were introduced, blades and handles from different manufacturers were not necessarily compatible. Current standard designs have green bands in the handle and blade to show compatibility between manufacturers (Figure 17.6).

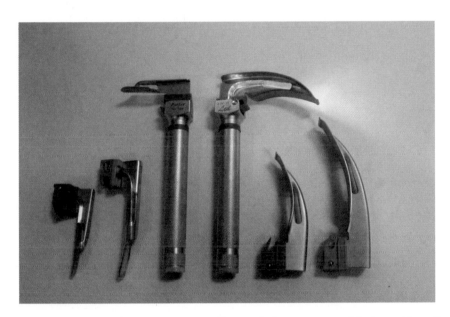

Figure 17.6 Green bands show compatibility between the fibreoptic laryngoscope blade and handle
Children's Health Queensland/CC BY 4.0

Despite improvements in the light source, laryngoscope batteries can and do go flat, so like all emergency equipment they should be regularly checked and a spare available.

Tracheal tubes (or endotracheal tubes)

Traditionally it has been taught that uncuffed tubes should be used in paediatrics. Improvements in materials and design, and modern studies of paediatric airway anatomy, have led to a gradual change in this view, such that cuffed tubes are generally recommended for infants and children in an emergency as their use increases the chance of selecting the correct size of tube at the first intubation attempt.

An appropriately sized, uncuffed tube should give a relatively gas-tight fit in the larynx but should not be so tight that no leak is audible when inflation is continued to pressures slightly over the maximum normal inflation pressure. Failure to observe this condition may lead to damage to the mucosa at the level of the cricoid ring and to subsequent oedema following extubation. An uncuffed tube that is significantly too small will have a leak of gas around it, possibly leading to difficulty achieving adequate ventilation, as well as possible problems with capnometry. In this situation, the child may need to be reintubated with a more suitably sized tube.

If a cuffed tube is used there will be no audible leak of air during ventilation after the cuff is inflated. However, overinflation of the cuff to excessive pressure may lead to mucosal damage. To prevent this, when possible, cuff pressures should be monitored and limited according to the manufacturer's recommendations (usually less than 20 cmH$_2$O (less than 2 kPa)).

In the circumstance of resuscitation in a young child where the lungs are very 'stiff', for example in severe bronchiolitis, a cuffed tube rather than an uncuffed tube may be preferred but the possible risk of airway damage from the cuff must be balanced against the risk of failure to inflate the lungs.

To estimate ETT size for emergency intubation use the following formula for an uncuffed tube:

$$\text{Internal diameter } (\text{mm}) = (\text{Age}/4) + 4$$

The age is in whole years, so the formula is appropriate for ages over 1 year. If a cuffed tube is chosen it may be appropriate to calculate the size using:

$$\text{Internal diameter } (\text{mm}) = (\text{Age}/4) + 3.5$$

(NB: some manufacturers place an age guide on the endotracheal tube pack.)

Neonates under 3 kg usually require an uncuffed tube of size 3.0 or 3.5 mm. Preterm neonates may require a smaller tube.

- Age 6 months: size 4
- Age 1 year: size 4.5

Note that for historical reasons ETTs are sized by the internal diameter of the tube, not the overall diameter, which will be affected by the wall thickness; this may vary slightly between manufacturer and tube type. Alternative tubes, one half-size larger and one half-size smaller, should always be immediately available, for example 5.0 ± 4.5 and 5.5.

To estimate ETT length, use:

$$\text{Length } (\text{cm}) = (\text{Age}/2) + 12 \text{ for an oral tube}$$

$$\text{Length } (\text{cm}) = (\text{Age}/2) + 15 \text{ for a nasal tube}$$

Knowledge of the predicted length may be of use following intubation to check that the tube has been inserted to approximately the correct length from the lips. This does not replace clinical checks of correct tube placement.

There is a risk in cutting a tube to shorten it to the predicted length. A tube that has been cut to a length that is inappropriately short for a patient may, at best, only enter the trachea for a short distance, and hence be at risk of accidentally slipping out of the trachea. At worst the tube may be too short to even reach the vocal cords, and hence be useless. For emergency use, therefore, an uncut, non-shortened tube should be used.

Tracheal tube introducers

Tracheal tube introducers should not be used to force a tracheal tube into position. While these are not routinely necessary, intubation may be facilitated by the use of a stylet or introducer, placed through the lumen of the tracheal tube. This is used to alter the shape of the tube, but can easily damage the tissues if allowed to protrude from the end of the tracheal tube.

It is wise to apply lubrication to the introducer before insertion into the ETT. This reduces the chance of being in the situation of having achieved tracheal placement of the ETT, but being unable to withdraw the introducer.

Tracheal tube connectors

In adults, the proximal end of the tube connector is of standard size, based on the 15–22 mm system, ensuring that they can be connected to a standard self-inflating bag.

The same standard system exists for children, including neonates. Smaller 8.5 mm connectors may be used in some intensive care units (in infants) but should be avoided in the resuscitation setting because of the risk of incompatibility with standard resuscitation equipment.

Magill forceps

Magill forceps are angled to allow a view around the forceps when in the mouth. They may be useful to help position a tube through the cords by lifting it anteriorly, or to remove pharyngeal or supraglottic foreign bodies.

Suction devices

In the resuscitation room the usual suction device is the pipeline vacuum unit. It consists of a suction hose inserted into a wall terminal outlet, a controller (to adjust the vacuum pressure), a reservoir jar, suction tubing and a suitable sucker nozzle or catheter. In order to aspirate vomit effectively, it should be capable of producing a high negative pressure and a high flow rate, although these can be reduced in non-urgent situations so as not to cause mucosal injury.

The Yankauer sucker is available in both adult and paediatric sizes. It may have a side hole, which can be occluded by a finger, allowing greater control over vacuum pressure. Lack of awareness of the existence of such a side hole may give the impression of suction failure. Vigorous blind sweeping with the hard Yankauer sucker may lead to intraoral damage. Partly for this reason, in small infants, a soft suction catheter and a Y-piece are often preferred, but are less capable of removing vomit.

Portable suction devices are required for resuscitation in remote locations, and for transport to and from the resuscitation room. These are usually battery powered, but foot- and hand-powered versions are also available.

Tracheal suction may be required after intubation to remove bronchial secretions or aspirated fluids. In general, the appropriate size in French gauge of the required catheter is numerically twice the internal diameter of the ETT in millimetres, for example for a 3 mm tube the correct suction catheter is French gauge 6. Use of an excessively large tracheal suction catheter may occlude the tracheal tube, such that all the suction pressure is transmitted to the lungs, encouraging atelectasis.

Equipment for difficult intubations

Occasionally, for example in the presence of craniofacial abnormalities, it may be difficult to visualise the vocal cords by direct line of sight. Management of the airway should be maintained by a face mask with a supraglottic airway (see Chapter 19) or LMA/i-gel®.

In videolaryngoscopes (e.g. the GlideScope®, Storz C-MAC™ system) the angled laryngoscope blade has a camera situated at the angle of the blade. The operator holds and manipulates the ETT in the normal manner, but while visualising the larynx on the device's monitor screen.

The AirTraq® device is akin to a laryngoscope, with a series of prisms in the laryngoscope blade that carry the view from the blade tip to an optical eyepiece, or to a monitor screen. A channel in the handle and blade of the device guides the ETT.

In fibreoptic intubating bronchoscopes, the ETT is initially placed over the flexible fibreoptic shaft. The shaft is then inserted through the mouth or nose, or alternatively inserted through an LMA that is already in place. The operator sees the view at the tip on a screen or though the bronchoscope eyepiece. Controls on the handle alter the configuration of the shaft while advancing it towards the vocal cords. Once the bronchoscope is through the vocal cords, the ETT is advanced over it into the trachea.

The above devices have a significant associated learning curve. So, while these are useful aids in experienced hands, there is no place for the uninitiated to 'have a go' for the first time once a real airway emergency has developed.

17.9 Monitoring an intubated patient

Immediately following intubation, the following checks should be performed. These checks should also be performed when taking over an intubated patient, such as following an out-of-hospital intubation.

- Attach a pulse oximeter (if not already in place)
- Connect a capnometer
- Auscultate the patient in both axillae and over the stomach
- Pulse oximetry assesses patient oxygenation, not ventilation. In the event of a misplaced (i.e. oesophageal) ETT, the saturations may only drop slowly, not immediately. Thus pulse oximetry has limited use as a rapid check of correct intubation
- Capnometers respond rapidly to falls in expired CO_2 and immediately indicate the absence of expired CO_2. Hence capnometry is the gold standard monitor for correct intubation: lack of expired CO_2 suggests oesophageal intubation

When monitoring a ventilated patient, a sudden drop in expired CO_2 to zero indicates an equipment problem such as a disconnection in the breathing system, extubation or ventilator failure.

A more gradual fall in expired CO_2 suggests a patient problem such as a drop in cardiac output due to cardiac arrest, inadequate external cardiac compressions or pulmonary embolism. As the lungs are still ventilated, expired CO_2 falls more slowly as CO_2 is washed out of the lungs over several breaths.

Limits of capnometry

- There may be little or no CO_2 output in low or zero cardiac output states
- Capnometry may not detect endobronchial intubation. Endobronchial intubation may be suspected by asymmetrical chest movement following intubation, and should be detected by auscultation
- Ventilation of a patient with an uncuffed ETT that is significantly too small may result in a large leak with expiration around the tube rather than through it, especially if PEEP is used. As no expired gases are flowing through the breathing system, the capnometer may give a misleadingly low or even zero reading
- Auscultation should be performed over both axillae, as in small patients breath sounds may transmit from one side of the chest to the other. Auscultation is also performed over the stomach, as the sound of air entry into the stomach may be misinterpreted as lung air entry unless the stomach is auscultated as well for comparison

Airway and ventilator problems in an intubated patient

The DOPES mnemonic may aid assessment of potential causes of airway and ventilator problems (Table 17.3) (Van de Voorde et al., 2021).

Table 17.3 DOPES mnemonic for airway and ventilator problems in intubated patients

DOPES	Problem		Action
D	Tracheal tube is endobronchial	Asymmetrical chest movements, unilateral breath sounds, SpO_2 falling	Slightly withdraw endotracheal tube (ETT), re-auscultate
	Tracheal tube is oesophageal	Capnometry – no end-tidal CO_2	Remove ETT, mask ventilate, prepare for reintubation
O	Kinked tube	Examine visible part of tube for kinks	Straighten tube, fix securely
	Plugged tube (mucus, blood)	Have high index of suspicion of tube plugging if patient with small ETT has been ventilated with non-humidified gases. Thick mucus plugs may form near tube tip	Suction full length of tube If not resolved: remove ETT, mask ventilate and prepare for reintubation
P	Tension pneumothorax	See Chapters 9 and 21	Needle decompression
		High peak ventilator pressure, rapid decline in SpO_2 and cardiac output	
E	Equipment problems	Check breathing system for disconnection, leaks, oxygen supply and ventilator function	If problem not immediately obvious, hand ventilate while equipment is checked
		Check for deflated ETT cuff	
S	Splinting from abdominal compartment	Decreasing tidal volumes with rising airway pressures	Insert a gastric tube (oral or nasal) or suction catheter to decompress the stomach
		Obvious abdominal distension	

D	Displaced (endobronchial or oesophageal) endotracheal tube
O	Obstructed endotracheal tube (blocked or kinked)
P	Pneumothorax
E	Equipment problems (may include ventilator problems, leaks, breathing system disconnection, oxygen supply failure or disconnection)
S	Stomach (abdominal compartment)

17.10 Management of a blocked tracheostomy

Many children with an established tracheostomy will improve when the blocked tube is removed, allowing them to breathe through the stoma prior to replacing the blocked tube with a new one. However, there are risks in removing the tube from a newly created tracheostomy as, until the stoma track is established, attempted replacement of a tracheostomy tube may be difficult and a blind-ending false track could be created.

Parents who routinely care for their child's tracheostomy at home may be more familiar with tube suction and tube changing for their child than hospital staff in medical areas where this is rarely performed.

A blocked tracheostomy should be managed as in the algorithm in Figure 17.7.

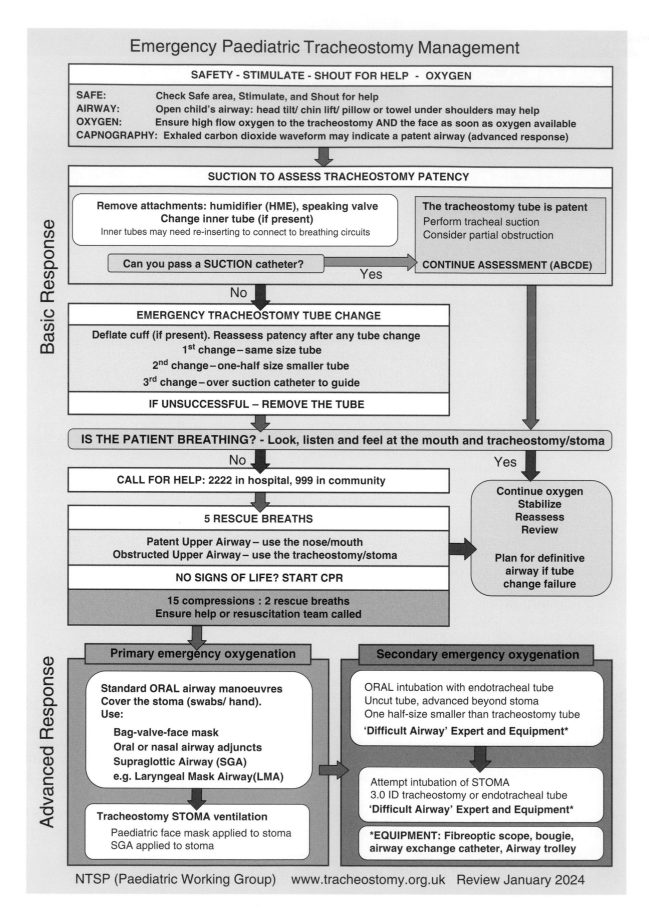

Figure 17.7 National Tracheostomy Safety Project paediatric tracheostomy emergency management algorithm
Reproduced with permission of National Tracheostomy Safety Project (NTSP) Paediatric Working Group

Procedure

Commence basic life support.

1. Stimulate the child.
2. Shout for help.
3. Open and check airway with a head tilt/chin lift. This exposes the tracheostomy tube and opens the upper airway.
4. Apply oxygen to the face *and* **tracheostomy**.
5. Assess patency of the tracheostomy using a suction catheter.
6. If you are unable to pass the suction catheter through the tracheostomy tube, then the tube must be changed immediately with the same size tube. If this fails to relieve the obstruction, or you cannot insert it:
   - Try a half size smaller tube
   - If it is not possible to insert this, thread a lubricated suction catheter through the size smaller tracheostomy tube. Insert the suction catheter into the stoma and then attempt to guide the new tracheostomy tube along the catheter and into the stoma
   - If this is unsuccessful then remove the tracheostomy tube
7. Check for breathing. Look, listen, feel: place the side of your face over the tracheostomy tube or patient's face to listen and feel for any breaths, and at the same time look at the child's chest to observe any breathing movement. If the child is breathing satisfactorily, place them in the recovery position and continue to assess. If the child is not breathing, you will have to give rescue breaths.
8. Give five rescue breaths.
9. If you have succeeded in removing the obstructed tracheostomy and replaced it with a patent tracheostomy tube you should attach a self-inflating bag and ventilate (or, if that is not available, perform mouth-to-tracheostomy ventilation).
10. If you have failed to replace the tracheostomy tube:
    - If the child has a fully or partially patent upper airway, occlude the tracheal stoma and provide rescue breaths via the mouth by bag–valve–mask or mouth-to-mouth ventilation
    - If the child does not have a patent upper airway these resuscitation breaths are applied directly to the stoma

---

Emergency equipment for tracheostomy change

- Usual size tracheostomy tube with tapes attached
- Half-size smaller tracheostomy tube with tapes attached
- Suction catheter of appropriate size
- Resuscitation trolley: self-inflating bag and face masks, oxygen sources, simple airway adjuncts such as oropharyngeal airways, nasopharyngeal airways and laryngeal mask airways
- Scissors
- Spare tape
- Gauze swab
- Gloves

For more information see the UK National Tracheostomy Safety Project: www.tracheostomy.org.uk (last accessed January 2023).

Surgical airway: cricothyroidotomy cannulae and ventilation systems

Purpose-made cricothyroidotomy cannulae are available, usually in three sizes: 12 gauge for an adult, 14 gauge for a child and 18 gauge for a baby. They are less liable to kinking than intravenous cannulae and have a flange for suturing or securing to the neck.

In an emergency, an intravenous cannula can be inserted through the cricothyroid membrane (Figure 17.8) and oxygen insufflated at 1 l/per year of age/min to provide some oxygenation (but no ventilation). A side hole can be cut in the oxygen tubing or a Y-connector can be placed between the cannula and the oxygen supply, to allow intermittent occlusion and achieve partial ventilation, as described in Chapter 19.

Needle crycothroidotomy is a technique of last resort to be used only in an emergency, and has a significant failure rate as the cricothyroid membrane is difficult to feel in young patients. Many ENT surgeons, if present, will prefer an open tracheostomy (see Chapter 19).

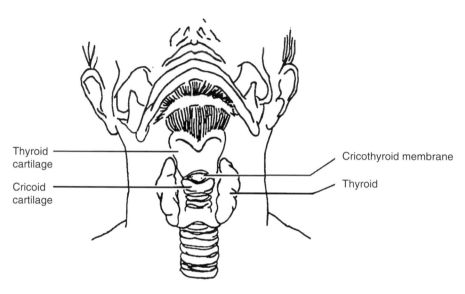

Figure 17.8 Surgical airway anatomy

17.11   Summary

This chapter has discussed how, along with control of catastrophic haemorrhage, the management of airway and breathing has priority in resuscitation. Effective resuscitation techniques must be applied quickly and in order of priority since respiratory function can deteriorate rapidly in children.

CHAPTER 18

Management of cardiac arrest

Learning outcomes

After reading this chapter, you will be able to:
- Assess the cardiac arrest rhythm and perform advanced life support

---

18.1 Introduction

Cardiac arrest has occurred when there is no effective cardiac output. Before any specific therapy is started, effective basic life support (BLS) must be established as described in Chapter 16. The cardiac arrest algorithm is shown in Figure 18.1.

Four cardiac arrest rhythms will be discussed in this chapter:

1. **Asystole.**
2. **Pulseless electrical activity (including electromechanical dissociation).**
3. **Ventricular fibrillation.**
4. **Pulseless ventricular tachycardia.**

The four are divided into two groups:

- Arrest rhythms that do not require defibrillation ('non-shockable'): asystole and pulseless electrical activity (PEA)
- Arrest rhythms that do require defibrillation ('shockable'): ventricular fibrillation (VF) and pulseless ventricular tachycardia (pVT)

Advanced Paediatric Life Support: A Practical Approach to Emergencies, Seventh Edition. Edited by Stephanie Smith.
© 2023 John Wiley & Sons Ltd. Published 2023 by John Wiley & Sons Ltd.

Management of cardiac arrest

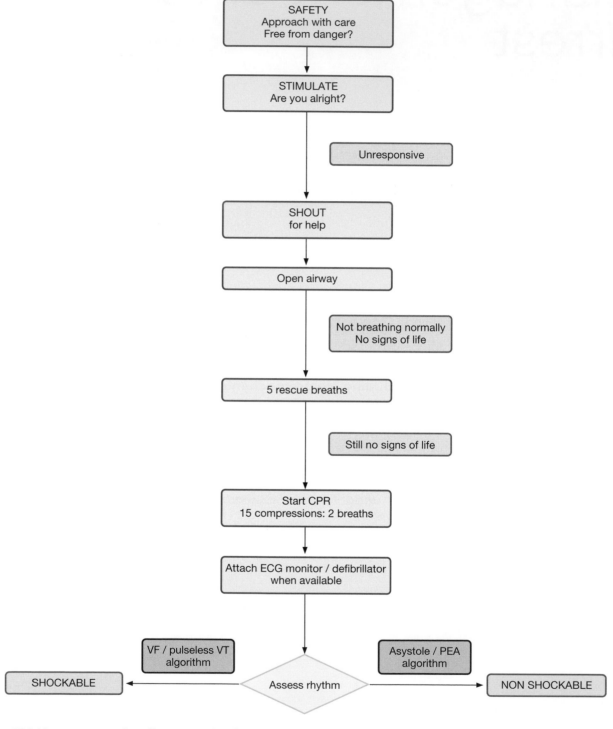

Figure 18.1 Management of cardiac arrest algorithm
CPR, cardiopulmonary resuscitation; ECG, electrocardiogram; PEA, pulseless electrical activity; VF, ventricular fibrillation; VT, ventricular tachycardia

18.2 Non-shockable rhythms

Asystole

Asystole is the most common arrest rhythm in children. The usual response of the young heart to prolonged severe hypoxia and acidosis is progressive bradycardia leading to asystole (Figure 18.2). An electrocardiogram (ECG) monitor will help distinguish asystole from VF, ventricular tachycardia and PEA. The ECG appearance of ventricular asystole is an almost straight line, though occasionally P waves may be seen. To ensure that the appearance (flat line) is not caused by an artefact (a loose wire or disconnected electrode), the gain (ECG size) should be turned up on the ECG monitor.

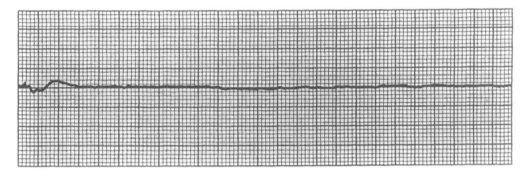

Figure 18.2 Asystole

Pulseless electrical activity

Pulseless electrical activity is suggested by the absence of signs of life or a palpable pulse despite the presence on the ECG monitor of recognisable complexes that would normally produce perfusion (Figure 18.3). PEA is treated in the same way as asystole and is often a 'pre-asystolic' state.

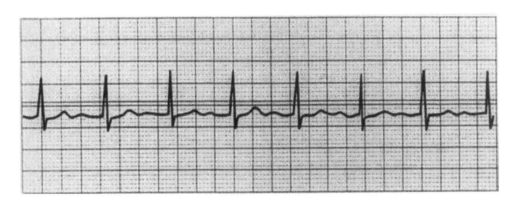

Figure 18.3 Pulseless electrical activity

PEA may be due to an identifiable and reversible cause. In children, the most common causes are hypovolaemia and hypoxia. In the setting of trauma, reversible causes of PEA include severe hypovolaemia, tension pneumothorax and pericardial tamponade. PEA is also seen in hypothermic patients and in patients with electrolyte abnormalities, including hypocalcaemia (e.g. from calcium channel blocker overdose). Rarely in children, PEA may be seen after massive pulmonary thromboembolus.

Management of asystole/PEA

The first essential step in the management of non-shockable cardiac arrest rhythms in infants and children is to continue high-quality cardiopulmonary resuscitation (CPR). Ventilations should be provided initially by bag–mask ventilation (BMV) with high-concentration oxygen. Airway position should be optimised (ensure patency), initially using an airway manoeuvre to open the airway and then stabilising it with an airway adjunct.

Effective chest compressions should be provided at a rate of 100–120 per minute with a compression : ventilation ratio of 15:2. The depth of compression should be at least one-third of the depth (anteroposterior diameter) of the patient's chest: at least 5 cm for a child and at least 4 cm in an infant. **The child should have an ECG monitor attached and the cardiac rhythm assessed.**

Although procedures to stabilise the airway and gain circulatory access are described sequentially, they are best undertaken simultaneously under the direction of a resuscitation team leader. The role of the team leader is to coordinate care and to anticipate problems in the sequence of resuscitation.

Adrenaline is the first line drug used for asystole and PEA. It acts through α-adrenergic-mediated vasoconstriction to increase aortic diastolic pressure during chest compressions, thus improving coronary perfusion pressure and the delivery of oxygenated blood to the heart. It also enhances the contractile state of the heart and stimulates spontaneous contractions. The adrenaline dose is 10 micrograms/kg (0.1 ml/kg of 1:10 000 solution) given IV or IO to a maximum of 1 mg per dose. If intravenous access does not already exist (nor is attainable within 1 minute), intraosseous access should be used. Central lines may provide more secure long-term access, but compared to intraosseous or peripheral intravenous access, offer no advantages during a resuscitation. Each adrenaline dose should be immediately followed by a 0.9% sodium chloride flush (2–5 ml).

As soon as is feasible, a skilled and experienced operator should intubate the patient's airway. Endotracheal intubation offers better control and protection of the airway and enables chest compressions to be given continuously, thus improving coronary perfusion. If endotracheal intubation cannot be rapidly attained, BMV should be continued to minimise interruptions to chest compressions. Both cuffed and uncuffed endotracheal tubes (ETTs) are acceptable for infants and children undergoing emergency intubation (see Chapters 17 and 19). Once the child has been intubated and compressions can continue uninterrupted, the ventilation rate should approximate the lower limit of normal rate for age:

- Infants: 25 breaths per minute
- Children 1–8 years old: 20 breaths per minute
- Children 8–12 years old: 15 breaths per minute
- Children older than 12 years old: 10–12 breaths per minute

It is important for the team leader to assess that the ventilations remain adequate when chest compressions are continuous. This may be best assessed by the person doing the chest compressions who can feel the chest moving when ventilated. The algorithm for asystole and PEA is shown in Figure 18.4.

During and following the administration of adrenaline, chest compressions and ventilations should continue.

> It is vital that chest compressions and ventilations continue with minimal interruptions during advanced life support as they form the basis of the resuscitative effort

The only reasons to briefly interrupt CPR include:

- To deliver a direct current (DC) shock (if needed)
- To reassess the cardiac rhythm
- To perform rapid endotracheal intubation

Performing chest compressions is fatiguing, so the person performing compressions should be rotated every 2 minutes. Providing feedback on CPR quality can improve outcomes.

Asystole/PEA

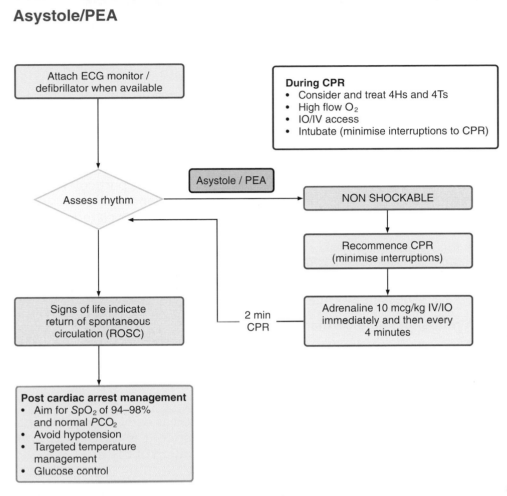

Figure 18.4 Asystole and pulseless electrical activity (PEA) algorithm
CPR, cardiopulmonary resuscitation; ECG, electrocardiogram

At intervals of 2 minutes, chest compressions should be briefly paused to assess the cardiac rhythm on the monitor. If asystole remains, CPR should be continued (again checking the electrode position and contacts). If a more organised rhythm is seen, the patient should be checked for signs of life and for a pulse. If there is a return of spontaneous circulation (ROSC), chest compressions may be discontinued and the ventilation rate may be increased to approximate the lower limit of normal rate for age: 25/min (infants), 20/min (over 1 year), 15/min (over 8 years), 10/min (over 12 years). Post-resuscitation care should commence, aiming for controlled oxygenation, normocapnia, normoglycaemia, targeted temperature management and avoidance of hypotension.

If there are no signs of life and no pulse, CPR should immediately recommence and the asystole/PEA algorithm should be continued. Adrenaline should be administered every 4 minutes at a dose of 10 micrograms/kg (0.1 ml of 1:10 000 solution, max. 1 mg/dose).

Reversible causes

During CPR, possible reversible causes of the cardiac arrest should be considered (based on the history of the event, known underlying illness in the child and any clues that are found during resuscitation) and corrected as they are found. The causes of cardiac arrest in infancy and childhood are multifactorial but the two most common pathways are through hypoxia and hypovolaemia.

Contributing factors may be conveniently remembered as the **4Hs and 4Ts**:

- **H**ypoxia is a leading cause of cardiac arrest in childhood and correction of hypoxia is key to successful resuscitation
- **H**ypovolaemia is common in arrests associated with trauma, anaphylaxis and sepsis and requires rapid restoration of intravascular volume (with crystalloid fluid or blood) (see Chapter 8)
- **H**yperkalaemia, hypokalaemia, hypocalcaemia and other metabolic abnormalities may be suggested by the patient's underlying condition (e.g. renal failure), blood tests taken during the resuscitation or by clues given in the ECG (see Appendices A and B). Intravenous 10% calcium gluconate 0.5 ml/kg (max. 20 ml/dose) may be used to treat hyperkalaemia, hypocalcaemia and calcium channel blocker overdose
- **H**ypothermia is associated with drowning incidents and requires particular care. A low reading thermometer should be used for accurate detection (see Appendix H)
- **T**ension pneumothorax and cardiac **T**amponade are especially associated with PEA and should be suspected in a cardiac arrest as a result of trauma (see Chapter 9)
- **T**oxic ingestion following accidental or deliberate overdose or following an iatrogenic drug error may require specific antidotes (see Appendix F)
- **T**hromboembolic phenomena are rare events in children

Adrenaline use in non-shockable cardiac arrest rhythms

Although there have (to date) been no randomised controlled trials examining the use of adrenaline in paediatric cardiac arrest, several observational studies have found that early administration of adrenaline is associated with better outcomes in paediatric in-hospital cardiac arrest (IHCA) and out-of-hospital cardiac arrest (OHCA).

In non-shockable rhythms, adrenaline should be administered as early as possible after collapse – if possible, within 3 minutes – then every 3–5 minutes thereafter. It is advisable to prepare several doses as soon as possible to avoid any delay in the administration of the drug.

Alkalising agents

Children with asystole will usually be acidotic, as cardiac arrest will have been preceded by respiratory arrest or shock. However, the routine use of alkalising agents has not been shown to be of benefit.

Sodium bicarbonate is the most common alkalising agent currently available. The IV dose is 1 mmol/kg (1 ml/kg of an 8.4% solution). If it must be used:

- Bicarbonate must not be given in the same intravenous line as calcium because precipitation will occur
- Sodium bicarbonate inactivates adrenaline and dopamine and therefore the line must be flushed with 0.9% sodium chloride if these drugs are subsequently given

These agents should be considered only in cases where profound acidosis is likely to adversely affect the action of adrenaline. Sodium bicarbonate therapy also increases intracellular carbon dioxide (CO_2) levels. Therefore, administration of sodium bicarbonate should only be considered for the patient with prolonged cardiac arrest and only after adequate ventilation and effective CPR. In addition, sodium bicarbonate is recommended in the treatment of patients with hyperkalaemia (see Appendix B) and tricyclic antidepressant overdose (see Appendix F).

In the arrested patient, arterial pH correlates poorly with tissue pH. Mixed venous or central venous pH should be used to guide any further alkalising therapy and it should always be remembered that effective CPR is more effective than alkalising agents at raising myocardial pH.

Calcium

In the past, calcium was recommended in the treatment of PEA and asystole, but there is no evidence for its efficacy and there is some evidence of harmful effects. Therefore, the routine use of calcium in the treatment of cardiac arrest in infants and children is not recommended. Calcium is indicated only for treatment of documented hypocalcaemia, calcium channel blocker overdose, hyperkalaemia and hypermagnesaemia.

Atropine

Atropine has no place in the management of cardiac arrest. It may be used to combat excessive vagal tone causing bradycardia in the non-arrested patient.

18.3   Shockable rhythms

Shockable arrhythmias (VF and pVT) are less common in children but may be suspected in sudden collapse, in those suffering from hypothermia, in those poisoned by tricyclic antidepressants and in those with underlying cardiac disease. ECGs showing VF and pVT are shown in Figures 18.5 and 18.6, respectively.

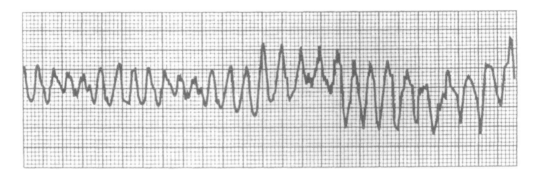

Figure 18.5 Ventricular fibrillation

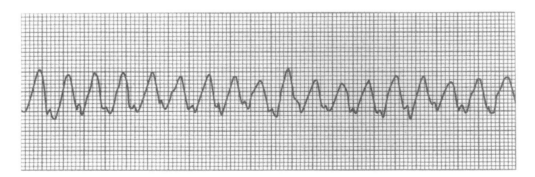

Figure 18.6 Pulseless ventricular tachycardia

The management algorithm for VF and pulseless VT is the same and is shown in Figure 18.7.

The guidance provided is for non-experts in paediatric cardiology. In the paediatric cardiac intensive care unit, theatre or catheter laboratory, patient treatment should be individualised appropriately. If the patient is being monitored, the rhythm can be identified before significant deterioration. With immediate identification of VF/pVT, asynchronous electrical defibrillation of 4 joules per kilogram (J/kg) should be carried out immediately and the protocol continued as below.

Ventricular fibrillation and pulseless ventricular tachycardia

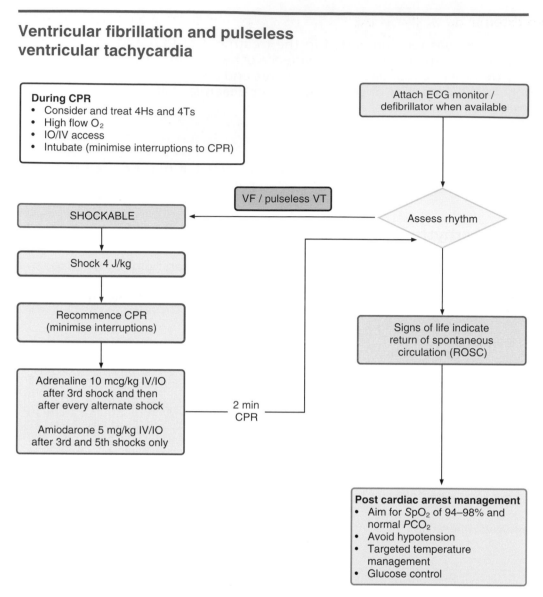

Figure 18.7 Ventricular fibrillation (VF) and pulseless ventricular tachycardia (VT) algorithm
CPR, cardiopulmonary resuscitation; ECG, electrocardiogram

In unmonitored children, CPR should be started in response to the collapse and the identification of VF/pVT will occur only once cardiac monitoring is applied. An asynchronous shock of 4 J/kg should be given immediately and CPR immediately resumed (without reassessing the rhythm or feeling for a pulse). Immediate resumption of CPR is vital because there is a pause between successful defibrillation and the appearance of a rhythm on the monitor. Prolonged pauses of chest compressions reduce the chance of a successful outcome if further shocks are needed. No harm results from 'unnecessary' compressions.

Appropriately sized adhesive defibrillation pads should be used. The recommended sizes are 4.5 cm for children weighing less than 10 kg and 8–12 cm for children more than 10 kg. One pad is placed over the apex of the heart in the mid-axillary line and the other is applied immediately below the clavicle just to the right of the sternum. If only adult pads are available or if the pads are too large for the infant/child (and they overlap on application), one pad should be placed on the upper back (below the left scapula) and the other on the front (below the clavicle and to the left of the sternum) in an anteroposterior configuration.

Automated external defibrillators (AEDs) are now commonplace. Most AEDs can detect VF/pVT in children of all ages and differentiate 'shockable' from 'non-shockable' rhythms with a high degree of sensitivity and specificity.

In children over 8 years, if a manual defibrillator is not available, an AED with standard adult shock doses may be used. For children under 8 years, attenuated paediatric pads should preferably be used with the AED.

In an infant (less than 1 year), a manual defibrillator that can be adjusted to give the correct shock is recommended. However, if an AED is the only defibrillator available, its use should be considered, preferably with paediatric attenuation pads. Many AEDs now have a setting for adult or paediatric use. The paediatric setting lowers the joule output from the AED without having to change the pads. The order of decreasing preference for defibrillation in the infant is as follows:

1. Manual defibrillator.
2. AED with dose attenuator or paediatric switch.
3. AED without dose attenuator.

If the shock fails to defibrillate, attention must revert to supporting coronary and cerebral perfusion as in asystole. Although procedures to stabilise the airway and gain circulatory access are described sequentially, they are best undertaken simultaneously under the direction of a resuscitation team leader.

Continuing high-quality CPR with minimal interruptions is vital for optimal outcome.

As soon as is feasible, a skilled and experienced operator should intubate the patient's airway. Endotracheal intubation offers better control and protection of the airway and enables chest compressions to be given continuously, thus improving coronary perfusion. If endotracheal intubation cannot be rapidly attained, BMV should be continued to minimise interruptions to chest compressions. Capnography monitoring should be used when ventilating.

Circulatory access should be secured. If intravenous access does not already exist (nor is attainable within 1 minute), intraosseous access should be used. Central lines may provide more secure long term access, but compared to intraosseous or peripheral intravenous access, offer no advantages during a resuscitation.

Two minutes after the first shock, chest compressions should be paused briefly to allow assessment of the cardiac rhythm on the monitor (and to change the person providing compressions). If VF/pVT is still present, a second shock of 4 J/kg should be administered and CPR resumed immediately (commencing with chest compressions). Reversible causes (4Hs and 4Ts) should be considered and corrected while continuing CPR for a further 2 minutes.

Chest compressions should be paused briefly again to allow assessment of the cardiac rhythm. If the rhythm is still VF/pVT, a third shock of 4 J/kg should be given and CPR resumed immediately. After the third shock, adrenaline 10 micrograms/kg (0.1 ml/kg of 1:10 000 solution) IV or IO to a maximum of 1 mg per dose and amiodarone 5 mg/kg IV or IO (max. 300 mg/dose) should be administered. Each drug dose should be immediately followed by a 0.9% sodium chloride flush (2–5 ml). After completion of a further 2 minutes of CPR, compressions should be again paused briefly to check the monitor and if the rhythm is still VF/pVT, an immediate fourth shock of 4 J/kg should be administered and CPR resumed.

After a further 2 minutes of CPR, compressions should be again paused briefly for a rhythm check and if the rhythm is still shockable, a fifth shock of 4 J/kg should be given and CPR recommenced immediately. After the fifth shock, a second adrenaline dose of 10 micrograms/kg (0.1 ml/kg of 1:10 000 solution) IV or IO to a maximum of 1 mg per dose and a second amiodarone dose of 5 mg/kg IV or IO (max. 150 mg/dose) should be administered.

After completion of each subsequent 2 minutes of CPR, compressions should be pause briefly to allow checking of the cardiac rhythm on the monitor. Further shocks of 4 J/kg should be administered every 2 minutes for shockable rhythms, minimising the interruptions to CPR as much as possible. Further doses of adrenaline 10 micrograms/kg (0.1 ml/kg of 1:10 000 solution) IV or IO should be provided after every alternate shock (i.e. every 4 minutes).

During CPR consider and correct reversible causes of the cardiac arrest based on the history of the event and any clues that are found during resuscitation. These factors are remembered as the 4Hs and 4Ts (see full list earlier in the chapter).

If at any time the patient should show signs of life, such as regular respiratory effort, coughing, eye opening or a sudden increase in end-tidal CO_2, CPR should be paused and the cardiac rhythm reviewed:

- If still VF/pVT, the sequence above should be continued
- If asystole, further management should follow the asystole/PEA algorithm (Figure 18.4)
- If organised electrical activity is seen, the infant/child should be examined for signs of life and a pulse. If there is ROSC, post-resuscitation care should be commenced. If there is no pulse (or a pulse rate below 60 beats/min with no signs of circulation) and no other signs of life, further management should follow the asystole/PEA algorithm

Adrenaline use in shockable cardiac arrest rhythms

Although there have (to date) been no randomised controlled trials examining the use of adrenaline in paediatric cardiac arrest, several observational studies have found that early administration of adrenaline is associated with better outcomes in paediatric IHCA and OHCA.

In non-shockable rhythms, adrenaline should be administered as early as in shockable rhythms, the first dose of adrenaline should be administered after the third shock (about 4–5 minutes after start of CPR) – then every 3–5 minutes (after every second shock) thereafter.

Antiarrhythmic drugs

Amiodarone is the antiarrhythmic drug of choice in shock-resistant VF and pVT. The dose of amiodarone for VF/pVT is 5 mg/kg (max. 300 mg/dose) via rapid intravenous bolus.

In VF/pVT caused by an overdose of an arrhythmogenic drug, the use of amiodarone should be omitted. Expert advice should be obtained from a poisons centre. Amiodarone is likely to be unhelpful in the setting of VF caused by hypothermia, but may be used nevertheless.

Lidocaine (lignocaine) is an alternative to amiodarone. A recent, retrospective, comparative cohort study found no difference in outcome for either drug. The dose is 1 mg/kg IV or IO (do not exceed 3 mg/kg over the first hour).

DC cardioversion, not the action of antiarrhythmic drugs, converts the heart back to a perfusing rhythm. The purpose of antiarrhythmic drugs is to stabilise the converted rhythm. Adrenaline is used to improve myocardial oxygenation by increasing coronary perfusion pressure. Adrenaline also increases the vigour and intensity of ventricular fibrillation, which increases the success of defibrillation.

Magnesium 25–50 mg/kg (max. 2 g) is indicated in children with hypomagnesaemia or with polymorphic VT (torsades de pointes), regardless of cause.

Shock resistant VF/pVT

If there is still resistance to defibrillation, different paddle positions or another defibrillator may be tried. In the infant in whom paediatric paddles have been used, larger paddles applied to the front and back of the chest may be an alternative.

If the rhythm initially converts and then deteriorates back to VF or pVT then the sequence should continue to cycle, omitting a further dose of amiodarone if two have already been given. If further amiodarone is thought necessary, an infusion of 0.3–1.5 mg/kg/h (max. 1.2 g in 24 hours) may be administered.

Automatic external defibrillators

The use of AEDs in the pre-hospital setting (and especially for public access) significantly improves the outcome for VF/pVT cardiac arrest in adults. In the pre-hospital setting, AEDs are commonly used in adults to assess cardiac rhythm and to deliver defibrillation. Most AEDs can detect VF/pVT in children of all ages and differentiate 'shockable' from 'non-shockable' rhythms with a high degree of sensitivity and specificity. Thus, if an AED is the only defibrillator available, its use should be considered (preferably using the paediatric setting or with the paediatric pads) as described earlier.

Many devices have paediatric attenuation pads that decrease the energy to a level more appropriate for the child (1–8 years) or leads reducing the total energy to 50–80 joules. For infants, a manual defibrillator that can be adjusted to give the desired shock (4 J/kg) is preferred. However, if an AED is the only defibrillator available, its use should be considered, preferably with paediatric attenuation pads.

Modern defibrillators now use biphasic waveforms. Defibrillation appears to be as effective at lower energy doses as conventional waveforms in adults and the biphasic waveform appears to cause less myocardial damage than monophasic shocks. Both monophasic and biphasic wave form defibrillators are acceptable for use in childhood.

Capnography

Monitoring of end-tidal CO_2 ($ETCO_2$) can be helpful in managing cardiac arrest as long as the operator appreciates that the absence of a waveform is more likely to be due to absent or very poor pulmonary perfusion than to tube misplacement. The presence of exhaled CO_2 during CPR is encouraging evidence of efficacy of the CPR and a sudden improvement may indicate ROSC. Adrenaline will decrease and bicarbonate increase the measured CO_2. Levels of less than 2 kPa (15 mmHg) should prompt attention to chest compression adequacy.

Oxygen use

Use of 100% oxygen (when available) is recommended during the resuscitation process outside the delivery room. However, once ROSC is achieved, hyperoxia can be detrimental to recovering tissues. Pulse oximetry should be used to monitor and adjust for oxygen requirement after a successful resuscitation. Oxygen delivery should then be titrated to maintain oxygen saturation levels between 94% and 98%.

Targeted temperature management

Recent evidence suggests that post-arrest hypothermia (core temperatures of 32–34°C) may have beneficial effects on neurological recovery in children. Current paediatric post-arrest recommendations are to either cool to 32–34°C for 24–72 hours (mild hypothermia) or actively maintain normothermia (36–37.5°C) depending on hospital resources. Importantly, increased core temperature increases metabolic demand by 10–13% for each degree centigrade increase in temperature above normal. Therefore, in the post-arrest patient, hyperthermia should be treated with active cooling to maintain a core temperature of less than 37.5°C. Shivering should be prevented as it increases metabolic demand. Sedation may be adequate to control shivering, but neuromuscular blockade may also be needed. See also Appendix H on drowning.

Hypoglycaemia

All children, but especially infants, can become hypoglycaemic when seriously ill. Blood glucose should be checked frequently and hypoglycaemia corrected carefully and rapidly (see Chapter 5). It is important not to cause hyperglycaemia as this will promote an osmotic diuresis. Both hypoglycaemia and hyperglycaemia are associated with a worse neurological outcome in animal models of cardiac arrest.

Resuscitation of the newborn outside the delivery room

There are significant differences in the recommendations for resuscitation at birth (newborn resuscitation) and resuscitation of the infant and child (paediatric resuscitation). This may cause a dilemma for the clinician confronted with the collapsed newborn outside the delivery room as to which algorithm should be used. Current guidance is to recommend that providers use the resuscitation algorithm with which they (and their team members) are most familiar, for example the newborn algorithm in the neonatal intensive care unit (NICU) and the paediatric algorithm in other areas (paediatric critical care unit (PCCU), emergency department, etc.). The newborn with a probable cardiac aetiology for the arrest is the exception, as this group should be resuscitated using the paediatric algorithm.

18.4   When to stop resuscitation

Resuscitation efforts are unlikely to be successful and cessation can be considered if there is no return of spontaneous circulation (ROSC) at any time with up to 20 minutes of cumulative life support and in the absence of recurring or refractory VF/pVT. Exceptions are patients with a history of poisoning or a primary hypothermic insult in whom prolonged attempts may occasionally be successful. In these circumstances, expert advice should be sought from a toxicologist or paediatric intensivist. Importantly, there is no single predictor that reliably indicates when resuscitation efforts should best be stopped.

18.5   Family presence during resuscitation

In general, family members/carers should be offered the opportunity to be present during the resuscitation of their child. Evidence suggests that family presence at the child's side during resuscitation allows family members to gain a realistic understanding of the efforts made to help their child and they subsequently may show fewer symptoms of anxiety and depression.

Important points:

- A staff member should be designated to be the parents' support and interpreter of events at all times
- The team leader, not the parents, is responsible for the decision to stop the resuscitation
- If the presence of the family members is impeding the progress of the resuscitation (a rare situation), they should sensitively be asked to leave
- After the resuscitation, a debriefing session to support staff and reflect on practice is very beneficial

18.6   Summary

This chapter is consistent with the International Liaison Committee on Resuscitation (ILCOR) guidelines, *Resuscitation 2021*, and there are an enormous number of references that have informed this process. These are available on the ALSG website.

The management of overall cardiac arrest is shown in Figure 18.8.

Management of cardiac arrest (expanded)

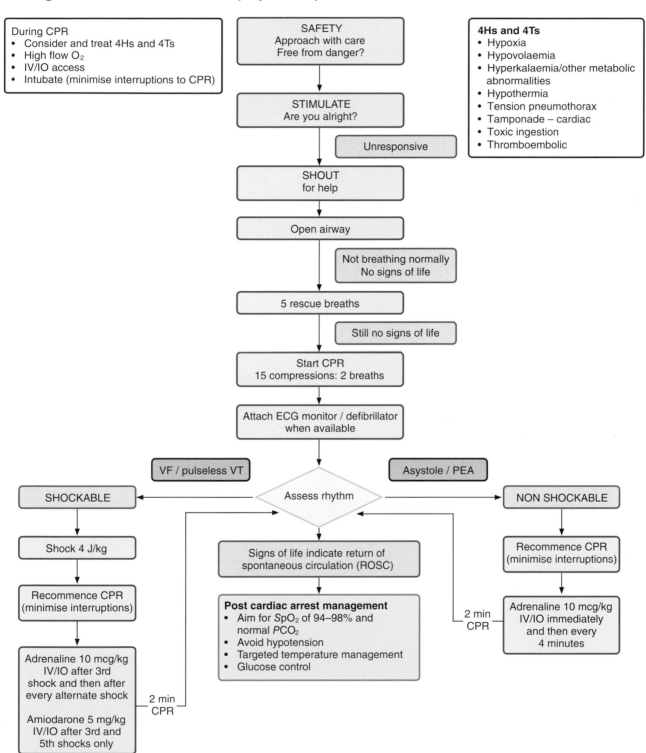

During CPR
- Consider and treat 4Hs and 4Ts
- High flow O_2
- IV/IO access
- Intubate (minimise interruptions to CPR)

4Hs and 4Ts
- Hypoxia
- Hypovolaemia
- Hyperkalaemia/other metabolic abnormalities
- Hypothermia
- Tension pneumothorax
- Tamponade – cardiac
- Toxic ingestion
- Thromboembolic

SAFETY
Approach with care
Free from danger?

STIMULATE
Are you alright?

Unresponsive

SHOUT
for help

Open airway

Not breathing normally
No signs of life

5 rescue breaths

Still no signs of life

Start CPR
15 compressions: 2 breaths

Attach ECG monitor / defibrillator
when available

VF / pulseless VT

Asystole / PEA

Assess rhythm

SHOCKABLE

NON SHOCKABLE

Shock 4 J/kg

Recommence CPR
(minimise interruptions)

Signs of life indicate return of
spontaneous circulation (ROSC)

Recommence CPR
(minimise interruptions)

Post cardiac arrest management
- Aim for SpO_2 of 94–98% and normal PCO_2
- Avoid hypotension
- Targeted temperature management
- Glucose control

Adrenaline 10 mcg/kg
IV/IO after 3rd
shock and then after
every alternate shock

Amiodarone 5 mg/kg
IV/IO after 3rd and
5th shocks only

2 min
CPR

Adrenaline 10 mcg/kg
IV/IO immediately
and then every
4 minutes

2 min
CPR

Figure 18.8 Management of overall cardiac arrest
CPR, cardiopulmonary resuscitation; ECG, electrocardiogram; PEA, pulseless electrical activity; VF, ventricular fibrillation; VT, ventricular tachycardia

PART 5

Practical application of APLS

CHAPTER 19

Practical procedures: airway and breathing

Learning outcomes

After reading this chapter, you will be able to identify the equipment for and describe the following procedures:

- Ventilation without intubation:
  - Mouth-to-mask
  - Bag–mask
- Oropharyngeal airway insertion
- Nasopharyngeal airway insertion
- Tracheal intubation and rapid sequence induction
- Supraglottic airway insertion
- Surgical airway

This chapter should be read in conjunction with Chapter 17. After all interventions, the patient should be reassessed to ascertain success or failure of the intervention.

19.1   Ventilation without intubation

Mouth-to-mask ventilation

Procedure

1. Pocket masks and similar devices will need pushing into shape before use. A filter, if present, may be attached to the mask before use to decrease the risk of aerogenic cross-infection.
2. Apply the mask to the face with both hands, using a jaw thrust grip, with either thumbs or thumbs and index finger holding the mask. If using a shaped mask, it should be the right way up in children (Figure 19.1a) or upside down in infants (Figure 19.1b). Ensure a neutral head position in infants, and a more extended one in older children.
3. Ensure an adequate seal.
4. Blow into the mouth port, observing the resulting chest movement.
5. Ventilate and adjust the rate according to age. If using the mask for cardiopulmonary resuscitation (CPR), then use 2 ventilations to 15 compressions.
6. Attach oxygen to the face mask if available.

Advanced Paediatric Life Support: A Practical Approach to Emergencies, Seventh Edition. Edited by Stephanie Smith.
© 2023 John Wiley & Sons Ltd. Published 2023 by John Wiley & Sons Ltd.

(a)

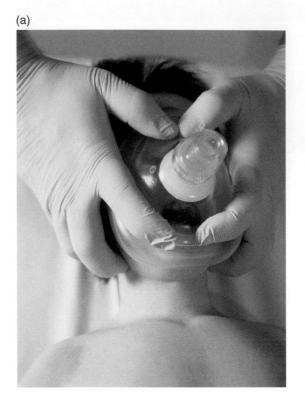

(b)

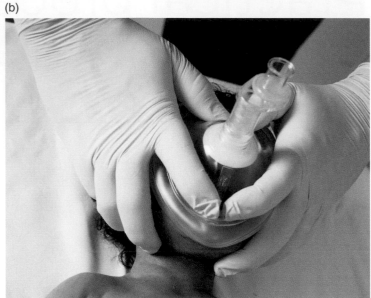

Figure 19.1 Mask position for mouth-to-mask ventilation in (a) a child, and (b) an infant, using both thumbs and index finger
Children's Health Queensland/CC BY 4.0

Bag–mask ventilation

Bag–mask ventilation with a self-inflating bag is the core skill of emergency airway management. It is sometimes described as both simple and routine. In fact, it is a skill that takes practice and experience to acquire; this applies particularly to single-operator use. This piece of equipment has a one-way valve, which must be open for oxygen to be delivered. It does not supply wafting oxygen. If used in a spontaneously breathing patient, they must be able to generate sufficient respiratory effort to open the valve, therefore a non-rebreather oxygen mask is preferable in the sponataneously breathing patient who does not require ventilatory support.

Procedure

1. Select the appropriate size and connect the bag to an oxygen supply at 15 l/min.
2. Ensure the correct head position and apply the mask to the face. The thumb and first finger are placed on top of the mask in a 'C' shape; the third, fourth and fifth fingers are spread over the mandible from the angle of the jaw to the chin (Figure 19.2). The jaw and chin are then lifted, pulling the face up into the mask to obtain a seal. Pushing the mask down into the face results in neck flexion and obstructs the airway.
3. Squeeze the bag, looking for chest movement, misting of the mask and end-tidal carbon dioxide (ETCO$_2$) if available. If the chest is not moving, consider adjusting the head extension to one appropriate to the size of the patient, repositioning the mask, using an airway adjunct or employing a two-person technique.
4. Ventilate and adjust the rate according to age or a ratio of 2 ventilations to 15 chest compressions if performing CPR.
5. Continually reassess the efficacy of oxygenation and ventilation.

(a)   (b)

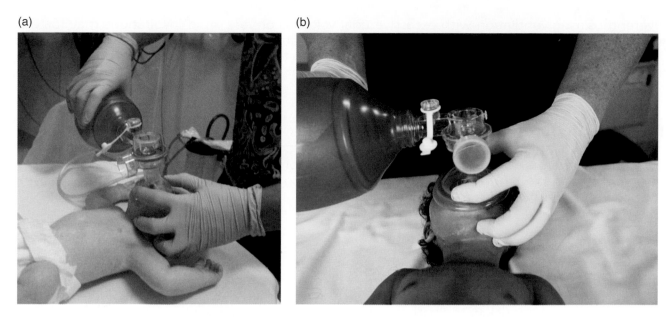

Figure 19.2 Bag and mask ventilation in (a) an infant, and (b) a child
Children's Health Queensland/CC BY 4.0

A two-person technique (Figure 19.3) makes obtaining a seal around the mask easier, with both hands of one rescuer holding the mask. The thumbs are used on top of the mask and the first fingers used to perform a jaw thrust. The other rescuer supports and squeezes the bag. In conjunction with an oropharyngeal airway this is an extremely effective method for airway management in an unconscious apnoeic patient. Self-inflating bags are used to hand ventilate apnoeic patients. Although spontaneous breathing is possible, these systems are not designed to support spontaneously breathing patients or give positive end-expiratory pressure (PEEP). This is done with anaesthetic circuits such as the Ayres T-piece (in a child weighing less than 20 kg) or Waters circuit.

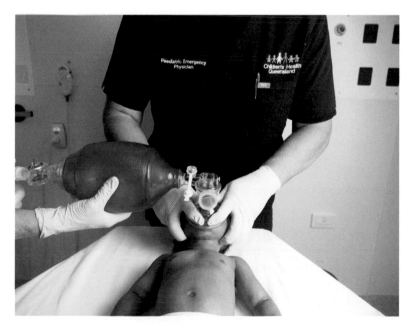

Figure 19.3 Two-person bag–mask ventilation
Children's Health Queensland/CC BY 4.0

Overenthusiastic ventilation with excessive tidal volumes or very rapid inspirations may force air into the stomach. The resulting gastric distension may inhibit ventilation and encourage regurgitation, with the risk of aspiration of stomach content into the airways. Using an airway adjunct and inserting a nasogastric tube, with intermittent manual suction (usually using a 50 ml syringe), reduces this risk.

19.2   Oropharyngeal airway insertion

The oropharyngeal airway prevents obstruction by the tongue. It is extremely effective but can only be used in unconscious or very obtunded patients with no gag reflex due to the potential to provoke vomiting and laryngospasm.

Procedure

1. Select the appropriate size airway (see Chapter 17).
2. Extend the neck slightly if it is safe to do so and open the mouth. In trauma patients, open the mouth with a jaw thrust, avoiding excessive neck movement. (In most resuscitations, however, hypoxia is of greater risk to the patient than a slight neck movement.)
3. In older children and adults, the airway is usually inserted upside down and then rotated through 180° as it is passed between the tongue and soft palate. In smaller children and infants, it is often easier to insert the airway the right way up. The use of a tongue depressor or laryngoscope blade might help pass the airway over the tongue. Avoid pushing the tongue back during insertion.
4. When in position, the curve of the oropharyngeal airway follows the natural curve of the tongue and pharynx (Figure 19.4), and the device will sit naturally in place, with the flange just above the lip.
5. Be prepared to change to a different size if no airway improvement is achieved.

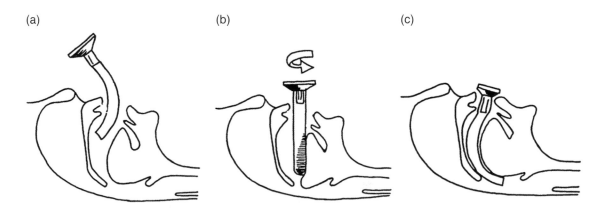

(a)　　　　　　　　　　(b)　　　　　　　　　　(c)

Figure 19.4 (a–c) Airway insertion using the rotational technique

19.3   Nasopharyngeal airway insertion

The nasopharyngeal airway can be useful to relieve airway obstruction in children who have a reduced level of consciousness but are not obtunded enough to tolerate an oropharyngeal airway (Figure 19.5). It may be of use in a fitting child if the mouth is difficult to open. It is relatively contraindicated when basal skull fracture is suspected. However, trismus and vomiting are common in head injury and a nasopharyngeal airway may provide the only route for oxygenation and suction.

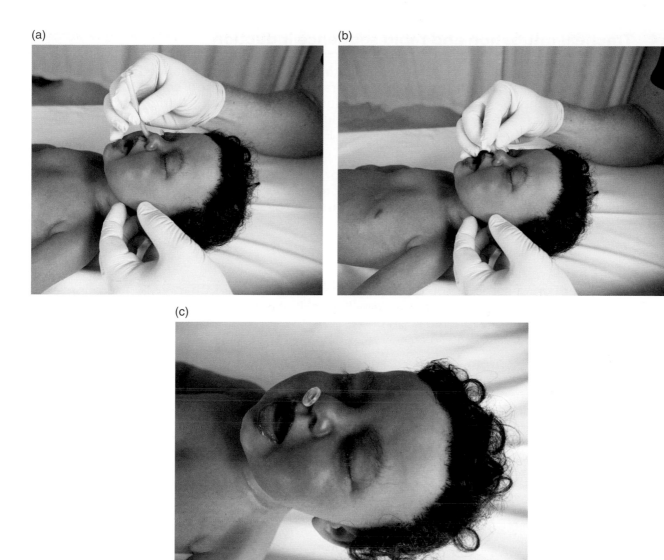

Figure 19.5 (a–c) Insertion of of the nasopharyngeal airway
Children's Health Queensland/CC BY 4.0

Therefore, the benefits of careful insertion in head injury may outweigh the risks. There is a risk of causing a nosebleed, which can seriously complicate airway management.

Procedure

1. Select an appropriate size airway (see Chapter 17). An endotracheal tube cut to a suitable length can also be used.
2. Lubricate the airway with a water-soluble lubricant.
3. Insert the tip into the nostril and direct it posteriorly along the floor of the nose (not upwards).
4. Gently pass the airway past the turbinates with a slight rotating motion. As the tip advances into the pharynx, there should be a palpable 'give'.
5. Continue until the flange rests on the nostril.
6. If there is difficulty inserting the airway, consider using the other nostril or a smaller size from the original estimate. Do not use excessive force or have repeat attempts.
7. Reassess airway and breathing, provide oxygen and commence ventilation if necessary.

19.4   Tracheal intubation and rapid sequence induction

Intubation must be performed only by appropriately trained and experienced practitioners. All children should be anaesthetised and preferably paralysed before laryngoscopy. There are very few exceptions to this, although intubation may be performed without drugs during cardiopulmonary arrest and muscle relaxant may be omitted if gas induction is performed in theatre for upper airway obstruction, as part of a team-based approach with ENT specialists.

The whole team should understand the steps involved in the process of induction of anaesthesia and intubation, and there must be an agreed plan for failed intubation. Role allocation aided by the use of a checklist is helpful (see the example in Figure 19.6). Equipment and drugs must be organised, readily available and regularly checked in all areas of the hospital that may treat a critically ill child.

Laryngoscopy

There is a description of some of the equipment for laryngoscopy in Chapter 17. The priority is to visualise the vocal cords, pass an endotracheal tube into the trachea and to confirm correct placement. Expert providers are increasingly choosing to use video-laryngoscopes over conventional laryngoscopes for primary intubation.

Inspection of chest wall movement, auscultation and $ETCO_2$ measurement (capnometry) are mandatory components of confirming tracheal placement. Later, a chest X-ray may be performed to confirm tube tip placement in the mid-trachea at the level of T1, or the midpoint between the tip of the clavicles and the carina.

In all young children, the epiglottis is horseshoe-shaped and projects posteriorly at 45°, making tracheal intubation more difficult. This, together with the fact that the larynx is high and anterior (at the level of the second and third cervical vertebrae in the infant, compared with the fifth and sixth vertebrae in the adult), means that it is often easier to intubate an infant using a straight-blade laryngoscope. The cricoid ring is oval in shape, and thus passage of a round endotracheal tube will almost always result in a leak around the tube. In fact, if there is not a leak at pressures of approximately 20 cmH$_2$O, it is likely that that tube is too large. Although uncuffed endotracheal tubes have been used preferentially in children, there is increasing evidence that cuffed endotracheal tubes may be advantageous in many settings. However, the use of a cuffed tube requires meticulous attention to size, to cuff pressure and to exact placement of the endotracheal tube in the correct position.

Rapid sequence induction

Traditionally, the delivery of emergency anaesthesia was in the form of a rapid sequence induction (RSI). It is a core skill for anaesthetists and emergency physicians and involves:

1. Pre-oxygenation with 100% oxygen for at least 3 minutes.
2. Induction of anaesthesia.
3. Application of cricoid pressure by a skilled assistant. The aim of cricoid pressure is to compress the oesophagus against the vertebral body behind, theoretically preventing passive regurgitation of gastric contents.
4. Administration of a rapid-acting muscle relaxant, normally suxamethonium or rocuronium.
5. Intubation of the trachea, followed by the release of cricoid pressure once correct intubation is confirmed.

This technique was intended to prevent aspiration of the gastric contents after induction and before intubation. However, there is little evidence that RSI reduces this small risk, and it is associated with a high incidence of hypoxia. This is because ventilation is not performed after the induction of anaesthesia until the airway is secured, and the incidence of failed intubation is higher in the presence of cricoid pressure, which can distort airway anatomy.

Emergency induction checklist (Paediatric)

Prepare for difficulty

- ☐ Are any specific complications anticipated?
  - ☐ previous difficult airway
  - ☐ rapid desaturation
  - ☐ circulatory collapse / need for ECMO
- ☐ If the airway is difficult, could we wake the patient up?
- ☐ If the intubation is difficult, how will you maintain oxygenation? (facemask/supraglottic airway and adjuncts, front of neck access)
- ☐ Is the relevant equipment, including alternative airway, immediately available?

Prepare equipment

- ☐ What monitoring is applied?
  - ☐ ECG
  - ☐ Blood pressure (cycling)
  - ☐ Saturations
  - ☐ Capnography
- ☐ What equipment is checked and available?
  - ☐ Self-inflating bag/T-piece
  - ☐ Facemask and adjuncts
  - ☐ Suction
  - ☐ Correctly sized ET tubes -cuffed or uncuffed?
  - ☐ 2 laryngoscopes +/– CMAC
  - ☐ Stylet/Bougie
- ☐ Do you have all the drugs required, including vasopressors (dilute adrenaline) and IV fluid boluses?

Prepare patient

- ☐ Is pre-oxygenation optimal?
- ☐ Is the patient's position optimal?
- ☐ NG tube considered?
- ☐ Is iv access adequate?
- ☐ Can the patient's condition be optimised any further before intubation?
- ☐ How will anaesthesia be maintained after induction?

Prepare team

- ☐ Who is ...?
  - ☐ Team leader
  - ☐ First Intubator
  - ☐ Second Intubator
  - ☐ Cricoid Manipulation
  - ☐ Intubator's Assistant
  - ☐ Drugs
  - ☐ MILS (if indicated) (Manual InLine Stabilisation)
- ☐ How do we contact further help if required?

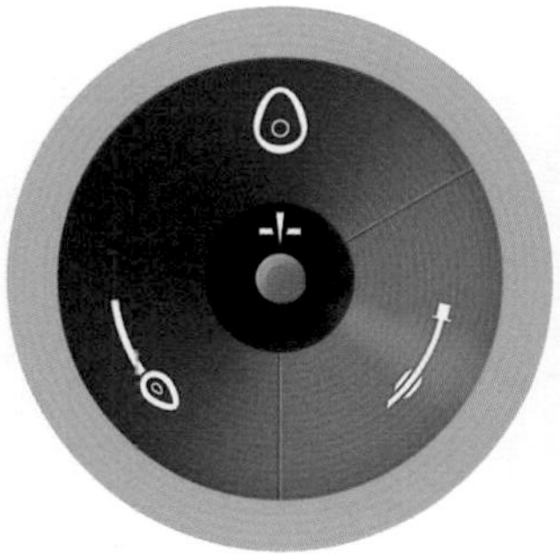

Bristol Royal Hospital For Children

RTIC Severn

This Checklist is not intended to be a comprehensive guide to preparation for induction

Figure 19.6 Example of paediatric intubation checklist
Courtesy of Bristol Royal Hospital for Children and RTIC Severn
ECG, electrocardiogram; ECMO, extracorporeal membrane oxygenation; ET, endotracheal; MILS, manual in line stab lisation; NG, nasogastric

Hypoxia is a greater threat to children than aspiration during the induction of anaesthesia, and for this reason classic RSI should be avoided. Ventilation should be maintained after induction and cricoid pressure omitted, although the intubator may use external laryngeal manipulation during laryngoscopy to improve the view of the vocal cords.

Controlled RSI procedure

1. Insert a nasogastric tube either before induction of anaesthesia or as soon as possible afterwards. Aspirate the stomach contents and leave a 50 ml syringe attached.
2. Use a 20° head-up position and preoxygenate for 3 minutes if possible, either using face mask oxygen with a reservoir bag, high-flow nasal cannula or Ayres T-piece.
3. Administer the induction agent (e.g. ketamine 1 or 2 mg/kg) followed by a muscle relaxant (e.g. rocuronium 1–2 mg/kg).
4. Maintain oxygenation with bag–mask ventilation. Use the least pressure required for effective oxygenation. Keep the stomach decompressed with intermittent aspiration of the nasogastric tube.
5. Intubate the trachea (usually about 1 minute after the muscle relaxant).

Tracheal intubation

This is performed after pre-intubation checks have been performed, and the child is anaesthetised and paralysed.

Procedure

1. The head is brought forward (into the sniffing position) by flexing the neck and extending the head. A pillow in older children or shoulder roll in infants may help achieve this and reduce head movement. A head ring is sometimes used for infants. If there are strong grounds to suspect cervical spine injury, then the neck should be manually immobilised by an assistant (this makes the vocal cords harder to visualise and a bougie or secondary intubation technique may be required). A cervical collar, if present, may need removing and replaced by manual in-line stabilisation if it is impeding the process of intubation.
2. The laryngoscope should be held in the left hand and is inserted down the right side of the mouth using it to sweep the tongue to the left of the blade. The intubator will often hold the occiput with their right hand at this point, to control the head and apply the optimal degree of extension.
3. The tip of the blade is brought into the midline and either rests in the vallecula (curved blade) or picks up the epiglottis (straight blade) (Figure 19.7). Failure to keep the blade in the midline is a common cause of difficulty in visualisation of the larynx.
4. The handle is then pulled upwards without rotating to reveal the vocal cords, that is, pulled in the direction of the laryngoscope handle. Inexperienced operators often lever the blade onto the top gum or teeth, which can cause trauma and should be avoided. In a baby, it is common to advance the laryngoscope blade well beyond the epiglottis and then slowly withdraw it until the vocal cords come into view.
5. The tube should then be passed from the right side through the vocal cords. Most tubes have a black line that should rest at the level of the cords. The intubator should take a note of the tube length at the lips. Do not cut the endotracheal tube before intubation.
6. The tube position should be confirmed by inspecting the chest for symmetrical movement and auscultation in both axillae for equal air entry, and over the stomach to confirm lack of air entry. The definitive test is the measurement of $ETCO_2$ ($ETCO_2$ capnography) which must be used for all intubations. If in doubt, remove the tube and reinstitute bag–mask ventilation. (NB: these checks should also be performed when taking over the care of an intubated patient from another team.)
7. If intubation is not achieved quickly (less than 30 seconds), then oxygenation should be re-established before a further attempt. Hypoxia due to prolonged or multiple intubation attempts should be avoided. Bradycardia and desaturation are late signs of hypoxia. There should not usually be a fall in oxygen saturations during intubation.

8. Inflate the cuff to the appropriate pressure, sufficient to obtain a seal. (If cuff pressure is measured, this is usually 20 cmH$_2$O although it may need to be more if high ventilation pressures are required.) Cuffed endotracheal tubes are increasingly used in paediatric critical care, The ability to eliminate a leak confers several advantages including reduced need for reintubation, ability to use higher ventilation pressures if required and protecting against aspiration. Specially designed cuffed tubes are available for use in patients weighing more than 3 kg.

9. Secure the tube at the correct length. Sticky tape may not be adequate if the face is wet with saliva, blood or vomit, in which case the tube can be tied.

10. A chest X-ray is usually performed later to ensure the tip is appropriately positioned below the vocal cords but above the carina.

(a)   (b)

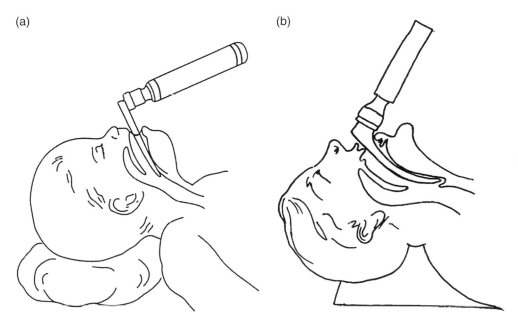

Figure 19.7 **Technique using (a) a straight-blade laryngoscope, and (b) a curved-blade laryngoscope**

19.5 Drugs

Induction agents

Ketamine is the induction agent of choice for anaesthesia in paediatric critical care. The dose is 1 or 2 mg/kg. The lower dose should be chosen when there is established circulatory shock. Ketamine causes the least cardiovascular instability of all induction agents, due to stimulation of endogenous catecholamine release. It is a bronchodilator, which is helpful in children with acute severe asthma. Studies have shown that ketamine does not increase intracranial pressure as previously thought and can be used safely in head-injured patients. It is also an anticonvulsant. An induction dose provides about 20 minutes of anaesthesia, which is useful time for ongoing resuscitation and vascular access before ongoing sedation needs to be commenced.

Ketamine is the safest drug to use in the vast majority situations, however other drugs are sometimes considered:

- **Thiopentone (1–5 mg/kg)** is sometimes used to terminate a prolonged seizure, as described in the status epilepticus algorithm (see Chapter 6). **Propofol (0.5–2 mg/kg)** also has anticonvulsive properties. Both these drugs are sometimes used to treat patients with raised intracranial pressure. However, thiopentone and propofol can cause profound hypotension or even cardiac arrest when used to induce anaesthesia in critically ill patients and should be avoided in patients with signs of shock. When a seizure is associated with cardiovascular compromise, ketamine is a safer choice of induction agent and is an effective anticonvulsant

- **Sevoflurane (or halothane)** may be preferred by anaesthetists managing the airway of a child with upper airway obstruction in theatre with ENT specialists. These are examples of volatile anaesthetic gases, which can also cause severe hypotension, especially if used at similar doses as during induction for elective surgery
- **Etomidate** (0.3 mg/kg) causes less hypotension but is used less often because of the side effect of adrenal suppression
- **Fentanyl** (1 microgram/kg) is sometimes used with ketamine for induction of anaesthesia, although it should be avoided in the presence of shock. It is also commonly used by neonatologists to facilitate intubation (often in combination with atropine and suxamethonium). It is given slowly to avoid the complication of chest wall rigidity

Muscle relaxants

A muscle relaxant is given after induction and makes both bag–mask ventilation and intubation easier. Rapid acting agents are preferable in critical care scenarios. **Suxamethonium** (1–2 mg/kg) and **rocuronium** (1–2 mg/kg) are commonly used and both give good intubating conditions within approximately 1 minute. Higher doses are likely to lead to faster onset of optimal intubating conditions. Atracurium (0.3–0.6 mg/kg) is an alternative. Suxamethonium depolarises muscle causing visible fasciculations to occur before the onset of paralysis. It is rapidly metabolised by plasma cholinesterase in most people and its effects last for just a few minutes. Suxamethonium is contraindicated after burns or spinal cord injury, when the serum potassium is high and when there is a personal or family history of malignant hyperthermia. Rocuronium and atracurium are non-depolarising muscle relaxants. A single dose will last for about 20–30 minutes. They have fewer side effects than suxamethonium and are often preferred.

Whichever drugs are used at induction, the team must be prepared for cardiovascular collapse, especially in shocked patients. Boluses of balanced crystalloid should be prepared.

It is useful to have resuscitation doses of adrenaline (0.1 ml/kg of 1:10000) immediately available. One of these adrenaline doses can be diluted in 0.9% sodium chloride to a volume of 10 ml, giving a solution of 1 microgram/kg/ml. Boluses of 0.5–1 ml (0.5–1 micrograms/kg) can be given to treat significant hypotension before inotrope or vasopressor infusions are prepared and commenced. Morphine and/or midazolam infusions are commonly used for (analgo)-sedation, although α_2-agonists (clonidine or dexmedetomidine) are increasingly preferred to midazolam.

19.6 Intubation algorithm

Most children are easy to intubate. The overall incidence of paediatric difficult airways is very low (about 0.28%) and mostly occurs in children under 1 year of age. However, airway management can be especially stressful during critical illness and trauma scenarios, and it is very important that all team members are empowered to predict and prepare for the next steps. Intubation algorithms are a useful tool for this, and an example is given in Figure 19.8.

The common principles of failed intubation algorithms are:

- Early recognition
- Limited attempts at laryngoscopy
- Early progression to advanced techniques

Video-laryngoscopes (which incorporate fibreoptic technology to help visualise the vocal cords) are now widely available for use in children. Some experts argue that video-laryngoscopes (such as McGrath™, Storz C-MAC™ or GlideScope®) should be used for the first intubation attempt rather than when intubation has failed with a conventional laryngoscope. Whichever approach is used, team discipline is required to avoid multiple attempts at intubation, which causes trauma to the airway and can turn a 'cannot intubate, can oxygenate' situation into a much more time-critical 'cannot intubate, cannot oxygenate' scenario, potentially requiring emergency front of neck access. This is associated with very poor outcomes.

Failed intubation

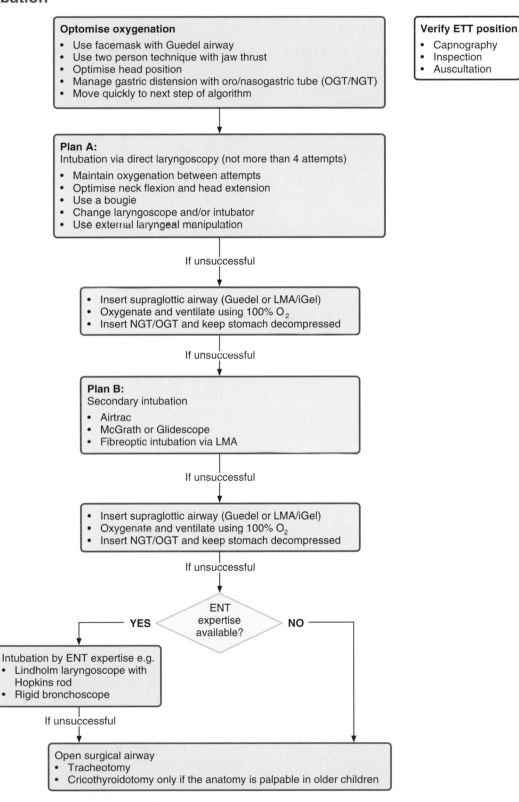

Optomise oxygenation
- Use facemask with Guedel airway
- Use two person technique with jaw thrust
- Optimise head position
- Manage gastric distension with oro/nasogastric tube (OGT/NGT)
- Move quickly to next step of algorithm

Verify ETT position
- Capnography
- Inspection
- Auscultation

Plan A:
Intubation via direct laryngoscopy (not more than 4 attempts)
- Maintain oxygenation between attempts
- Optimise neck flexion and head extension
- Use a bougie
- Change laryngoscope and/or intubator
- Use external laryngeal manipulation

If unsuccessful

- Insert supraglottic airway (Guedel or LMA/iGel)
- Oxygenate and ventilate using 100% O$_2$
- Insert NGT/OGT and keep stomach decompressed

If unsuccessful

Plan B:
Secondary intubation
- Airtrac
- McGrath or Glidescope
- Fibreoptic intubation via LMA

If unsuccessful

- Insert supraglottic airway (Guedel or LMA/iGel)
- Oxygenate and ventilate using 100% O$_2$
- Insert NGT/OGT and keep stomach decompressed

If unsuccessful

ENT expertise available?

YES — Intubation by ENT expertise e.g.
- Lindholm laryngoscope with Hopkins rod
- Rigid bronchoscope

If unsuccessful

NO

Open surgical airway
- Tracheotomy
- Cricothyroidotomy only if the anatomy is palpable in older children

Figure 19.8 Failed intubation algorithm
ENT, ear, nose and throat; ETT, endotracheal tube; LMA, laryngeal mask airway; NGT, nasogastric tube; OGT, orogastric tube

In contrast to elective anaesthesia, in critical illness and injury there may not be an option to abandon intubation and wake the patient up. The steps in the intubation algorithm are moved through methodically until the airway is secured. Team-based simulation training improves performance managing these rare scenarios.

Complications of intubation and their recognition are discussed in Chapter 17.

19.7   Supraglottic airway

The laryngeal mask airway (LMA) is a supraglottic airway (as is the similar i-gel®). It is a popular choice for elective anaesthesia, to rescue the airway after failed intubation and sometimes as the airway of choice in pre-hospital care. They are relatively easy to insert but require some training and experience to know that they are sitting correctly. Once in position, placement should be confirmed in a similar way as an endotracheal tube (although of course endobronchial placement is not possible).

It is difficult to ventilate stiff lungs with an LMA as there will be a leak around the cuff at pressures much above 20 cmH$_2$O. Intubation through an LMA, with or without a flexible bronchoscope, is possible (see Chapter 17).

Insertion of the classic laryngeal mask airway

Insertion of LMAs is rapid and blind (no laryngoscopy is required). LMAs can easily become displaced, however, and are not a definitive long-term airway. They do not protect completely from aspiration.

Equipment

- Appropriate size LMA (see Chapter 17)
- Syringe for LMA cuff inflation
- Water-soluble lubricant
- Stethoscope
- Tape to secure the LMA

Procedure

1. Whenever possible, pre-oxygenate with 100% oxygen before inserting the LMA.
2. Check the LMA, in particular checking there is cuff inflation with no leak, and check the tube for blockage or loose objects; have lubricant and suction to hand.
3. Deflate the cuff and lightly lubricate the back and sides of the mask. Avoid excessive amounts of lubricant. In children, it may be preferred to have the cuff partially inflated for insertion.
4. Tilt the patient's head back (if safe to do so), open the mouth fully and insert the tip of the mask along the hard palate with the open side facing, but not touching, the tongue (Figure 19.9a). A jaw thrust performed by an assistant may aid placement.
5. Slide the mask further, along the posterior pharyngeal wall, with your index finger initially providing support for the tube. Eventually resistance is felt as the tip of the LMA lies at the upper end of the oesophagus.
6. Fully inflate the cuff, which makes the LMA rise up slightly (Figure 19.9b).
7. Secure the LMA with adhesive tape and check its position during ventilation as for a tracheal tube: good equilateral chest rise, no leak and capnometry if available.

It is sometimes easier to insert an LMA rotated 90° or 180° from its final position. The mask is then quickly rotated into its natural position as it passes into position.

(a)

(b)

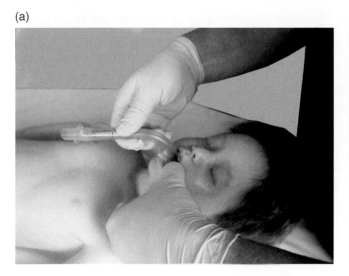
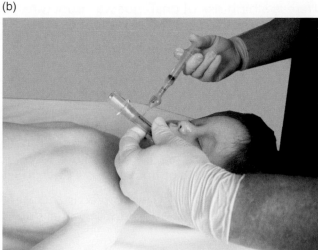

Figure 19.9 (a, b) Insertion of a laryngeal mask airway
Children's Health Queensland/CC BY 4.0

Complications of laryngeal mask airway use

- The epiglottis can get caught by the LMA and displaced over the larynx. This results in obstruction of the airway
- The tip of the LMA may fold over during insertion

If either of the above problems occurs, or if the airway is unsatisfactory for another reason, withdraw the LMA and reinsert.

- Rotation of LMAs may occur after insertion, more commonly with smaller LMAs and particularly while the breathing system or self-inflating bag is attached

I-gel® insertion

The principles of insertion are broadly similar to the LMA. The i-gel® is supplied in a protective cradle and has a non-inflatable gel cuff. A small blob of water-soluble lubricant jelly can be placed onto the cradle to facilitate light lubrication of the back, sides and front of the gel cuff. The device is inserted into the mouth, sliding it backwards along the hard palate until a clear resistance is felt. It is not necessary to insert fingers into the patient's mouth during insertion. A jaw thrust by the assistant may aid insertion if early resistance is felt, or, alternatively, insertion 'upside down' followed by rotation may aid insertion.

With both LMA and i-gel® insertion, the device is in place when definitive resistance is felt. Repeated to-and-fro pushing and pulling when this resistance is felt is not necessary.

19.8 Surgical airway

In an emergency *'cannot intubate, cannot oxygenate'* (CICO) situation, it is necessary to achieve front of neck access to the airway. This is an absolute last resort but, when indicated, should be performed without delay. Needle and open techniques entering at either the cricothyroid membrane or the trachea are described. There is debate about which techniques are optimal for children and guidelines vary. Needle cricothyroidotomy has historically been the first choice, especially in the absence of an ENT specialist. However, a national UK audit reported a high failure rate, even in adults. Children have smaller and much more compressible airways than adults. The cricothyroid membrane is very difficult to palpate in children under the age of 5, and nearly impossible to feel in infants. Most CICO events happen under the age of 1 year. At this age, the relationship between the mandible and trachea means a very steep angle is required for needle puncture of the airway and there is a high risk of posterior wall puncture. It is therefore recommended that needle techniques should be avoided in children under 5 years.

- Children up to 1 year of age should have an emergency surgical tracheotomy, with direct visualisation of the tracheal wall
- Between the ages of 1 year and 5 years either emergency surgical tracheotomy or cricothyroidotomy may be performed, but the latter only if the cricothyroid membrane can be confidently identified
- In older children and adolescents, needle cricothyroidotomy is more achievable than in small children, but surgical techniques may have a higher success rate and allow better protection of the airway. Current adult guidelines recommend surgical cricothyroidotomy using scalpel and bougie. The relevant anatomy is shown in Figure 19.10

An ENT specialist should be involved in the management of difficult airways as early as possible and is likely to be the most appropriately qualified team member to perform a surgical airway.

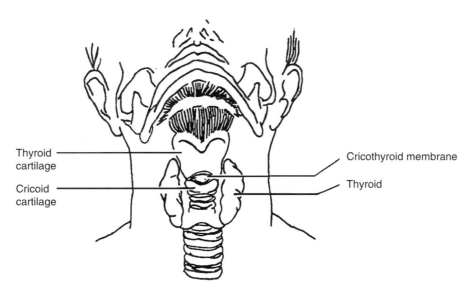

Thyroid cartilage

Cricoid cartilage

Cricothyroid membrane

Thyroid

Figure 19.10 Surgical airway anatomy

Needle cricothyroidotomy

Procedure

1. Consider extending the neck to improve access. (This technique is only performed in a dire 'cannot intubate, cannot oxygenate' emergency: protection of the cervical spine is of secondary importance at this stage.)
2. Clean the skin with antiseptic.
3. Stabilise the larynx with the non-dominant hand, and with the other hand identify the cricothyroid membrane by palpation between the thyroid and cricoid cartilages.
4. Use a cricothyroidotomy cannula-over-needle (or 14- or 16-gauge intravenous cannula) attached to a 5 ml syringe and aim in a caudal direction, at an angle to the skin of about 45°, aspirating on the syringe while advancing (Figure 19.11). Always ensure the needle is advanced in the midline.
5. Confirm position by the aspiration of air, then advance the cannula over the needle. Half-filling the syringe with 0.9% sodium chloride might aid the visualisation of air bubbles. Attach the hub of the cannula to either an oxygen flow meter via a Y-connector, a three-way stopcock or an adjustable pressure-limiting device. (NB: the pressure relief valve on an anaesthetic machine means that the common gas outlet on the machine is unsuitable as the gas supply.)
6. If using a Y-connector or three-way stopcock, set the flow rate (starting flow in litres/min = age in years). If this is insufficient, cautiously increase the flow rate (in increments of 1 litre with a maximum of 10–12 l/min) or inflation pressure to achieve observable chest expansion using an inspiration time of 1 second.

7. Maintain upper airway patency, allowing roughly 4 seconds for exhalation. (NB: expiration occurs through the patient's upper airway, *not* through the cannula.)
8. Constantly check the neck to exclude cannula misplacement, that is, swelling from the injection of gas into the tissues rather than the trachea.
9. Secure the equipment to the patient's neck.
10. Arrange to proceed urgently to a more definitive airway procedure such as an emergency surgical tracheostomy once more skilled help has arrived. Using the needle cricothyroidotomy may be a transiently life-saving technique in terms of temporarily oxygenating the child in the 'cannot intubate, cannot oxygenate' situation, but does not prevent hypercapnia and is not suitable for ventilation..

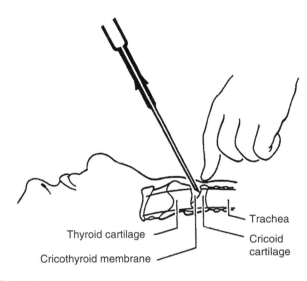

Thyroid cartilage

Cricothyroid membrane

Trachea

Cricoid cartilage

Figure 19.11 Needle cricothyroidotomy

Surgical cricothyroidotomy

Procedure

1. Place the patient in a supine position.
2. Consider extending the neck to improve access. Otherwise, maintain a neutral alignment.
3. Identify the cricothyroid membrane.
4. Prepare the skin and, if the patient is conscious, infiltrate with local anaesthetic.
5. Place the non-dominant hand on the neck to stabilise the cricothyroid membrane and to protect the lateral vascular structures from injury.
6. Make a vertical incision in the skin and press the lateral edges of the incision outwards, to minimise bleeding.
7. Make a transverse incision through the cricothyroid membrane, being careful not to damage the cricoid cartilage.
8. Insert a tracheal spreader or bougie.
9. Insert an appropriately sized endotracheal or tracheostomy tube.
10. Ventilate the patient and use capnography to confirm correct placement. Confirmation of ETCO$_2$ is mandatory and will be present even during CPR.
11. Secure the tube to prevent dislodgement.

Emergency tracheotomy

Procedure

1. Place the patient in a supine position.
2. Consider extending the neck to improve access. Otherwise, maintain a neutral alignment if possible.
3. Palpate the trachea (the laryngeal cartilages are difficult to palpate in smaller children).

4. Place the left thumb and index finger firmly on the neck either side of the trachea from above to stabilise the trachea and to protect the lateral vascular structures from injury.
5. Make a low, vertical, midline incision in the skin, above the suprasternal notch, maintaining pressure and stabilising the trachea with the left hand thumb and index finger. Pressure and remaining in the midline will minimise bleeding and damage to lateral structures.
6. The incision should be midline through the strap muscles and thyroid isthmus (if encountered) and directly onto the tracheal wall.
7. Make a vertical incision through the tracheal rings (rings 3–5 if possible), being careful not to damage the cricoid cartilage or innominate artery (which may cross the trachea inferiorly).
8. Insert an appropriately sized cuffed endotracheal or tracheostomy tube with an introducer or use a bougie.
9. Ventilate the patient and use capnography to confirm correct placement (see surgical cricothyroidotomy).
10. Secure the tube to prevent dislodgement.
11. Having completed emergency airway management, stabilise the patient, transfer to theatres, address haemostasis and place lateral tracheal stay sutures.

Postoperative care

- Perform a chest X-ray
- Check and monitor the cuff pressure
- Inform staff how to use the stay sutures
- A tracheostomy tube care box should be kept at the bedside containing an introducer, spare tracheostomy tube of the same dimensions, one size smaller tracheostomy tube, suction catheters, tapes, non-adherent dressings, scissors and lubricant jelly
- A small artery clip or tracheal dilator should be available at the bedside

Complications of tracheotomy or cricothyoroidotomy

- Subglottic oedema or stenosis
- Haemorrhage
- Pneumothorax or pneumomediastinum
- Damage to lateral structures such as the recurrent laryngeal nerves, carotid sheath or oesophagus
- Pulmonary oedema
- Tracheostomy tube problems such as displacement and blockage
- Subcutaneous emphysema
- Swallowing difficulties
- Local infection
- Aspiration
- False passage

19.9   Management of a blocked tracheostomy

The equipment list, algorithm and checklist are detailed in Chapter 17.

19.10   Summary

This chapter has covered the basic practical procedures that you need to be familiar with to manage problems with airway and breathing.

CHAPTER 20

Practical procedures: circulation

Learning outcomes

After reading this chapter, you will be able to identify the equipment for and describe the following procedures:

- Intraosseous access
- Peripheral venous access:
  - upper and lower extremity veins
  - scalp veins
  - external jugular vein
  - umbilical vein
  - venous cut-down
  - midline access
- Central venous access:
  - peripherally inserted central catheter
  - femoral vein
  - internal jugular vein
  - subclavian vein
- Arterial cannulation:
  - Radial artery cannulation
- Defibrillation

20.1 Introduction to vascular access

Access to the circulation is a crucial step in delivering advanced paediatric life support. Many access routes are possible: intraosseous, peripheral venous, central venous and/or arterial cannulation. The one chosen will reflect both clinical need and the skills of the operator.

If fluids are to be given, infusion pumps or paediatric infusion sets should be used. This avoids inadvertent overperfusion in small children.

Advanced Paediatric Life Support: A Practical Approach to Emergencies, Seventh Edition. Edited by Stephanie Smith.
© 2023 John Wiley & Sons Ltd. Published 2023 by John Wiley & Sons Ltd.

20.2 Intraosseous access

Indications

Intraosseous access should be used in an infant or child where intravenous access has failed and emergency medications and fluids are time critical. It is the recommended technique for vascular access in cardiac arrest.

Contraindications

- Fracture of the target bone or a proximal ipsilateral bone
- Infection at the area of insertion
- Excessive tissue or absence of adequate anatomical landmarks
- Inability to identify landmarks
- IO access or attempted IO access in the target bone within the previous 48 hours
- Prosthesis or orthopaedic procedure near the insertion site

The proximal tibia is the recommended site in paediatrics due to the easier identification of the landmark (Figure 20.1). The landmarks for the upper and lower tibial, lower femoral and humerus sites are shown in Figures 20.1, 20.2, 20.3 and 20.4, respectively.

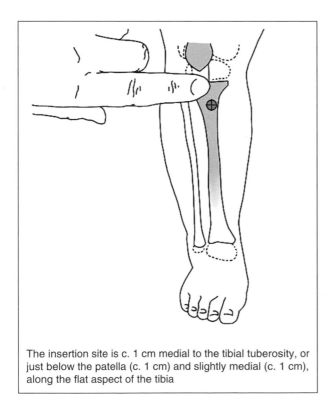

The insertion site is c. 1 cm medial to the tibial tuberosity, or just below the patella (c. 1 cm) and slightly medial (c. 1 cm), along the flat aspect of the tibia

Figure 20.1 Proximal tibia in the infant/child

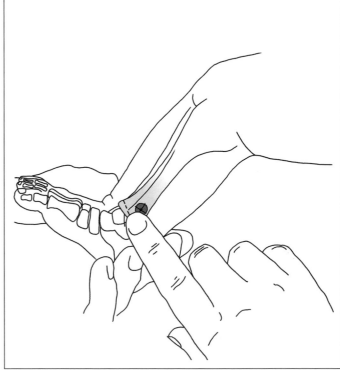

Figure 20.2 Distal tibia in the infant/child

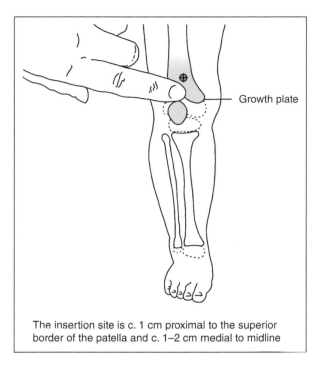

The insertion site is c. 1 cm proximal to the superior border of the patella and c. 1–2 cm medial to midline

Figure 20.3 Distal femur in the infant/child

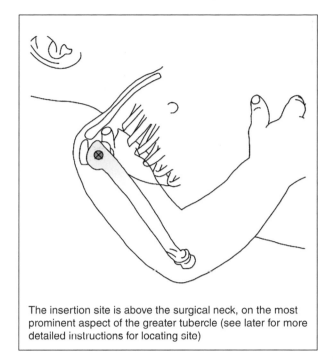

The insertion site is above the surgical neck, on the most prominent aspect of the greater tubercle (see later for more detailed instructions for locating site)

Figure 20.4 Proximal humerus in the infant/child

Tibial access

Procedure using a handheld needle

The handheld technique is the preferred technique in neonates.

1. Extend the leg. Pinch the tibia between the fingers to identify the medial and lateral borders; identify the site.
2. Clean the skin over the chosen site, maintaining aseptic technique.
3. Insert the needle at 90° to the skin and emphasise the rotational motion.
4. Continue to advance the needle until a clear give is felt as the cortex is penetrated.
5. Attach the 5 ml syringe and aspirate or infuse to confirm correct positioning with as minimal movement as possible. Flush with 2–5 ml 0.9% sodium chloride.
6. Secure with a dressing.

Procedure using a powered device

The EZ-IO® drill is a powered device that enables the rapid insertion of an intraosseous needle. The same landmarks are used as for manual insertion and the procedure is less painful for the conscious victim due to its rapidity.

The EZ-IO® needle sets (Figure 20.5) occur in three sizes:

- 15 mm needle – may be suitable for neonates and young infants
- 25 mm needle – for infants and younger children
- 45 mm needle – for older children and use for humeral access at any age

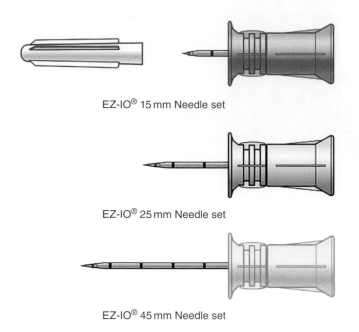

EZ-IO® 15 mm Needle set

EZ-IO® 25 mm Needle set

EZ-IO® 45 mm Needle set

Figure 20.5 EZ-IO® needle sets
Teleflex Medical Australia & New Zealand

The procedure for insertion is as follows:

1. Use universal precautions, maintaining aseptic technique. Prime the connection line.
2. Identify the infusion site and clean it.
3. Choose an appropriate size needle and attach it to the drill – it will fix magnetically.
4. Hold the drill and needle at 90° to the bone surface and push through the skin without drilling, until bone is felt. **The 5 mm mark must be visible above the skin for confirmation of an adequate needle set length** (Figure 20.6). If not, use a longer needle.
5. Push the drill button and drill continuously and push until there is loss of resistance – there is a palpable give as the needle breaches the cortex.
6. Remove the drill and unscrew the trochar (holding the needle in place with as minimal movement as possible).
7. Aspirate the marrow if possible. Failure to aspirate does not mean the insertion has failed. Placement can also be confirmed by observing flash back of blood, or by flushing fluids without difficulties or signs of extravasation.
8. Blood samples for analysis can be drawn; samples must be identified as blood.
9. Use an EZ-Stabilizer® dressing to secure the needle and stabilise the extremity.
10. Attach a preprepared (primed with 0.9% sodium chloride) connection tube and flush with 2–5 ml 0.9% sodium chloride.
11. Proceed with the required therapy.

With the needle set inserted through the soft tissue and touching bone, the 5 mm mark (at least one black line) must be visible outside the skin for confirmation of adequate needle set length prior to drilling.

Verify placement/patency prior to all infusions. Compartment syndrome, which can result from undetected infiltration/extravasation, is a serious complication. The intraosseous insertion site should be monitored frequently for signs of infiltration/extravasation. Other complications include infection and fracture (both very rare).

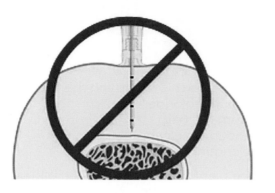
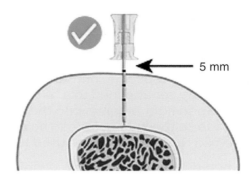

5 mm

Figure 20.6 Needle set length confirmation
Teleflex Medical Australia & New Zealand

Humeral access

Procedure

1. Place the patient's hand over the umbilicus, which causes medial rotation of the elbow and humerus and provides greater prominence of the insertion site (Figure 20.7a).
2. Place your palm on the patient's shoulder anteriorly.
   - The area that feels like a 'ball' under your palm is the general target area
   - You should be able to feel this ball, even on obese patients, by pushing deeply
3. Place the ulnar aspect of your hand vertically over the axilla and the ulnar aspect of your other hand along the midline of the upper arm laterally.
4. Place your thumbs together over the arm; this identifies the vertical line of insertion on the proximal humerus.
5. Palpate deeply up the humerus to the surgical neck. This may feel like a golf ball on a tee – the spot where the 'ball' meets the 'tee' is the surgical neck.
6. The insertion site is above the surgical neck, on the most prominent aspect of the greater tubercle (Figure 20.7b).
7. Follow steps 4–11 of the procedure using a powered device as in the tibial access section.

(a)   (b)

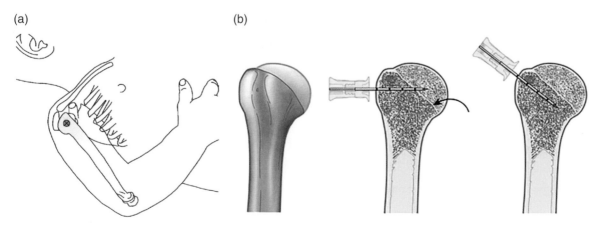

Figure 20.7 (a, b) Humeral access
(b) Teleflex Medical Australia & New Zealand

Intraosseous fluid infusion

Procedure

- Fluid will not run through the intraosseous access device by gravity
- Attach a three-way tap to the primed connection piece. To this tap attach the filled 50 ml syringe and a fluid giving set attached to a bag of 0.9% sodium chloride:
  - Turn the tap so fluid is drawn into the syringe from the bag
  - Turn the tap so the fluid bolus can be pushed though the cannula
- A pressure bag device can also be used to ensure continuous flow

It should be noted that rapid infusion of fluid may be painful for the conscious patient and if this proves to be the case 0.5 mg/kg of 2% lignocaine (adult dose 20–40 mg) may be infused slowly prior to medication/fluid administration to combat this.

Removal of the intraosseous needle

1. Remove the extension set and dressing.
2. Stabilise the catheter hub and attach a Luer lock syringe to the hub.
3. Maintaining axial alignment, twist clockwise and pull straight out (Figure 20.8).
4. Do not rock the syringe.
5. Dispose of the catheter with the syringe attached into sharps container.
6. Apply pressure to the site as needed to control bleeding and apply a dressing as indicated.

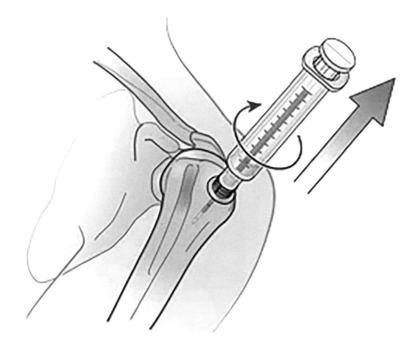

Figure 20.8 Removal of the intraosseous needle
Teleflex Medical Australia & New Zealand

Complications of intraosseous infusion

- Compartment syndrome
- Infection (rare)
- Fracture

20.3 Peripheral venous access

Obtaining vascular access can be difficult in awake children. Reducing anxiety and pain is the goal. This can be achieved by non-pharmacological techniques such as oral sucrose, distraction, parental presence or pharmacological techniques such as topical patches or intranasal analgesia. Local warming, transillumination techniques (under 2 years) and ultrasound guidance may facilitate placement.

Upper and lower extremity veins

Veins on the dorsum of the hand, the elbow, the dorsum of the feet and the saphenous vein at the ankle can be used for cannulation. Standard percutaneous techniques should be employed if possible.

Scalp veins

The frontal superficial, temporal posterior, auricular, supraorbital and posterior facial veins can be used. This option is mostly used in infants.

The technique is close to standard percutaneous techniques, except for the inability to use a tourniquet. Gentle pressure proximal to the puncture site with a taut piece of tubing, rubber band, bandaging or finger can help distend the vein. The direction of cannulation should be towards the heart.

External jugular vein

Equipment

- Skin-cleansing swabs
- Appropriate cannula
- Tape

Procedure

1. Place the child in a 15–30° head-down position (or with padding under the shoulders so that the head hangs lower than the shoulders).
2. Turn the head away from the site of puncture.
3. Clean the skin.
4. Identify the external jugular vein, which can be seen passing over the sternocleidomastoid muscle at the junction of its middle and lower thirds (Figure 20.9). If skilled, use ultrasound.
5. Have an assistant place their finger at the lower end of the visible part of the vein just above the clavicle. This stabilises it and compresses it so that it remains distended.
6. Puncture the skin and enter the vein.
7. When a free flow of blood is obtained, ensure no air bubbles are present in the tubing and then attach a giving set.
8. Tape the cannula securely in position.

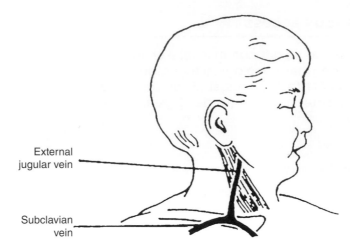

Figure 20.9 Course of the external jugular vein

Umbilical vein

Venous access via the umbilical vein is a rapid and simple technique. It can be used during resuscitation at birth.

Equipment

- Skin-cleansing swabs
- Umbilical tape
- Scalpel
- Syringe and 0.9% sodium chloride
- Catheter

Procedure

1. Loosely tie the umbilical tape around the base of the cord.
2. Cut the cord with a scalpel, leaving at least a 1 cm strip distal to the tape.
3. If there is bleeding from the vein, gently tighten the tape to stop it.
4. Identify the umbilical vein. Three vessels will be seen in the stump: most of the time two will be small and contracted (the arteries) and one will be dilated (the vein) (Figure 20.10a). If this is not the case, the arteries usually sit above the Wharton's jelly whilst the vein is pendulous at the level of the stump.

(a)   (b)

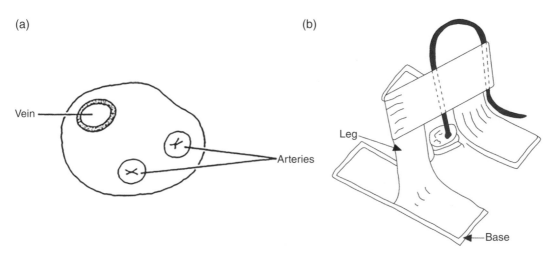

Figure 20.10 (a) Umbilical cord cross-section, and (b) a catheter bridge

5. Fill a 5 French gauge umbilical catheter with 0.9% sodium chloride.
6. Insert the catheter into the vein with gentle caudal stretch and advance it approximately 5 cm. Verify a backflow of blood.
7. Tighten the umbilical tape to secure the catheter and use tape to create a bridge affixed to the abdominal wall (Figure 20.10b).

Venous cut-down

This technique may be useful in situations where peripheral access is difficult or impossible, and time is available. A surgical consult should be obtained before performing this procedure. The saphenous vein is most often used.

Midline access

Midline access (Figure 20.11) is useful in prolonged (antibiotic) treatments. The midline catheter, which is about 6–12 cm long, is inserted in the deep veins of the arm under ultrasound guidance. The tip of the catheter is located in a peripheral vein which distinguishes it from a PICC.

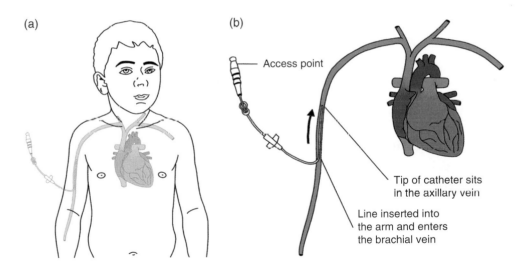

Figure 20.11 (a, b) Midline access

20.4 Central venous access

Central venous access can be obtained through the femoral, internal jugular, external jugular and subclavian veins. In non-urgent situations a peripherally inserted central catheter (PICC) can be use via the deep arm veins. The Seldinger technique is safe and effective. The UK National Institute for Health and Care Excellence (NICE) guidelines recommend ultrasound-guided insertion to increase the success rate as well as to decrease the complications. The femoral vein is often used as it is relatively easy to cannulate away from the chest during cardiopulmonary resuscitation (CPR). Central venous access via the neck veins is not without risk and may be difficult in emergency situations. The course of the central veins of the neck is shown in Figure 20.12.

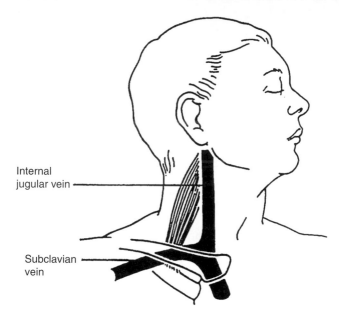

Figure 20.12 Course of the central veins of the neck

Peripherally inserted central catheter

Access using a PICC (Figure 20.13) is obtained by putting a specifically designed central catheter in one of the deep arm veins – the basilic, brachial or cephalic – with the tip lying in the junction of the superior vena cava and right atrium. In contrast to the midline, this is a central line.

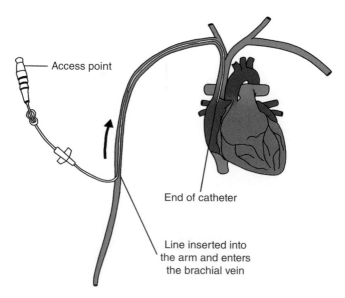

Figure 20.13 Peripherally inserted central catheter

Femoral vein

This procedure can be carried out with or without ultrasound guidance. The two techniques are described here.

Equipment

- Skin-cleansing swabs
- Lidocaine 1% for local anaesthetic with a 2 ml syringe and 23 gauge needle
- Syringe and 0.9% sodium chloride
- Seldinger cannulation set:
  - Syringe
  - Needle
  - Seldinger guidewire
  - Cannula
- Suture material
- Prepared paediatric infusion set
- Tape

Procedure with ultrasound guidance

1. If the child is responsive to pain, provide adequate pain relief either by infiltrating the area with 1% lidocaine (be aware of maximum doses for your patient) or IV/intranasal analgesia.
2. Place the child supine with the groin exposed and leg slightly abducted at the hip.
3. Clean the skin at the appropriate site.
4. Use a sterile probe cover or prep all around the probe once it is positioned and use a sterile no-touch technique with the injecting hand.
5. Hold a linear probe in the non-dominant hand, placing it transversely, with the centre over the femoral artery pulse at the level of the groin skin crease (Figures 20.14 and 20.15). A cross-sectional view of the vessels and nerve will be obtained.

(a) (b)

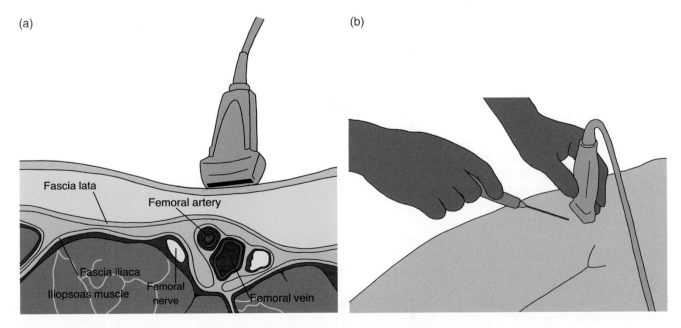

Figure 20.14 (a, b) Ultrasound-guided needle approach to femoral vein access

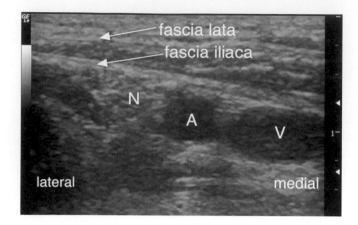

Figure 20.15 Ultrasound image of the femoral region
A, artery; N, nerve; V, vein

6. Identify the pulsating femoral artery and move the probe so that the vein is in the middle of the ultrasound view.
7. Identify the puncture site. The vein lies directly medial to the artery.
8. Attach the needle to the syringe.
9. Penetrate the skin with the needle and identify the tip in the images. Move the probe slightly proximal and advance the needle until the tip can be visualised again. Repeat this step several times until the needle is seen to penetrate the vein.
10. Check the needle's position by aspirating blood. If blood flows back into the syringe, take the syringe off the needle.
11. Insert the Seldinger wire into the needle, and into the vein.
12. Withdraw the needle along the wire, ensuring that the wire is not dislodged from the vein.
13. Advance the dilator over the wire through the skin and vessel wall into the vein. Remove the dilator while making sure the wire is not removed as well.
14. Place the catheter over the wire and advance it through the skin, into the vein. Make sure the end of the wire is sticking out of the end of the catheter before advancing the catheter through the skin.
15. Withdraw the wire, immediately occluding the end of the cannula to prevent blood loss.
16. Confirm correct placement by drawing blood from all the lumina, immediately flush and lock the catheter afterwards.
17. Suture the catheter in place.
18. Attach the infusion set.

Procedure without ultrasound guidance

1. If the child is responsive to pain, provide pain relief.
2. Place the child supine with the groin exposed and leg slightly abducted at the hip.
3. Clean the skin at the appropriate site.
4. Identify the puncture site. The femoral vein is found by palpating the femoral artery. The vein lies directly medial to the artery.
5. Attach the needle to the syringe.
6. Keeping one finger on the artery to mark its position, introduce the needle at a 45° angle pointing towards the patient's head directly over the femoral vein. Keep the syringe in line with the child's leg. Advance the needle, intermittently pulling back on the plunger of the syringe all the time.
7. As soon as blood flows back into the syringe, take the syringe off the needle. Immediately occlude the end of the needle to prevent blood loss.

8. If the vein is not found, withdraw the needle to the skin, locate the artery again and advance as in point 6 above.
9. Insert the Seldinger wire into the needle, and into the vein.
10. Withdraw the needle along the wire, ensuring that the wire is not dislodged from the vein.
11. Advance the dilator over the wire through the skin and vessel wall into the vein. Remove the dilator while making sure the wire is not removed as well.
12. Place the catheter over the wire and advance it through the skin, into the vein. Make sure the end of the wire is sticking out of the end of the catheter before advancing the catheter through the skin.
13. Withdraw the wire, immediately occluding the end of the cannula to prevent blood loss.
14. Confirm correct placement by drawing blood from all the lumina, immediately flush and lock the catheter afterwards.
15. Suture the catheter in place.
16. Attach the infusion set.
17. Tape the infusion set tubing in place.

Internal jugular vein

Equipment

This is the same as for the femoral vein cannulation.

Procedure

1. If the child is responsive to pain, provide pain relief.
2. Place the child in a 15–30° head-down position.
3. Turn the head away from the side that is to be cannulated.
4. Clean the skin at the appropriate side of the neck.
5. Under ultrasound guidance (if available) identify the puncture site. This is found at the apex of the triangle formed by the two lower heads of the sternomastoid and the clavicle.
6. Attach the needle to the syringe and puncture the skin at the appropriate place.
7. Penetrate the skin with the needle and identify the tip in the images. Move the probe slightly distally and advance the needle until the tip is visualised again. Repeat this step several times until the needle is seen to penetrate the vein.
8. Check the needle's position by aspirating blood. If blood flows back into the syringe, take the syringe off the needle.
9. Insert the Seldinger wire into the needle, and into the vein.
10. Withdraw the needle along the wire, ensuring that the wire is not dislodged from the vein.
11. Advance the dilator over the wire through the skin and vessel wall into the vein. Remove the dilator while making sure the wire is not removed as well.
12. Place the catheter over the wire and advance it through the skin, into the vein. Make sure the end of the wire is sticking out of the end of the catheter before advancing the catheter through the skin.
13. Withdraw the wire, immediately occluding the end of the cannula to prevent air embolism.
14. Confirm correct placement by drawing blood from all the lumina, immediately flush and lock the catheter.
15. Suture the catheter in place.
16. Attach the infusion set.
17. Tape the infusion set tubing in place.
18. Obtain a chest radiograph in order to see the position of the catheter and to exclude a pneumothorax. The ideal tip location of the central venous catheter is near the superior vena cava and right atrium junction.

Subclavian vein

Equipment

This is the same as for the femoral vein and internal jugular vein positions.

Procedure without ultrasound

1. If the child is responsive to pain, provide pain relief.
2. Place the child in a 15–30° head-down position.
3. Turn the head away from the site that is to be cannulated and restrain the child as necessary.
4. Clean the skin over the upper side of the chest to the clavicle.
5. Identify the puncture site. This is 1 cm below the midpoint of the clavicle.
6. Attach the needle to the syringe and puncture the skin at the appropriate place. This is found at the apex of the triangle formed by the two lower heads of the sternomastoid and the clavicle.
7. Direct the needle under the clavicle, 'stepping down' off the bone.
8. Once under the clavicle, direct the needle towards the suprasternal notch. Advance the needle, pulling back on the plunger of the syringe all the time and staying as superficial as possible.
9. As soon as blood flows back into the syringe, take the syringe off the needle. Immediately occlude the end of the needle to prevent air embolism.
10. If the vein is not found, slowly withdraw the needle, continuing to pull back on the plunger. If the vein has been crossed inadvertently, free flow will often be established during this manoeuvre.
11. If the vein is still not found repeat steps 7–10, aiming at a point a little higher in the sternal notch.
12. Insert the Seldinger wire into the needle, and into the vein.
13. Withdraw the needle along the wire, ensuring that the wire is not dislodged from the vein.
14. Place the catheter over the wire and advance it through the skin, into the vein. Make sure the end of the wire is sticking out of the end of the catheter before advancing the catheter through the skin.
15. Withdraw the wire, immediately occluding the end of the cannula to prevent air embolism.
16. Confirm correct placement by drawing blood from all the lumina, immediately flush and lock the catheter.
17. Suture the catheter in place.
18. Attach the infusion set.
19. Tape the infusion set tubing in place.
20. Obtain a chest radiograph in order to see the position of the catheter and to exclude a pneumothorax.

There are several techniques for placing a central venous access device in the subclavian vein with ultrasound. Mostly these are out-of-plane techniques like that described for the femoral and internal jugular veins, except advancing from lateral to medial. This technique allows you to see the top of the lung, making it easier to avoid puncturing it accidentally. Another technique uses a supraclavicular view while placing the needle into the vessel with an in-plane view. This technique is harder to master so training in a controlled environment under supervision is recommended.

Complications of central venous line insertion

- Arterial puncture
- Catheter malposition
- Pneumothorax or hemothorax
- Subcutaneous hematoma

20.5 Arterial cannulation

Arterial cannulation is used to monitor arterial blood pressure, guide dosage adjustments in shock and hypertensive crisis, obtain blood samples for respiratory and acid–base status, and calculate cerebral perfusion pressure. It should not be performed in sites where there is skin infection or interruption, or absent collateral circulation. In children, the possible sites include the radial, posterior tibial, dorsalis pedis, brachial and femoral arteries. The site should remain visible and not be prone to contamination. In neonates, the umbilical artery can be used. Ultrasound guidance improves the success rate and reduces complications.

Radial artery cannulation

Equipment

- Skin-cleansing swabs
- (Heparinised) syringe
- Cannula:
  - Preterm: 24 gauge
  - Infant/pre-school: 22–24 gauge
  - School age: 20–22 gauge
  - Adolescent to adult: 18–20 gauge
- T-connector or three-way tap with extension
- Gauze, pad and tapes
- Transparent sterile dressing
- Flushed infusion set (with 0.9% sodium chloride) with pressure infusion bag or pump
- Pressure transducer and monitor

Procedure

1. Before using the radial artery check that the ulnar artery is present and patent. Occlude both arteries at the wrist and then release the pressure on the ulnar artery; circulation should return to the hand. (It will flush pink.) If this does not happen, do not proceed with a radial puncture on that side.
2. If the child is responsive to pain, provide pain relief.
3. Keep the wrist hyperextended and restrained and palpate the radial artery (usually located in the middle of the lateral third of the wrist).
4. Clean the skin. If needed, infiltrate with local anaesthetic.
5. Insert the cannula over the artery at 45° to the skin and advance it slowly. When the artery is punctured, blood will be seen to pulsate into the syringe.
6. Advance the cannula over the needle into the artery and remove the needle whilst compressing the artery proximal to the position of the cannula tip.
7. Connect the T-connector or three-way tap with extension, ready flushed with 0.9% sodium chloride to test cannula patency.
8. Tape the cannula securely in place and cover with a transparent dressing.
9. Connect the infusion set and calibrate the monitoring equipment.

Complications of cannulation

- Arteriospasm
- Haematoma
- Thrombosis
- Bacterial colonisation and sepsis (very rare)

20.6 Defibrillation

In order to achieve the optimum outcome, defibrillation must be performed quickly and efficiently. This requires the following:

- Correct electrode pad/paddle selection
- Correct electrode pad/paddle placement
- Good electrode pad/paddle contact
- Correct energy selection

Many defibrillators are available. Providers of advanced paediatric life support should make sure that they are familiar with those they may have to use.

Correct electrode pad/paddle selection

Defibrillators for paediatric use should be supplied with two sets of electrode pads/paddles – adult and paediatric.

- Adult electrode pads can be used for children aged 8 years and above and paediatric electrode pads for the younger child. Children vary in size so there is some discretion
- Adult paddles are 13 cm diameter. If available, paddles of 4.5 cm diameter are used in infants. The paediatric/infant paddles usually will be clipped over or hidden under the adult paddles

Electrode pads/paddles are usually labelled pictorially to show placement positions.

Correct electrode pad/paddle placement

Pads have become the method of choice, but paddles may be encountered in low and middle income countries. Pads have become mainstream because once placed they save time, resulting in less interruption to chest compressions and time to defibrillation, and they are also safer. They promote charging during compressions which decreases hands-off chest time.

The usual placement of both paddles and pads is anterolateral. One is put over the apex in the mid-axillary line (a finger breadth below the left nipple) and the other is placed just to the right of the sternum (a finger breadth below the right clavicle) (Figures 20.16 and 20.17a). Ensure they are at least 2 cm apart to prevent arcing.

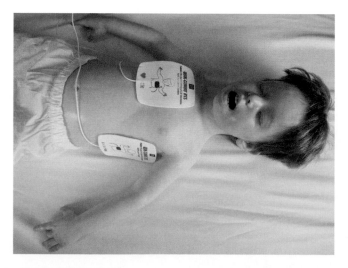

Figure 20.16 Standard anterolateral pad placement
Children's Health Queensland/CC BY 4.0

(a)   (b)

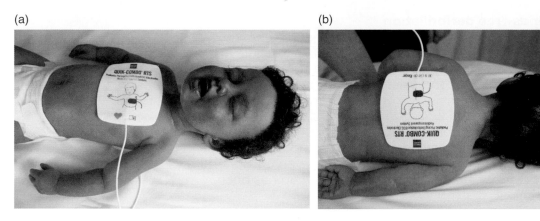

Figure 20.17 Anteroposterior pad placement (a) front, and (b) back
Children's Health Queensland/CC BY 4.0

In the infant where anterolateral is not feasible (e.g. when pads/paddles are too close to each other), the anteroposterior placement is used: one is placed just to the left side of the sternum and the other in the middle of the back between the scapulae (Figure 20.17b).

Good electrode pad/paddle contact

Electrode pads should be placed on dry skin and smoothed on to guarantee good contact and ensure effective energy delivery. Gel pads or electrode gel should always be used in conjunction with manual paddles (if the latter, care should be taken not to join the two areas of application). Firm pressure should be applied to the paddles.

Correct energy selection

The recommended levels are given in Chapters 18 and 20.

Automated external defibrillators (AEDs) are now commonplace. The standard adult shock is used for children over 8 years. For children under 8 years, attenuated paediatric pads should be used with the AED. For an infant of less than 1 year, a manual defibrillator which can be adjusted to give the correct shock is recommended. However, if an AED is the only defibrillator available, its use should be considered, preferably with paediatric attenuation pads. The order of decreasing preference for defibrillation in the under 1-year-olds is as follows:

1. Manual defibrillator.
2. AED with dose attenuator.
3. AED without dose attenuator.

Many AEDs can detect ventricular fibrillation/ventricular tachycardia (VF/VT) in children of all ages and differentiate 'shockable' from 'non-shockable' rhythms with a high degree of sensitivity and specificity.

Safety

A defibrillator delivers enough current to cause cardiac arrest. The user must ensure that other rescuers are not in physical contact with the child (or the trolley) at the moment the shock is delivered. When using paddles, the defibrillator should only be charged when the paddles are either in contact with the child or replaced properly in their storage positions. When using electrode pads, it is advisable to charge whilst compressions are ongoing.

Procedure: hands-free defibrillation

Basic life support should be interrupted for the shortest possible time (steps 6–9).

1. Apply adhesive monitoring electrodes to the correct positions whilst compressions continue.
2. Turn on the defibrillator and select the energy required whilst compressions continue.
3. Shout 'Charging, oxygen away, continue compressions'.
4. Press the charge button whilst compressions continue.
5. Wait until the defibrillator is charged.
6. Shout 'Rhythm check, stop compressions, stand clear'.
7. If VF/pulseless VT is confirmed, shout 'Shock, everybody stand back'.
8. Check all personnel are clear and that the oxygen has been removed.
9. Deliver the shock.
10. Recommence CPR.

Procedure: manual defibrillation

Basic life support should be interrupted for the shortest possible time (steps 4–10 below).

1. Apply gel pads or electrode gel whilst compressions continue.
2. Select the correct paddles.
3. Turn on the machine and select the energy required.
4. Interrupt briefly to confirm VF/pulseless VT, then immediately recommence compressions.
5. Shout 'Stand back'.
6. Remove the paddles from the machine, place the paddles onto the gel pads and apply firm pressure.
7. Shout 'Charging' whilst pressing the charge button.
8. Wait until the defibrillator is charged.
9. Check that all other rescuers are clear.
10. Shout 'Shock, stand clear' and deliver the shock.
11. Recommence CPR.

20.7 Summary

This chapter has covered the basic practical procedures that you need to be familiar with to manage problems with circulation.

CHAPTER 21

Practical procedures: trauma

Learning outcomes

After reading this chapter, you will be able to identify the equipment for and describe the following procedures:

- Tourniquet
- Pelvic binder
- Cervical spine immobilisation:
  - Application of head blocks and straps
  - 20° tilt
- Chest decompression:
  - Needle thoracocentesis
  - Finger thoracostomy
  - Chest drain placement
- Pericardiocentesis
- Femoral nerve block

21.1   Tourniquet

Tourniquets are an effective means of arresting life-threatening external haemorrhage from a limb injury (Figure 21.1). There are a wide variety of commercial tourniquets available, and in a hospital setting it may also be possible to use a pneumatic tourniquet from theatres to allow monitoring and control of pressure settings. The tourniquet is designed to completely and consistently occlude arterial blood flow. The UK Defence Medical Services selected the Combat Application Tourniquet® (North American Rescue Products, Inc., USA) after experimental studies showed 100% effectiveness in occluding distal arterial flow using human volunteers (King et al., 2006).

In civilian practice it is rare to encounter catastrophic external haemorrhage from a limb, but these scenarios can be encountered in the context of stabbings, firearms incidents, industrial accidents and major incidents.

Advanced Paediatric Life Support: A Practical Approach to Emergencies, Seventh Edition. Edited by Stephanie Smith.
© 2023 John Wiley & Sons Ltd. Published 2023 by John Wiley & Sons Ltd.

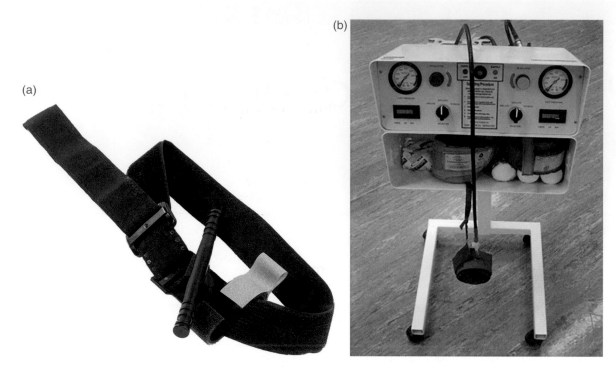

Figure 21.1 (a) The Combat Application Tourniquet®, and (b) pneumatic tourniquet
(a) An-T/Adobe Stock

Indications for use

1. Extreme life-threatening limb haemorrhage or limb amputation/mangled limb with multiple bleeding points, to allow immediate management of airway and breathing.
2. Life-threatening limb haemorrhage when simple methods fail to control the haemorrhage.
3. Major incident or multiple casualties with extremity haemorrhage.
4. Where the benefits of preventing death from hypovolaemic shock by cessation of ongoing external haemorrhage are greater than the risk of limb damage or ischaemia caused by tourniquet use (Lee et al., 2007).

Procedure

1. The tourniquet should be placed as distal as possible, but at least 5 cm proximal to the injury.
2. Spare the joints as much as possible.
3. Apply directly to the skin to avoid slipping.
4. The effectiveness is determined by the cessation of external haemorrhage and not by the presence or absence of a distal pulse.
5. If bleeding persists, a second tourniquet can be placed just proximal to the first.
6. The time of application must be recorded.

Complications

1. Permanent nerve injury.
2. Permanent muscle injury (including contractures, rhabdomyolsis and compartment syndrome).
3. Vascular injury.
4. Skin necrosis (Wakai et al., 2001).

Removal

Assuming that the tourniquet has been applied for the correct indications, a decision will need to be made regarding its continued use. It is possible that after a period of time of reduced arterial blood flow from tourniquet use, clotting will have occurred sufficiently to arrest haemorrhage, allowing simpler methods to be effective and reducing the complications from continued tourniquet use. Before release of the tourniquet, the clinician should have secured wound packing and application of direct pressure over the bleeding point. The torniquet must be replaced with a pneumatic torniquet as soon as possible as they are much more controllable and safer to use. This decision will be taken depending on multiple factors including the haemodynamic status of the child, the medical resources available and the time to definitive treatment in the operating room.

21.2   Pelvic binder

Stabilisation of a pelvic injury before uncompensatable haemorrhage has occurred and clotting mechanisms are still intact should be done as early as possible after the injury. A pelvic splint should thus be applied during the circulatory element of primary survey. The binder should be used in children with a suspected rotational or vertically unstable pelvic fracture.

When assessing a child in a trauma situation, the pelvis should not be palpated for instability or pain. A conscious child may be able to give information about pain in the lower back, groin or hips. Once a splint has been applied, analgesia may be provided to a haemodynamically stable child prior to transfer.

Procedure

1. Undress the patient fully, or if not possible, remove all objects form the child's pockets and pelvic area.
2. Check the patient for the following:
   - Pulses
   - Pockets
   - Phones
   - Genitalia
3. Where possible, use a splint applicator to reduce friction and patient movement.
4. Slide the pelvic splint under the patient at the level of the greater trochanters.
5. Once in place, remove the upper applicator in the same direction that it was inserted.
6. Ensure the splint is still located at the greater trochanter level, and then fasten as per the manufacturer's directions (Figure 21.2).

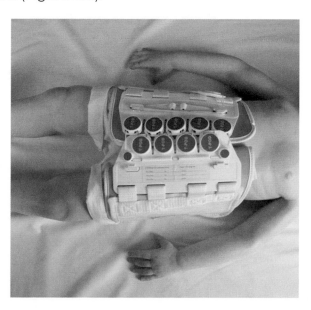

Figure 21.2 Pelvic binder
Children's Health Queensland/CC BY 4.0

In young children where commercially available binders do not fit it has been suggested that circumferential pelvic sheeting is an option. A folded sheet should be placed underneath the patient between the iliac crests and greater trochanters. Two team members should cross the sheet across the pubic symphysis and pull the sheet firmly. Twist the ends together and secure with a plastic clamp where possible

Complications

- Increased blood loss
- Misplaced binder

Removal

Currently there is no standards guidance on the removal of the pelvic binder within the emergency department, however this should be carried out on the advice of a paediatric pelvic specialist.

21.3 Cervical spine immobilisation

All children with serious trauma must be treated as though they have a spinal injury. It is only when an adequate examination and history is taken and appropriate investigations have been performed that the decision to remove the spinal protection can be made. This should be as soon as possible. Specialist consultation may be needed prior to this decision. Where there is risk of neck injury, manual in-line cervical stabilisation should be continued until the head blocks and tape have been applied or the cervical spine has been cleared clinically (Figure 21.3).

(a)   (b)

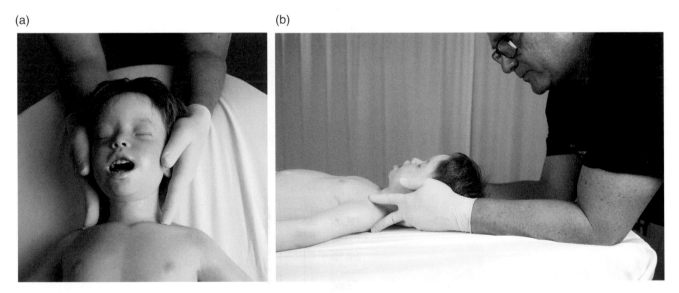

Figure 21.3 (a, b) Manual in-line stabilisation (MILS)
Children's Health Queensland/CC BY 4.0

Once the head blocks are in place, the neck may be obscured. Before application of the head blocks, look for the following signs quickly and without moving the neck:

- Distended veins
- Tracheal deviation
- Wounds
- Laryngeal crepitus
- Subcutaneous emphysema
- Visible blood at external auditory meatus

Application of head blocks and tape

Equipment

- Two head blocks
- Attachment system

Procedure

1. Ensure in-line cervical stabilisation is maintained by a second person throughout.
2. Place a head block either side of the head.
3. Apply the forehead strap and attach it securely to the trolley.
4. Apply the lower strap across the chin and attach it securely to the trolley.

Exceptions

An injured child may be uncooperative for many reasons including fear, pain and hypoxia. Manual immobilisation should be maintained and the contributing factors addressed. Overzealous immobilisation of the head and neck may paradoxically increase the leverage on the neck as the child struggles. Children with traumatic torticollis should be manually immobilised in their current position.

20° tilt

In order to minimise the chances of exacerbating unrecognised spinal cord injury and disruption of a clot in major abdominal trauma, non-essential movements of the spine must be avoided until adequate examination and investigations have excluded them. If manoeuvres that might cause spinal movement are essential (e.g. during examination of the back in the course of the secondary survey) or the child needs to be removed from a scoop stretcher, then the 20° tilt should be performed. The aim of the 20° tilt is to maintain the alignment of the spine during turning of the child. The basic requirements are an adequate number of carers and good control.

Procedure

1. Gather together enough staff to tilt the child. In larger children, four people will be required; three will be required in smaller children and infants (Figures 21.4 and 21.5).
2. Place the staff as shown in Table 21.1.
3. Ensure each member of staff knows what they are going to do, as shown in Table 21.2.
4. Carry out the essential manoeuvres as quickly as possible.

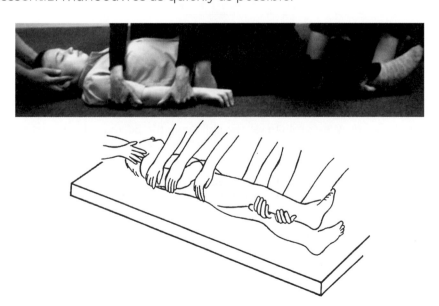

Figure 21.4 20° tilt (four-person technique)

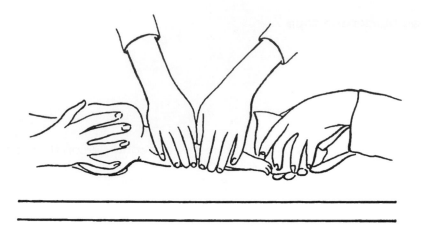

Figure 21.5 20° tilt (three-person technique)

Table 21.1 Position of staff for the 20° tilt		
	Position of staff for:	
Staff member no.	**Smaller child and infant**	**Larger child**
1	Head	Head
2	Chest	Chest
3	Legs and pelvis	Pelvis
4		Legs

Table 21.2 Tasks of individual members of staff	
Staff member: position	**Task**
Head	Hold either side of the head (as for in-line cervical stabilisation) and maintain orientation of the head with the body in all planes during turning. Control the 20° tilt by telling other staff when to roll and when to lay the child back onto the trolley
Chest	Reach over the child and carefully place both hands under the chest. When told to roll the child, support the weight of the chest and maintain stability. Watch the movement of the head at all times and roll the chest at the same rate
Legs and pelvis	This only applies to smaller children and infants. If it is not possible to control the pelvis and legs at the same time, get additional help immediately Place one hand either side of the pelvis over the iliac crests. Cradle the child's legs between the forearms. When told to roll the child, grip the pelvis and legs and move them together. Watch the movement of the head and chest at all times, and roll the pelvis and legs at the same rate
Pelvis	Place one hand over the pelvis on the iliac crest and the other under the thigh of the far lower limb. When told to roll the child, watch the movement of the head and chest at all times and roll the pelvis at the same rate
Legs	Support the weight of the far leg by placing both hands under it. When told to roll the child, watch the movement of the chest and pelvis and roll the leg at the same rate

21.4   Needle thoracocentesis

This procedure can be life saving and can be performed quickly with minimum equipment. It should be followed by chest drain placement.

Minimum equipment

- Alcohol swabs
- Large over-the-needle intravenous cannula (14 or 16 gauge or commercial devices are available for this procedure)
- Syringe: 20 ml

Procedure

1. Administer high-flow oxygen.
2. Identify the second intercostal space in the mid-clavicular line on the side of the pneumothorax.
3. Swab the chest wall with surgical preparation solution or an alcohol swab.
4. Attach the syringe to the cannula. Fluid in the syringe will assist in the identification of air bubbles.
5. Insert the cannula perpendicular to the chest wall while aspirating the syringe, just superior to the third rib (to avoid the neurovascular bundle that runs along the inferior aspect of ribs (Figure 21.6).
6. Once air is aspirated, stop advancing the needle, and advance the cannula over the needle while withdrawing the needle and syringe.
7. Tape the cannula in place and proceed to chest drain insertion as soon as possible.

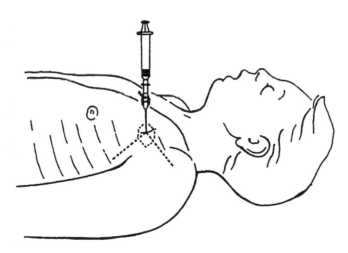

Figure 21.6 Needle thoracocentesis

Alternative method

1. Administer high-flow oxygen.
2. Attach a 10 ml syringe with 2 ml of sodium chloride to the rear of the cannula and needle.
3. Identify the fifth intercostal space in the mid-axillary line on the side of the suspected tension pneumothorax. This lateral approach provides a larger zone of safety than the anterior approach – but access may restrict its use.
4. Clean the skin and insert the cannula into the skin, just superior to the sixth rib. Once through the skin flush the needle with the sodium chloride – to expel any skin plug.
5. Remove the syringe plunger from the barrel of the syringe.
6. Advance the needle and cannula to pierce the pleura; draining of sodium chloride out of the syringe suggests penetration of the pleura.
7. Bubbling in the syringe indicates the presence of a tension pneumothorax.

8. Advance the cannula over the needle into the pleural space.
9. The cannula or needle may need flushing due to occlusion with a tissue.
10. Tape the cannula in place and proceed to chest drain insertion as soon as possible.
11. If needle thoracocentesis is attempted, and the patient does not have a tension pneumothorax, the risk of causing a pneumothorax is 10–20%. Patients who have had this procedure must have a chest radiograph, and will require chest drainage if ventilated.

In trauma, it may be better to perform an immediate slit or finger thoracostomy rather than a needle thoracocentesis. This is a more reliable and definitive method of reducing a tension pneumothorax.

21.5   Finger thoracocentesis followed by chest drain placement

The procedure for finger thoracocentesis is the same as the initial steps (steps 1–6 below) undertaken using the open technique for placing a chest drain that is described here. Be aware that in infants and small children, it may not be possible to clear a path using a finger sweep (step 6). In general, the largest size drain that will pass between the ribs should be used, as a guide use size 4 × endotracheal tube size.

Minimum equipment

- Gloves
- Skin preparation and surgical drapes
- Scalpel
- Blunt dissecting forceps
- Large clamps ×2
- Suture and tape
- (Local anaesthetic)
- Scissors
- Chest drain tube
- Underwater seal

Procedure

Finger thoracostomy (steps 1–6)

1. Decide on the insertion site (usually the fifth intercostal space in the mid-axillary line) on the side with the pneumothorax/fluid (Figure 21.7).
2. Swab the chest wall with surgical preparation or an alcohol swab.

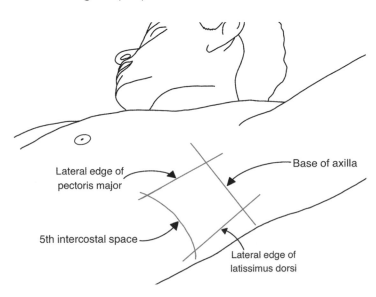

Figure 21.7 Chest drain insertion – landmarks

3. Use local anaesthetic if necessary.
4. Make a 2–3 cm skin incision along the line of the intercostal space, just superior to the rib below.
5. Using the dissecting forceps, bluntly dissect through the subcutaneous tissues through the incision just made until you puncture the parietal pleura.
6. Clear a path into the pleura (Figure 21.8). This can usually be done using a gloved finger but may not be possible in infants and small children when just forceps should be used.

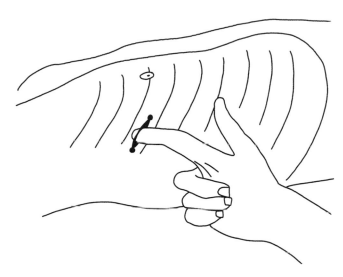

Figure 21.8 Chest drain insertion – clearing the path

Chest drain placement (steps 7–11)

7. Advance the chest drain tube into the pleural space during expiration. Using a clamp on the tip of the drain may be helpful to guide the drain through the track. Advance the tube until all the holes are in the pleural cavity.
8. Ensure the tube is in the pleural space by listening for air movement, and by looking for fogging of the tube during expiration.
9. Connect the chest drain tube to an underwater seal.
10. Suture the drain in place, and secure with tape.
11. Obtain a chest radiograph.

21.6   Clamshell thoracotomy

This is a life-saving procedure that may need to be performed in children presenting in cardiac arrest after chest trauma, usually penetrating trauma. The definitive intervention should be performed within 10 minutes of loss of cardiac output. This technique should only be performed by those with expertise and therefore it is not described in detail within these practical procedures.

21.7   Pericardiocentesis

The removal of a small amount of fluid from the pericardial sac can be life saving. The procedure is not without risks and the electrocardiogram (ECG) should be closely monitored throughout. An acute injury pattern (ST segment changes or a widened QRS) indicates ventricular damage by the needle. In traumatic cardiac arrest following penetrating injury, clamshell thoracotomy should be performed immediately if indicated rather than pericardiocentesis.

If point of care ultrasound is available, this can confirm the presence of pericardial fluid and guide needle aspiration.

Minimum equipment

- Skin preparation and surgical drapes
- ECG monitor
- (Local anaesthetic)
- Syringe: 20 ml
- Large over-the-needle cannula (16 or 18 gauge)

Procedure

1. Swab the xiphoid and subxiphoid areas with surgical preparation or an alcohol swab.
2. Use local anaesthetic if necessary.
3. Assess the patient for any significant mediastinal shift if possible.
4. Attach the syringe to the needle.
5. Puncture the skin 1–2 cm inferior to the left side of the xiphoid junction at a 45° angle (Figure 21.9).
6. Advance the needle towards the tip of the left scapula, aspirating all the time (Figure 21.10).
7. Watch the ECG monitor for signs of myocardial injury.
8. Once fluid is withdrawn, aspirate as much as possible (unless it is possible to withdraw limitless amounts of blood, in which case a ventricle has probably been entered).
9. If the procedure is successful, remove the needle, leaving the cannula in the pericardial sac. Secure in place and seal with a three-way tap. This allows later repeat aspirations should tamponade recur.

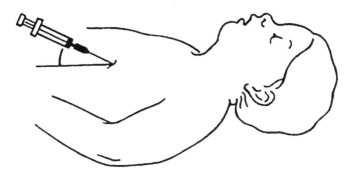

Figure 21.9 Needle pericardiocentesis – angle

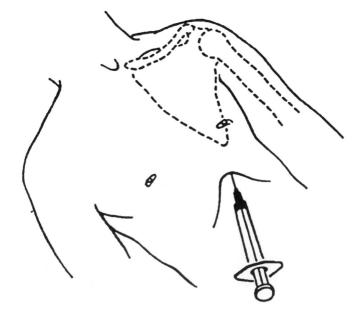

Figure 21.10 Needle pericardiocentesis – direction

21.8 Femoral nerve block

The femoral nerve supplies the femur with sensation, and a block is useful in cases of femoral fracture. The technique may also be of benefit when analgesic agents would interfere with the management or assessment of other injuries. A long-acting local anaesthetic agent should be used so that radiographs and splinting can be undertaken with minimal distress to the child.

Equipment

- Antiseptic swabs to clean
- Lidocaine 1%: up to 0.3 ml/kg
- Syringe (2 ml) and a 25 gauge needle
- Syringe (5 or 10 ml) and a 21 gauge needle
- Bupivacaine 0.25%: 0.8 ml/kg of 0.25% (maximum 2 mg/kg)

Femoral nerve block with ultrasound guidance (preferred technique)

Sterile technique for ultrasound

Prepare the groin skin with antiseptic solution. Use a sterile probe cover or, for a single shot block, prep all around the probe once it is positioned, and use a sterile no-touch technique with the injecting hand.

Procedure

1. Hold a 7–10 MHz linear probe in your non-dominant hand, placing it transversely, with the centre over the femoral artery pulse at the level of the groin crease (Figure 21.11). A cross-sectional view of the vessels and nerve will be obtained.
2. Identify the pulsating femoral artery and move the probe so it is in the middle of the ultrasound view.
3. The femoral nerve is an oval, white, honeycomb-like structure, located lateral to the artery. A good ultrasound view of the nerve is dependent on angling the probe to ensure the beam transects the nerve at 90° (anisotropy). It may be extremely difficult to visualise the nerve if the probe is angled incorrectly. Tilt the probe towards the head and the feet until you optimise your view (Figure 21.12).

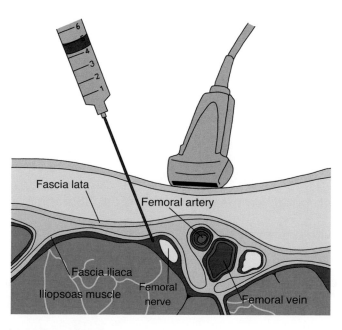

Figure 21.11 Ultrasound-guided needle approach

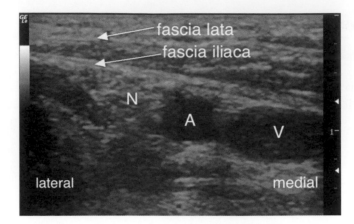

Figure 21.12 Ultrasound image of the femoral region
A, artery; N, nerve; V, vein

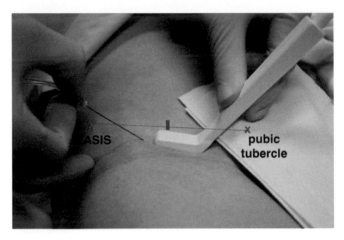

Figure 21.13 Ultrasound-guided block.
ASIS, anterior superior iliac spine

4. Sterile prep as above.
5. With your dominant hand insert a short bevel block needle, entering the skin at the lateral end of the probe (without touching it, to ensure sterility). Advance the needle slowly, keeping it parallel to and in the middle of the probe so the tip can be seen advancing towards the nerve, but stop just lateral to the nerve (to minimise the risk of intraneural injection). You may feel and see the needle breaching the fascia lata and the fascia iliaca (Figure 21.13).
6. Have an assistant inject the local anaesthetic, watching it surround the nerve, and reposition the needle if necessary to ensure good spread.

Landmark technique (if ultrasound not available)

1. Move the fractured limb gently so that the femur lies in abduction and the ipsilateral groin is exposed.
2. Swab the groin clean with antiseptic solution.
3. Identify the femoral artery and keep one finger on it. The femoral nerve lies immediately lateral to the artery.
4. Using the 2 ml syringe filled with lidocaine and a 25 gauge needle, infiltrate the skin just lateral to the artery.

5. Using the 5 or 10 ml syringe attached to the 21 gauge needle, insert the needle through the anaesthetised area at a 60° angle to the skin, aiming for the ipsilateral nipple. Advance the needle slowly, aspirating the syringe frequently to ensure that the needle is not in a vessel. Once a double pop has been felt, stop advancing the needle.
6. Aspirate the syringe to ensure the needle is not in a vessel, then inject the bupivacaine around the nerve, taking care not to puncture the artery or vein.
7. Wait until anaesthesia occurs (bupivacaine may take up to 20 minutes to have its full effect).

21.9 Summary

This chapter has covered the basic practical procedures that you need to be familiar with to manage traumatic injuries.

CHAPTER 22

Imaging in trauma

Learning outcomes

After reading this chapter, you will be able to:

- Describe the risks of ionising radiation in children
- Identify the areas to image
- Discuss which imaging modality to use
- Recognise when to ask for more senior/specialist support
- Define the basics of imaging interpretation

22.1   Introduction

This chapter provides an overview of the use of emergency imaging in major trauma in children. It gives an evidence-based approach for those involved in imaging decisions for paediatric trauma. It covers the different modalities of imaging available and also provides an introduction to basic radiological interpretation, as appropriate, for the clinician involved in managing paediatric trauma in the resuscitation room.

Principles

Injury patterns in children differ vastly from those in adults. Spinal and pelvic injuries, for example, are exceedingly rare in pre-adolescent children. Paediatric trauma is more likely to be blunt than penetrating. It is more likely to be a fall (particularly from a low height) than a road traffic collision. Due to these factors, significant bony injury to the cervical spine is rare and to the pelvis even rarer.

UK Trauma Audit Research Network (TARN) data for the paediatric population in 2018 shows that head injury is the commonest injury in major trauma, followed by injuries to the extremities and then to the abdomen. A common combination is that all three areas are injured. However, data suggest that areas in between injured regions (e.g. the pelvis or cervical spine) are not commonly injured as part of the process and should not be routinely imaged just because they lie between two other body regions that are injured.

It has become increasingly clear that the cancer risk of computed tomography (CT) in childhood is real, significant and is higher in younger age groups. Younger maturing tissues are more radiosensitive and there is a cumulative radiation risk over a lifetime, with children exposed at a younger age having a longer time in which to express the increased relative risk.

> Exposure to ionising radiation should always be kept to a minimum and the 'ALARA' principle should be adhered to, keeping radiation 'as low as reasonably achievable'

A sensible approach is to ask 'Does this child need to be imaged at all?', and if so this should be followed by 'Which anatomical areas are genuinely at risk?' Lastly, 'How do I select the best imaging modality for that body region?'

Reference should be made to the Royal College of Radiologists *Paediatric Trauma Protocols* (https://www.rcr.ac.uk/publication/paediatric-trauma-protocols, last accessed January 2023). These guidelines were brought together in 2017 by an expert panel of clinicians from across specialities to make recommendations on the best use of imaging modalities in injured children based upon the latest evidence. This chapter is based upon those recommendations.

Paediatric major trauma team leaders have overall responsibility for making difficult decisions about an imaging strategy for any individual patient and should be familiar with these guidelines.

Previously, a basic radiological screen for major injuries would often incorporate a routine 'primary survey' imaging request of chest X-ray, cervical spine X-ray and pelvic X-ray.

The routine ordering of a 'primary survey' set of films is no longer considered as gold standard, however if timely CT is unavailable they may provide some useful information. The lateral cervical spine X-ray on its own does not exclude bony injury and if the assessment of the child is difficult (due to depressed level of consciousness, alcohol or drugs) the cervical spine cannot be safely 'cleared' anyway. The need for pelvic X-rays should be carefully considered in view of the mechanism of injury and the true risk of pelvic ring instability. Each body region imaged needs to be justified on a risk/benefit analysis.

If a CT is required (e.g. CT head), it is **not** mandated to perform a whole-body CT in order to exclude other injuries. This particularly applies to the cervical spine which can be cleared by use of clinical assessment alone or in conjunction with X-rays. Do **not** routinely request a CT C-spine (200 × the radiation dose of a three-view cervical spine X-ray is delivered to the developing thyroid gland) simply because a CT head scan is indicated.

Due to the pattern of childhood injuries sustained it is relatively common for a CT head and CT abdomen to be required in combination. Do **not** routinely request a CT chest (a radiation dose of approximately 400–500 chest X-rays depending on age) in these patients simply because the chest lies between the two injured areas. This is inappropriate in children where multisystem trauma is the exception, not the rule. A chest X-ray is a perfectly adequate investigation to rule out management-changing pathology. National Institute for Health and Care Excellence (NICE) Guideline NG39 *Major Trauma: Assessment and Initial Management* also recommends this approach.

Imaging decisions can always be made in conjunction with radiological advice if there is any doubt about what to image and how best to proceed. Radiological advice should also be sought for the definitive interpretation of results.

The radiology department is not a safe place for an unstable trauma patient without adequate clinical supervision. Imaging is largely under the control of a radiographer, who will not be able to supervise an ill patient. Complex investigations including ultrasound scanning (USS), CT and contrast studies take time, during which the child may deteriorate significantly without appropriate monitoring and treatment. A core component of the trauma team should accompany and monitor the child on any transfer in the hospital and this includes to radiology.

Whole-body versus selective use of computed tomography

The primary cause of death in trauma patients is bleeding. The modality of imaging for accurately detecting bleeding is still regarded as CT. However, the use of CT in children has to weigh the benefits of finding clinically important injuries versus the real risks of ionising radiation in significant doses. Therefore, the *routine use of whole-body* CT scans in children is *not* considered appropriate. Adult trauma protocols should not be followed.

In the scenario of a **severely, multiply injured child**, a whole-body CT scan will be appropriate. For *critically injured* paediatric patients with multisystem trauma, the scan will usually be a head-to-thigh CT. This incorporates all important body regions including the pelvis. National targets (for adults) state that this should be performed within 30 minutes of the patient's arrival in the emergency department. However, few paediatric patients sustain multisystem trauma so this approach cannot be justified as first line investigation in *all* situations.

CT scans should be selectively used where there are isolated area injuries or two areas are injured.

In the common scenario where a child has injuries to the head and potentially the abdominal region it may be appropriate to do a CT scan of both the head and the abdomen, but no more. It is not necessary to routinely CT scan the chest just because it lies anatomically in between two areas that are injured. It is better to exclude significant pathology by careful clinical examination (repeated as necessary), use of vital sign observation (repeated routinely) and interpretation of a chest X-ray. The value of a normal chest X-ray should not be underestimated. It is then reasonable to proceed to CT chest if any combination of findings indicates that a more significant issue may be developing within the chest, not least of all the use of vital sign observation trends.

The indications for a CT scan of the head and the cervical spine follow the NICE head injury guidelines CG176 (https://www.nice.org.uk/Guidance/CG176, last accessed January 2023). The indications for a CT scan of the abdomen follow the recommendations of the Royal College of Radiologists *Paediatric Trauma Protocols* (2014). Outside of polytrauma there are no defined indications for a CT scan of the chest other than an abnormal chest X-ray, however experts largely agree that significant penetrating injuries to the chest warrant imaging by CT over chest X-ray from the outset.

Use of ultrasound

The use of focused assessment with sonography for trauma (FAST) scanning should be considered separately from USS performed by a competent paediatric sonographer or radiologist.

FAST scanning in emergency department physician hands carries a 50% sensitivity for ruling out the presence of free intra-abdominal fluid or blood in the injured paediatric population. This is clearly not accurate enough to allow a safe exclusion of pathology. Rarity of the need to perform such scans also has a role to play in this as regular trauma USS is required in order to maintain this key skill.

Currently there is no place for FAST scanning in children in the management of major trauma.

In contrast, adult studies show formal ultrasound actually performs better than chest X-ray in the exclusion of pneumothoraces (sensitivity of 85% versus 52%). No evidence exists for the paediatric population but there is no reason why this would be expected to be significantly different.

For haemothoraces, both ultrasound and chest X-ray have low sensitivity at 37% and 61%, respectively, with a similar specificity of 96–100%. Neither is accurate enough to confidently exclude a haemothorax, but in adults chest X-ray performs better.

For these reasons the Royal College of Radiologists and NICE recommend the use of chest X-ray as a first line investigation in children with the addition of ultrasound if required. As with chest X-rays, abnormal USS should prompt further detailed imaging with a CT scan of the chest. Routine CT scanning of the chest is not recommended.

Ultrasound does have value in detecting pericardial fluid indicating an impending cardiac tamponade, or for assessing cardiac function. An established cardiac tamponade should be managed clinically, as with a tension pneumothorax, and confirmation by imaging is not necessarily indicated.

USS can also have a valuable role to play in the securing of vascular access in an otherwise difficult, peripherally shut down, paediatric trauma patient.

22.2   Specific body region imaging (top to bottom)

Head imaging

The following imaging recommendations are based on guidance from the Royal College of Radiologists (RCR) guidelines on paediatric trauma (https://www.rcr.ac.uk/publication/paediatric-trauma-protocols, last accessed March 2023).

Computed tomography is the primary investigation for imaging of the head in trauma. It is readily available, quick to access and displays high sensitivity and specificity for the identification of traumatic brain injury (Figure 22.1). The NICE head injury assessment is recommended and indications for head CT scan contained within this assessment are used. Indication for CT head does not on its own indicate CT of the cervical spine or any other body area.

The NICE evidence is extrapolated from adult practice as there are few studies to form a scientific basis for this guidance in the paediatric age group. CT brain scanning is the prime modality for excluding acute intracranial haemorrhage. A child with clinical suspicion of intracranial bleeding requires a CT scan, not a skull X-ray film, as intracranial bleeding in children often occurs without a skull fracture. Before the child is sent into the radiology department for a scan, they must be resuscitated, stabilised and supervised at all times by a doctor or appropriately trained senior nurse.

According to NICE guidelines NG41 *Spinal Injury: Assessment and Initial Management* (https://www.nice.org.uk/guidance/ng41/resources/spinal-injury-assessment-and-initial-management-1837447790533, last accessed March 2023), if a child has an indication for a head CT and when there is strong clinical suspicion of a neck injury, then the cervical spine is included at the same time (see next section on cervical spine imaging).

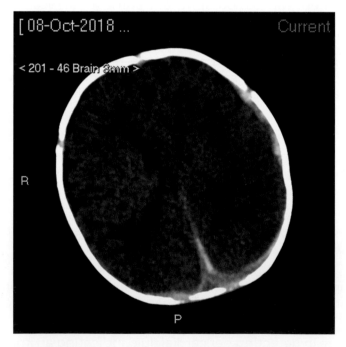

Figure 22.1 CT head showing subdural haematoma as a result of non-accidental injury
Alder Hey Radiology Department Teaching Library

Cervical spine imaging

The most common site of a 'missed' spinal injury is where a flexible part of the spine meets the fixed part. Unlike in adult spines, most paediatric cervical spine injuries occur either through the discs and ligaments at the cervicocranial junction (C1, C2, C3) or less commonly at the cervicothoracic junction (C7, T1).

The relatively large mass of the head, moving on a flexible neck with poorly supportive muscles, most commonly leads to injury in the higher cervical vertebrae. Children develop three patterns of spinal injury:

1. Subluxation or dislocation without fracture.
2. Fracture with or without subluxation or dislocation.
3. Spinal cord injury without radiographic abnormality (SCIWORA).

If significant cervical spine injury is suspected, cervical spine immobilisation should take place before any radiographs are performed. Cervical spine injuries should be imaged according to NICE guideline criteria. If sandbags rather than head blocks are used for immobilisation they may obscure bony landmarks.

Paediatric cervical spine injury is uncommon. Routine imaging of the cervical spine is therefore not indicated. Assess the child first. Most cervical spines can be cleared clinically. If there is difficulty in assessing the patient or very strong clinical suspicion of spinal injury, indicated by the following, then CT is the first line choice of imaging.

- Glasgow Coma Scale (GCS) score is less than13 on arrival
- Intubated patient
- Focal peripheral neurological signs
- Paraesthesia in the upper or lower limbs

Plain X-ray with three views (anteroposterior (AP), lateral and open mouth odontoid peg view (if possible)) are indicated for those where the index of suspicion is lower but is still present, such as with a dangerous mechanism. Dangerous mechanisms include falls from a significant height (more than 1 metre), axial loading to the head (e.g. diving accident), high-speed road traffic collision, rollover motor accident or ejection from a vehicle.

The lateral cervical spine X-ray should include the base of the skull to the junction of C7 and T1. The AP view should include C2 to T1. Peg views should be attained but may be very difficult in young children. These images should only be taken after immediately life-threatening injuries have been identified and treated.

Computed tomography of the cervical spine

If the plain films are unclear or abnormal or there is already a high-risk mechanism of injury the following is recommended:

- Under 10 years: the recommendation is for CT of the upper cervical spine (from the occipital condyles and foramen magnum down to C3) – this covers the craniocervical junction. This is the most common site of fracture in this age group and it excludes the radiosensitive thyroid gland from the scan
- Over 10 years: the recommendation is to image as for adults –from the occipital condyles down to the C7/T1 junction

Targeted CT of bony areas is often also carried out for further assessment of clinical spinal cord injuries.

However, bony injury in itself is not the prime concern in spinal injury. The main risk is actual or potential injury to the cord. Any unstable fracture, if inadequately immobilised, may lead to progressive cord damage.

MRI and spinal cord injury (any level)

Cervical spine X-rays and CT images may be falsely reassuring. They only show the position of bones at the time imaging was acquired and give no idea of the magnitude of the flexion and extension forces applied to the spine at the time of injury. The cord may be injured even in a child without any apparent radiographical abnormality on plain X-rays. For this reason, if there is strong clinical suspicion of significant cervical spine cord injury (paraesthesiae or neurological abnormalities) then magnetic resonance imaging (MRI) is the imaging modality of choice.

SCIWORA is said to have occurred when radiographic films are totally normal in the presence of significant cord injury. If the film is normal in a conscious child with clinical symptoms (such as pain, loss of function or paraesthesia in a limb), then neck protection measures should be continued and MRI should be obtained. In an unconscious child at high risk, a cord injury cannot be excluded until the patient is awake and has been assessed clinically, even in the presence of a normal cervical spine film. Adequate spinal precautions should be continued until the child is well enough to be assessed clinically or MRI has been carried out.

Chest imaging

In blunt chest trauma, the most useful initial investigation in terms of aiding immediate life-threatening problems in the emergency department is the chest X-ray. USS can also help and is actually more sensitive (in experienced hands) than X-rays for the detection of pneumothorax. X-rays can, however, be done quickly via a portable machine in the resuscitation room. Chest X-rays can also delineate rib fractures, gross mediastinal abnormalities and diaphragmatic injuries. If the chest X-ray is abnormal, then CT chest should be requested (Figure 22.2). If normal, then CT chest is **not** required if the child's clinical condition remains stable.

CT chest can be completely avoided in children with a normal chest X-ray, who are conscious and clinically stable.

In penetrating trauma, the first line investigation is CT scan of the chest with contrast to accurately enable detection of organ injury, the track of damage caused by knives, bullets, shrapnel, etc. and for detecting vascular injury.

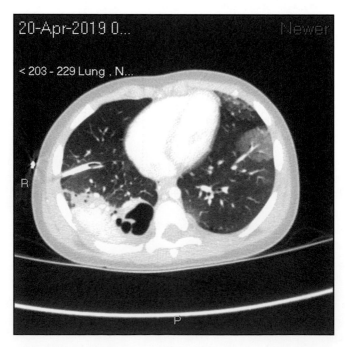

Figure 22.2 CT thorax showing pulmonary contusions
Alder Hey Radiology Department Teaching Library

Abdominal imaging

Abdominal ultrasound and FAST have been shown to have only 50% sensitivity in detecting haemoperitoneum in children. There is therefore no place for FAST scanning in the emergency department resuscitation room in children as it will not rule out free fluid or bleeding. A formal radiologist USS of the abdomen mat be helpful however.

Where indicated, contrast-enhanced CT is the modality of choice for the assessment of acute traumatic intra-abdominal injury (Figure 22.3). There is no mechanism of injury that mandates abdominal CT as an isolated investigation. Decisions should be based upon clinical history and examination findings. For example, in head injury where CT is to be performed, a reduced conscious level does not mandate CT abdomen as well. Children intubated and sedated prior to arrival at the emergency department or for transfer to another centre may require imaging as a reliable clinical assessment of tenderness cannot be undertaken.

The following criteria are all associated with intra-abdominal injury and indicate the need for CT with contrast:

- Lap belt injury/bruising
- Abdominal wall bruising
- Abdominal tenderness in a conscious patient
- Abdominal distension
- Clinical evidence of persistent hypovolaemia, such as persistent (unexplained) tachycardia
- Blood from the rectum or nasogastric tube
- Significant handle bar injuries (round handle bar end bruises)

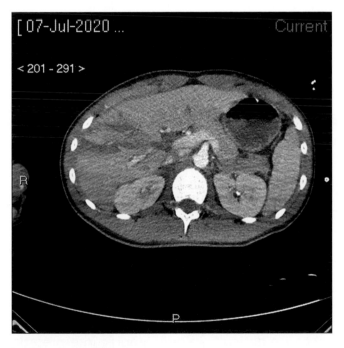

Figure 22.3 CT abdomen showing liver lacerations
Alder Hey Radiology Department Teaching Library

Pelvic imaging

Children rarely have significant pelvic ring disruption fractures (this excludes isolated pubic ramus fractures) and a routine pelvic X-ray is **not** required. Significant ring fractures should be clinically evident anyway and should be being treated, for example with fluids/blood and a pelvic brace. While pubic rami fractures are relatively common they do not cause significant bleeding or threat to life, organ or limb. If there is strong clinical suspicion of pelvic ring injury after clinical assessment then pelvic imaging is required, ideally CT.

It should be noted that pelvic fractures when present are often associated with multiorgan injuries and that the bony pelvis will be included on CT evaluation of the abdomen. Contrast-enhanced CT of the abdomen and pelvis will exclude pathology in either region if needed.

Interventional radiology may have a role to play in the management of complex pelvic fractures as well as for vascular injuries in limbs or within the abdomen and chest. This is generally a supraregional speciality and children requiring such procedures may have to be referred to a tertiary centre in a time-critical fashion.

Extremity imaging

Extremities should be imaged according to how likely the suspicion is for a fracture. Plain X-rays should be requested as the primary investigation for any region where clinical history and examination strongly suggest fracture. AP and lateral views of bones should be requested, including the adjacent joints.

Femoral fractures are particularly common. Plain films will be used again and the best images are generally obtained within the radiology department as opposed to mobile films within the resuscitation room. Resuscitation room films should be reserved for life-threatening primary survey problems – particularly chest and pelvis X-rays. Consideration should be given to a reassessment during a secondary survey later to ensure that more subtle fractures (e.g. to a wrist, foot or finger) are not missed. This is particularly common in children who present unconscious as they are unable to indicate pain in a particular area. A tertiary survey at a later date when appropriate (often on a paediatric critical care unit (PCCU) or a ward area) will help minimise the risk of missed injuries.

CT scans of injured extremities may be useful later for complex fracture management.

22.3   X-ray interpretation

Introduction

All major trauma centres and trauma units should have in place 'hot reporting' by a senior radiologist such that images (whether plain film or CT) are reported on a primary survey report form within 5 minutes. This documents all potentially life-threatening problems. Fuller, formal, written reporting should occur within 60 minutes of the scan. Important clinical decisions about management will usually be made on the radiologist report, particularly for CT scan images.

However, a basic understanding of anatomy on plain X-ray images is necessary for all clinicians. The main reason for performing a primary survey radiological image is to exclude a potentially life-threatening injury, so it is important to quickly review films that are obtained (pelvis and chest X-ray in particular) to assess for significant pathology such as a large haemothorax, a large pneumothorax that may proceed to a tension pneumothorax, or an unstable pelvic ring fracture that might signify large blood losses.

Be aware of equipment, for example sandbags may obscure cervical spine bony landmarks, and a pelvic brace may obscure important areas of the pelvic X-ray.

The child's positioning may cause difficulty in radiographic interpretation. The interpretation of a supine AP chest X-ray is notoriously more difficult than that of an erect posteroanterior (PA) film.

Discussing images with an experienced emergency physician or neuro-, trauma or orthopaedic surgeon may also help. An experienced emergency radiographer (technician) is a valuable asset to any department and, if they consider a film is abnormal, their comments should be carefully noted.

With all imaging, check that the image has the following information:

- Name of the patient
- Date and time that the image was taken
- Orientation (side marker position)
- Position that the X-ray was taken (e.g. supine/erect/decubitus)

Interpreting the chest X-ray

Adequacy can be assessed by considering both penetration and depth of inspiration. The film should be sufficiently penetrated to just visualise the disc spaces of the lower thoracic vertebrae through the heart shadow. At least five anterior rib ends should be seen above the diaphragm on the right side (Figure 22.4). An expiratory film may mimic consolidation. Beware of a large thymus gland mimicking a widened mediastinum.

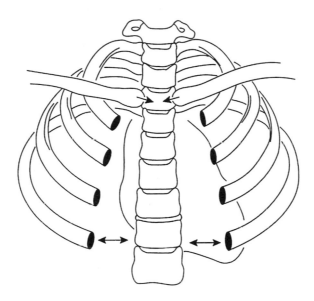

Figure 22.4 Assessing rotation – straight chest film

Alignment can be assessed by ensuring that the medial ends of both clavicles are equally spaced about the spinous processes of the upper thoracic vertebrae, as shown in Figure 22.4. Abnormal rotation may create apparent mediastinal shift. The trachea should be equally spaced between the clavicles.

Check the position of any apparatus, including:

- Tracheal tube
- Central venous lines
- Chest drains

Misplacement of the endotracheal tube (ETT) should be evident clinically, but may be seen on a chest film if you look for it. Do this first when reviewing any chest X-ray on an intubated patient. Malposition of an ETT can result in reduced ventilation and hypoxia. The ideal position for an ETT is below the clavicles and at least 1 cm above the carina. To find the carina, identify the slope of the right and left main bronchi – the carina is where the two lines meet in the midline.

The posterior, lateral and anterior aspects of each rib must be examined in detail. This can be done by tracing out the upper and lower borders of the ribs from the posterior costochondral joint to where they join the anterior costal cartilage at the mid-clavicular line. The internal trabecular pattern can then be assessed.

The ribs in children are soft and pliable and only break when subjected to considerable force. Even greater force is required to fracture the first two ribs or to break multiple ribs (Figure 22.5). Consequently, the presence of these fractures means you should look for other sites of injury both inside and outside the chest, including the cervical spine.

Finish assessing the bones by inspecting the visible vertebrae, the clavicles, scapulae and proximal humeri.

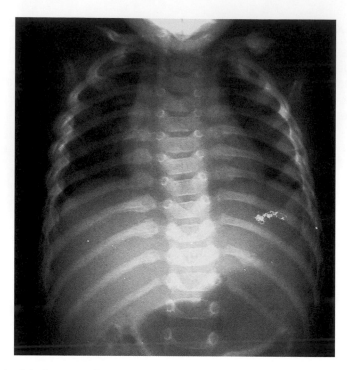

Figure 22.5 Healing rib and clavicle fractures in a newborn

Thoracic spine injuries may be overlooked on a chest radiograph. Abnormal flattening of the vertebral bodies, widening of the disc spaces or gaps between the spinous processes or pedicles may be seen. On AP views, increased vertical or horizontal distances between the pedicles or spinous processes indicate an unstable fracture.

If there are rib fractures in the first three ribs, these may be associated with major spinal trauma and great vessel injury.

A tension pneumothorax is a clinical diagnosis. A suspected tension pneumothorax should be treated in the emergency situation, without any confirmatory X-ray. On a supine film, the air in a simple pneumothorax rises anteriorly and may only be evident from an abnormal blackness or 'sharpness' of the diaphragm or of the cardiac border. The standard appearances of a pneumothorax, where there is a sharp lung edge and the vessels fail to extend to the rib cage and the lung edges, may not occur in the supine film. Air will not rise to cause an apical lucency.

The cardiac outline should lie one-third to the right of midline and two-thirds to the left of midline. If the film is not rotated, then mediastinal shift is due to the heart being either pushed to one side or pulled from the other. For example, mediastinal shift to the left may be due either to a pneumothorax, air trapping or effusion or blood on the right side, or to collapse of the left lung.

All major trauma radiographs will be taken in the supine position, often using portable X-ray machines. The tube is near to the patient and the heart is anterior with the film placed posteriorly. The heart in this situation appears abnormally magnified (widened) and the cardiothoracic ratio is difficult to assess on supine AP films.

A haemothorax will lie along the entire border of the posterior pleural space on a supine chest X-ray as the blood pools horizontally, so the classic fluid levels and blunted costophrenic or cardiophrenic angles described with an erect chest X-ray will not be seen.

The mediastinal cardiac outline should be clear on both sides. Any loss of definition suggests consolidation (de-aeration) of adjacent lungs. A 'globular' shape to the heart may suggest a pericardial effusion. Tamponade is managed clinically, not radiologically. A cardiac echo is useful in equivocal cases.

In the teenager, the mediastinum should appear as narrow as in an adult. In children under the age of 18 months, the normal thymus may simulate superior mediastinal widening (above the level of the carina). A normal thymus may touch the right chest wall, left chest wall, left diaphragm or right diaphragm, making it very difficult to exclude mediastinal pathology. Fortunately, mediastinal widening due to aortic dissection or spinal trauma is very rare in smaller children.

In cases of doubt, where there is a normal clinical examination, an opinion from a radiologist should be sought. In the older child involved in trauma, mediastinal widening may mean aortic dissection or major vessel or spinal injury. Ultrasound, CT or angiography may be required to resolve this when the child is stable.

The cardiophrenic and costophrenic angles should be clear on both sides. The diaphragms should be clearly defined on both sides and the left diaphragm should be clearly visible behind the heart. Loss of definition of the left diaphragm behind the heart suggests left lower lobe collapse, an abnormal hump suggests diaphragmatic rupture, and an elevated diaphragm suggests effusion, lung collapse or nerve palsy.

At the end of the systematic review of the X-ray, check again the key areas shown in the box.

- Behind the heart (left lower lobe consolidation or collapse, inhalation of foreign bodies)
- Apices for pneumothorax (erect films only), rib fractures and collapse/consolidation
- Costophrenic and cardiophrenic angles (erect films only) – fluid or haemothorax
- Horizontal fissure – fluid or elevation (upper lobe collapse)
- Trachea for foreign body (and ETT)

Interpreting the cervical spine X-ray

Adequacy can be assessed by checking that the whole spine can be viewed from the lower clivus down to the upper body of the T1 vertebra (Figure 22.6). If the C7/T1 junction is not seen initially then gentle traction should be applied by pulling the arms down, holding them above the elbow joint. If the child is conscious, they should be asked to relax their shoulders as traction is applied. If the child is on a spinal board then this must be stabilised by an assistant.

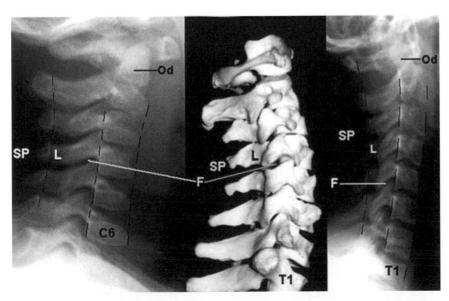
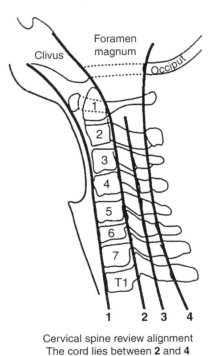

Figure 22.6 Lateral cervical spine showing the anatomy and three of the four review lines and disc spaces (facet joints and line not shown)
Courtesy of University of Hawaii
F, facet joint; L, lamina; Od, odontoid; SP, spinous process

Check the smooth continuity of the anterior vertebral line, the posterior vertebral line, the spinol-aminar line and the line joining the spinous processes posteriorly.These should all form a gentle lordosis curve. The presence of an abnormally straight cervical spine might indicate the placement of immobilisation or of 'splinting' from pain and muscular spasm and may in itself indicate significant injury.

Check for abnormal soft tissue swelling seen anterior to the vertebral bodies and in the retropharyngeal space at the higher cervical spine level. There should be less than 7 mm of space anterior to the body of C2 and less than 2 cm anterior to the vertebral body at the C7 level.

Trace around every vertebral body, lamina, facet joint and spinous process at every level in order to not miss subtle fractures. Check the peg (open mouth) view in order to fully assess the continuity of the 'ring' of C1.

Then check the AP view for vertebral height consistency and to assess symmetry of vertebral disc spacing (Figure 22.7).

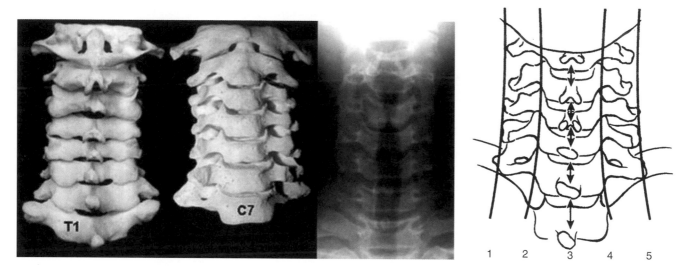

Figure 22.7 Anteroposterior cervical spine showing the anatomy and five review lines, discs and spinous processes
Courtesy of University of Hawaii

Interpreting the pelvic X-ray

Adequacy can be assessed by checking that the whole pelvis can be viewed from the pubic rami and the hips to the wings of the ilium and the lower lumbar spine. Check for rotation by assessing the shape of the ring made between the inferior and superior pubic rami on both sides and assess for symmetry. The tip of the coccyx should align with the symphysis pubis. See Figure 22.8 for a normal straight pelvis in a young child.

Check for the integrity of all the 'rings'. First check the main pelvic ring, then the obturator foramina (rings made by the superior and inferior pubic rami bilaterally), the ring formed around both hips and the integrity of the sacroiliac joints made where the pelvis joins the spinal column. Again assess for symmetry checking one side against the other.

An AP compression injury mechanism is very unusual in children. This can cause an open book type pelvic fracture. The pelvic ring will be disrupted anteriorly at the symphysis pubis, which will appear widened and posteriorly near the sacroiliac joints. It is this posterior disruption that can lead to significant venous bleeding, which can be catastrophic as a large volume of blood can then be accommodated in the increased volume of the opened up pelvis. This is the situation where a pelvic binder can be life saving.

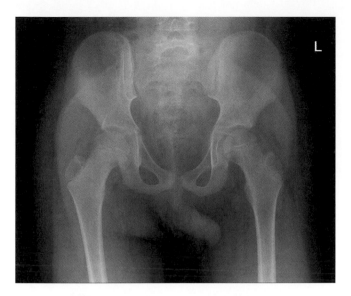

Figure 22.8 Normal straight pelvis in a young child

The type of injury more commonly seen in children is a lateral compression injury. With this, it is not uncommon to see pubic ramus fractures in children, often minor buckle fractures which are not significant in the context of major trauma or blood loss. They are painful and can affect mobilisation but are not life threatening. The sacroiliac joint can also be compressed but this is a stable injury and does not lead to catastrophic haemorrhage.

22.4 Summary

This chapter has covered the imaging that it is appropriate to carry out when managing trauma in children, and the importance of seeking radiological advice.

CHAPTER 23

Structured approach to stabilisation and transfer

Learning outcomes

After reading this chapter, you will be able to:

- Describe a structured approach to the stabilisation of a seriously ill or injured child
- Describe a structured approach to the transfer of a seriously ill or injured child

---

23.1   Stabilisation of the child

After successful resuscitation of the seriously ill or injured child, frequent clinical reassessment must be carried out in order to assess trends and detect any changes in the child's status. This is essential in order to provide the appropriate information to guide ongoing care. All children should have the following monitored:

- Oxygen saturation
- Carbon dioxide (CO_2) monitoring (if intubated)
- Pulse rate and rhythm
- Blood pressure (non-invasive)
- Urine output
- Core temperature
- Blood gases and lactate

Additionally, some children will require:

- Invasive blood pressure monitoring
- Central venous pressure (CVP) monitoring

The resources to measure some of these parameters may only be available in a static intensive care setting. The clinical team should carefully consider what surrogate signs they can consider where it is necessary to deviate from the ideal monitoring profile.

The investigations shown in Box 23.1 should be considered following successful resuscitation or during subsequent stabilisation.

Children who have been resuscitated from cardiorespiratory arrest may die hours or days later from multiple organ failure. In addition to the cellular and homeostatic abnormalities that occur during the preceding illness, and during the arrest itself, cellular damage continues after spontaneous circulation has been restored. This is called reperfusion injury.

Advanced Paediatric Life Support: A Practical Approach to Emergencies, Seventh Edition. Edited by Stephanie Smith.
© 2023 John Wiley & Sons Ltd. Published 2023 by John Wiley & Sons Ltd.

Box 23.1 Post-resuscitation investigations

- Blood glucose
- Chest radiograph
- Blood gases and lactate
- Full blood count
- Group and save serum for cross-match
- Sodium, potassium, calcium, urea and creatinine
- Clotting screen
- Liver function tests
- Blood culture and urine and cerebrospinal fluid (CSF) culture if indicated
- C-reactive protein or procalcitonin

Similarly, children resuscitated with serious illness or injury may suffer multisystem dysfunction as a result of hypoxia or ischaemia. Ongoing activation of inflammatory mediators, as occurs in serious sepsis or trauma, also contributes to multisystem organ failure. Post-resuscitation management aims to achieve and maintain homeostasis in order to optimise the chances of organ recovery. Management should be directed in a systematic way.

Airway and Breathing

Seriously ill children often exhibit an impaired conscious level and depressed airway reflexes. Intubation should always be considered and will usually have occurred during resuscitation. Any uncertainty regarding the indications for and against intubation should be discussed with a consultant intensivist or anaesthetist.

In some patients, the process of intubating and ventilating a child can lead to significant difficulty in ventilating (clearing CO_2) and oxygenating the child. The clinician managing the process should be ready for such an occurrence and be prepared to rapidly increase ventilator settings and ventilate by hand where necessary.

- The endotracheal tube (ETT) should, ideally, have a small leak. It should be secured according to local guidelines and ventilation should be monitored by continuous capnography and blood gases. The ETT should not be cut. A chest radiograph after intubation should be performed to confirm appropriate position of the ETT
- Ventilation settings should normally be maintained to keep end-tidal CO_2 (ETCO$_2$) between 4.0 and 5.5 kPa. Children with intracranial injuries should have their $PaCO_2$ maintained as close to 4.5–6.0 kPa (35–45 mmHg) as possible. The rational for this is to minimise increases in intracranial pressure (ICP) and cerebral oedema. If this is difficult because of airway or lung pathology, urgent advice should be obtained from a paediatric intensivist
- Sufficient inspired oxygen should be given to maintain SpO_2 at between 94% and 98% except for children with cyanotic cardiac lesions and chronic lung disease. The latter group will normally target an SpO_2 of 88–92% (provided their normal saturations are not significantly higher). If anaemia or carbon monoxide poisoning is suspected, inspired oxygen should be delivered at the highest possible concentration irrespective of the SpO_2 value. Specialist advice regarding target saturations should be sought from a paediatric intensivist or cardiologist for all children where a cardiac abnormality or significant chronic lung disease is either known or suspected

Circulation

If the child is intubated there may be a profound deterioration in cardiovascular function around the time of induction. This is due to the suppression of endogenous catecholamines, secondary to the induction agents used, and the physiological effect of positive pressure ventilation. A careful choice of induction agents can help reduce this risk and it may be helpful to gain advice from a specialist in order to optimise patient haemodynamics pre-induction.

Following resuscitation, there may be poor cardiac output, irrespective of the events around induction. This may be due to any combination of the following factors:

- An underlying cardiac abnormality
- The effects on the myocardium of hypoxia, acidosis and toxins, preceding and during any arrest
- Continuing acid–base or electrolyte disturbance
- Hypovolaemia

The following steps should be taken if there are signs of poor perfusion:

- Assess cardiac output clinically
- Infuse balanced fluids in doses of 10 ml/kg and reassess cardiac output clinically
- Aim for a normal arterial pH (more than 7.3) and good oxygenation. This may require the use of inotropic drug support with or without further fluid boluses
- Monitor ventilation and intervene with increased support when inadequate
- Identify and correct hypoglycaemia. Start to correct other electrolyte abnormalities

A CVP line may give useful information about the preload to the heart. This may assist in decisions about fluid infusion and inotropic support. A target value for the CVP should be discussed and established with an expert team. The CVP may be used in conjunction with heart rate and perfusion in assessing the response to a fluid challenge. In hypovolaemic patients CVP alters little with a fluid bolus, but in euvolaemia or hypervolaemia it usually shows a sustained rise. It is important to recognise that the maintenance of CVP should not be viewed as an isolated endpoint in itself; it must be interpreted and responded to within the overall clinical picture.

Drugs used to maintain perfusion following cardiac arrest or treatment of shock

There are no research data comparing one drug with another that show an advantage of any specific drug on outcome. In addition, the pharmacokinetics of these drugs vary from patient to patient and even from hour to hour in the same patient. Factors that influence the effects of these drugs include the child's age and maturity, the underlying disease process, metabolic state, acid–base balance, the patient's autonomic and endocrine response, and liver and renal function. Therefore, the recommended infusion doses are starting points; the infusions must always be adjusted according to patient response.

Wherever possible inotrope infusion should be administered via a central line. However, where this is not available, then intraosseous or peripheral infusions may be used. When this option is used, the site of infusion must be easily accessed for regular inspection. If there is any evidence of extravasation or ischaemia an alternative should be sought as a matter of urgency. In all cases intraosseous or peripheral inotrope infusions should be converted to central infusions at the earliest possible opportunity.

In the following text information is given on how to make up infusions customised to the child's weight. However, fixed concentration infusions may be used according to local protocols where available. Online calculators can be used in accordance with local guidelines.

Adrenaline

An adrenaline infusion is a good first line treatment for shock with poor systemic perfusion from any cause that is unresponsive to fluid resuscitation. Adrenaline is also a good first line treatment in patients with severe hypotensive shock; in very young infants in whom other inotropes may be ineffectual; or for speed if there is a rapid deterioration.

Infusion concentration: 0.3 mg/kg in 50 ml of 5% glucose or 0.9% sodium chloride will give 0.1 micrograms/kg/min if run at a rate of 1 ml/h. Use 1:1000 (1 mg/ml) adrenaline concentrate. The infusion may be run via a central intravenous line at 0.1–10 ml/h in order to deliver 0.01–1 micrograms/kg/min. To safely administer via a peripheral intravenous cannula or intraossesous needle, use 1/10th dilution: add 0.03 mg/kg in 50 ml or 0.3 mg/kg in 500 ml of 5% glucose or 0.9% sodium chloride, which will give 0.1 micrograms if run at a rate of 10 ml/h. The advantage of the latter is that given the bigger dilution, it is likely to reach the circulation more quickly and have a clinical effect sooner.

Noradrenaline

Noradrenaline can be considered as a first line treatment for warm shock, or as an additional inotrope for shock from any cause where adrenaline is already being used at high dose (more than 0.5 micrograms/kg/min). The infusion should be started at 0.1 micrograms/kg/min and should be titrated to response, increasing up to 1 microgram/kg/min (or even higher in rare cases) depending on clinical response.

Initial concentration: 0.3 mg/kg in 50 ml of 5% glucose or 0.9% sodium chloride will give 0.1 micrograms/kg/min if run at a rate of 1 ml/h. Use 1 mg/ml noradrenaline concentrate. The infusion may be run via a central intravenous line at 0.1–10 ml/h in order to deliver 0.01–1 micrograms/kg/min. To safely administer via a peripheral intravenous cannula or intraossesous needle, use 1/10th dilution: add 0.03 mg/kg to 50 ml or 0.3 mg/kg to 500 ml of 5% glucose or 0.9% saline, which will give 0.1 micrograms/kg/min if given at 10 ml/h. The advantage of the latter dilution is that running at a faster rate for the same dose, it is likely to reach the circulation more quickly and have a clinical effect sooner.

Hydrocortisone

If a patient is needing high doses of inotrope infusions to maintain blood pressure and cardiovascular stability, consider using hydrocortisone as an additional inotrope.

Dose: IV bolus or intermittent infusion:
- Neonate: initially 2.5 mg/kg repeated if necessary, after 4 hours then 2.5 mg/kg every 6 hours for 48 hours or until blood pressure recovers, then reduce dose gradually over at least 48 hours
- 1 month to 18 years: 1 mg/kg (maximum 100 mg every 6 hours)

Dopamine

Dopamine is an endogenous catecholamine with complex cardiovascular effects. It is usually only used at infusion rates of 5–10 micrograms/kg/min. Dopamine directly stimulates cardiac β-adrenergic receptors and releases noradrenaline from cardiac sympathetic nerves.

Dopamine infusions may produce tachycardia, vasoconstriction and ventricular ectopy. Infiltration of dopamine into the tissues can produce local tissue necrosis. Dopamine and other catecholamines are partially inactivated in alkaline solutions and therefore should not be mixed with sodium bicarbonate.

Infusion concentration: 15 mg/kg in 50 ml of 5% glucose or 0.9% sodium chloride to give 5 micrograms/kg/min if run at 1 ml/h. The infusion may then be run at 1–2 ml/h in order to deliver 5–10 micrograms/kg/min.

Kidneys

It is important both to maximise renal blood flow and to maintain renal tubular patency by maintaining urine flow. To achieve this, the following are necessary:

- Maintenance of an adequate blood pressure to drive renal perfusion
- Maintenance of adequate filling and a good cardiac output using inotropes and fluids as required
- Maintenance of good oxygenation
- Monitoring and normalisation of electrolytes (sodium, potassium, calcium, magnesium) and acid–base balance in blood should be undertaken as a supporting measure. Sodium bicarbonate should not be given without expert advice. Potassium should be given slowly and cautiously and only be given in small doses in oliguric or anuric patients

Liver

Hepatic cellular damage can become manifest up to 24 hours following an arrest or episode of hypoperfusion. Coagulation factors can become depleted, and bleeding may be worsened by concomitant ischaemia-induced intravascular coagulopathy. The patient's clotting profile and platelets should be monitored and corrected, as indicated, with fresh frozen plasma, cryoprecipitate or platelets. In complex coagulopathy, advice may be sought from a haematologist.

Brain

The aim of therapy is to protect the brain from further (secondary) damage. To achieve this, the cerebral blood flow must be maintained, normal cellular homeostasis must be achieved and cerebral metabolic needs must be reduced.

When intracranial pathology is present, cerebral autoregulation may not function correctly. In these circumstances, adequate cerebral blood flow may be achieved if the cerebral perfusion pressure (mean arterial pressure – intracranial pressure) is kept above 40–60 mmHg depending on age (lowest in infants). Maintenance of cellular homeostasis is helped by normalisation of the acid–base and electrolyte balances. Cerebral metabolic needs can be reduced by sedating and paralysing the child. Convulsions should be promptly treated and consideration given to their cause. Long-acting medication, such as levetiracetam or phenytoin, should be used if recurrent. Although a barbiturate coma reduces both cerebral metabolism and ICP, it has not been shown to improve neurological outcome.

Practical steps to minimise secondary brain injury are:

- Maintenance of good oxygenation
- Maintenance of adequate blood pressure using inotropes and fluids
- Intubation and maintenance of normal blood gases
- Nursing head up at 20° and in midline
- Using osmotic agents for acutely raised ICP such as sodium chloride 2.7% or 3% dose 3 ml/kg IV over 15 minutes or mannitol 250–500 mg/kg IV over 15 minutes
- Control of blood glucose avoiding both hypoglycaemia and hyperglycaemia
- Maintenance of good analgesia, sedation and paralysis (where indicated)
- Monitoring and normalisation of electrolytes and acid–base balance
- Control of seizures
- Maintenance of normothermia

The evidence does not support the use of post-arrest hypothermia (core temperatures of 32–34°C) in children and outside the newborn period. Studies have shown no beneficial effects on neurological recovery. Harm may occur, however, with raised core temperature, which increases metabolic demand by 10–13% for each degree centigrade increase in temperature above normal. Therefore, in a post-arrest patient either needing critical care or needing intubation, hyperthermia should be treated with active cooling to achieve a normal core temperature. Shivering should be prevented since it will increase metabolic demand. Sedation may be adequate to control shivering, but neuromuscular blockade is usually needed.

23.2   Principles of safe transfer and retrieval

After resuscitation and emergency treatment have been provided, consideration will need to be given to the best place to continue the child's care. This will usually involve a transfer to another unit, often another hospital. Critically ill children transferred by untrained personnel have been shown to be subjected to an excess of adverse events. These transfers have also been associated with a high incidence of serious transport-related adverse events. The impact of these events on long-term outcome is unknown and international practice has focused on minimising adverse events during transfer. It should be noted that even when the child only needs to be transported from the emergency department to another department within the same hospital, many of the same transfer risks are present and as such transfer should only be undertaken by appropriately trained staff.

In the UK, the Paediatric Critical Care Society has set a standard of practice for the transport of critically ill children (www.pccsociety.uk, last accessed January 2023). Where possible, it is recommended that transfers are undertaken by specialised paediatric critical care transfer teams. These teams can be contacted in the event of requests for the transfer of a child to a PCCU or a specialised facility such as a neurosurgical or burns unit. *Neonatal, Adult and Paediatric Safe Transfer and Retrieval: the Practical Approach* (NAPSTaR) (ALSG, 2016) is a sister publication to this manual that supports a practical course of the same name.

Transfers are undertaken to ensure that the child's care is of the highest possible standard at all times. To achieve this, the right child has to be taken at the right time, by the right people, to the right place, by the right form of transport, and receive the right care throughout. This requires a systematic approach that incorporates a high level of planning and preparation before the child is moved, for both acute and time critical transfers.

Differences between static and transport medicine

The medical care delivered on the move should, as far as possible, be identical to that delivered in the ward (static) environment. There are, however, limitations to this in that some therapies are not available in a mobile format and it is not always practical to take every piece of equipment that may be indicated even if it is suitable for the mobile environment. The team should be aware of the additional challenges faced during transport. These may be summarised through the acronym SCRUMP.

S	Shared assessment
C	Clinical isolation
R	Resource limitation
U	Unfamiliar equipment
M	Movement and safety
P	Physical and physiological changes

Shared assessment is included to highlight that in most instances of transfer, multiple teams are likely to be involved with the assessment and care of the child, at least one of which will be at a remote location. It is vital that each of these teams has access to all the key information they require in order to acquire and maintain their situation awareness. In practical terms this is achieved through fastidious, focused, closed-loop communication. This relies on all members of the team speaking up about information that they think is important and ensuring it is communicated to the other parties. It is also vital that team members are ready to speak up and request clarification on any aspect that is unclear to them because of confusing or incomplete information. Shared documentation and proformas will ensure this process is smooth and efficient.

Clinical isolation is perhaps the most obvious difference when a team works outside their normal clinical area. When planning the transfer it is important to recognise that physical isolation, with no additional supplies, equipment or personnel to hand, could mean no support whatsoever if communication devices fail, separating the team from their expert support. The team must therefore be fully self-sufficient by the time they move from the ward – a lift, stuck between floors, is, in many respects, no less isolating than an aircraft or ambulance on the road.

Resource limitation occurs by virtue of the isolation described. The team must ensure they carry sufficient consumables not only for the anticipated journey time, but also extra in case of delays. They must also pack appropriate supplies to address anticipated emergencies that might occur.

Unfamiliar equipment can present challenges at any time, but in the isolated environment of a transfer can present a major risk. Staff should never undertake transfers, however trivial, with equipment that they have not been trained to use.

Movement presents safety risks to the child, the transfer team and potentially the public when out on the roads. 'Make haste, not speed' is an idiom well applied to the transfer process. The process of moving the child from their bed to a stretcher or pod is the time when tubes and lines are most likely to be displaced. Plan all such moves, and brief the team before undertaking them. A discussion of the speed of travel is included later in this chapter.

Physical and physiological changes occur due to movement, particularly acceleration and deceleration forces on the road. They may also occur due to changes in atmospheric pressure when using air transport. These should be anticipated and wherever possible mitigated against.

Detailed discussions of these issues may be found in the NAPSTaR text and course.

ACCEPT: the systematic approach to the transfer of a child

One systematic approach to safe transfer and retrieval is the ACCEPT method, which is described in detail in the NAPSTaR text and course.

A	Assessment
C	Control
C	Communication
E	Evaluation
P	Preparation and packaging
T	Transportation

Assessment

When commencing the transfer process a formal (re)assessment of the situation must be undertaken. Sometimes the clinicians undertaking the transportation may have been involved in the care given up to that point. Increasingly, however, the transport team will have been brought in specifically for that purpose and will have no prior knowledge of the child's clinical history. The process of assessment and reassessment continues throughout the time of the transfer, continually monitoring for changes in the child's condition and taking remedial action where appropriate.

Control

Once the initial assessment is complete, the transport coordinator needs to take control of the situation. This requires:

- Identification of the clinical and logistical team leader(s)
- Identification of the tasks to be carried out
- Allocation of tasks to individuals or teams

The lines of responsibility must be established promptly. Ultimate responsibility is held jointly by the referring consultant clinician, the consultant clinician at the receiving centre and the transport personnel at different stages of the transport process. There should always be a clearly identified person with overall responsibility for organising the transport.

Communication

Moving ill children from one place to another requires cooperation and the involvement of many people. Key personnel need to be informed when transportation is being considered (Box 23.2).

Box 23.2 People who need to know about a transfer

Current (local) clinical team
- Consultant in charge
- Clinicians at bedside
- Referring doctor/nurse
- Nurse in charge
- Child's family

Transfer team
The transfer coordinator should disperse information to:
- Consultant in charge
- Clinician(s) undertaking transfer
- Ambulance providers
- Child's family

Receiving team
The transfer coordinator or receiving unit coordinator should disperse information to:
- Consultant accepting referral
- Other consultants who will need to be involved in care (paediatric critical care unit, surgical and anaesthetic teams)
- Receiving doctors
- Receiving nursing staff
- Child's family

Communication may take a long time to complete if one person does it all. It is therefore advisable to share the tasks between appropriate people, taking into account expertise and local policies. In all cases it is important that information is passed on clearly and unambiguously. This is particularly the case when talking to people over the telephone. It is useful to plan what to say before telephoning and to use the systematic summary shown below. It is also useful in complex conversations to summarise the situation and repeat what you need from the listener at the end.

The content of all discussions should be documented in the child's notes.

Key elements in any communication

- Who you are
- Contact details
- What the problem is (soundbite)
- What you need (from the listener)
- What you have done
- Effect of these actions
- Summarise agreed plans

Evaluation

The aim of evaluation is to confirm that transfer is appropriate for the child and, if so, what the clinical urgency is. Whilst evaluation is a dynamic process that starts from first contact with the child, it is usually only when the first phase of ACCEPT (that is, ACC) has been completed that enough information will have been gathered to fully evaluate the transport needs.

Is transport appropriate for this child?

Critically ill babies and children require transport because of the need for:

- Specialist treatment
- Specialist investigations that are unavailable in the referring hospital
- Specialist facilities that are unavailable in the referring hospital

The risks involved in transport must be balanced against the risks of staying and the benefits of care that can be given only by the receiving unit.

What clinical urgency does this child have?

Once it has been established that transfer is needed, the urgency must be evaluated. The degree of urgency for transfer and the severity of illness may be used to rank the child's transfer needs. This decision will determine both the personnel required and the mode and speed of transport.

Some children will require a time-critical transfer, when delays must be minimised to transport the child to where emergency definitive treatment can be delivered to prevent imminent deterioration and a poor outcome. An example of this may be a child with an expanding extradural haematoma that needs surgical evacuation. Although speed is essential, safety is paramount. All trauma receiving units should plan and have systems to be able to undertake such a transfer when required.

In other situations, a semi-elective transfer may be appropriate. An example of this may be a haemodynamically stable child with a liver or spleen laceration. This child should be transferred to a paediatric surgical centre for monitoring as they may require specialist intervention. As they are stable, there is time to plan transfer and use of the best resources.

Preparation and packaging

Both preparation and packaging have the aim of ensuring that transport proceeds uneventfully, with no deterioration in the child's condition. The first stage (preparation) involves the completion of stabilisation and preparation of transfer team personnel and equipment. The second stage (packaging) involves the final measures that need to be taken to ensure the security and safety of the child, equipment and staff during the transportation itself.

Child preparation

To reduce complications during any journey, adequate resuscitation and stabilisation should be carried out before transfer. This may involve carrying out procedures requested by the receiving hospital or unit. The standard airway, breathing, circulation, disability, exposure and family (ABCDEF) approach should be followed. The airway must be cleared and secured and appropriate respiratory support established. Two points of secure venous access are essential and may include a sutured multilumen central line as one point. Where two points cannot be achieved an IO line may be substituted for one lumen of access. The child must have received adequate fluid resuscitation to ensure optimal tissue oxygenation. Hypovolaemic children tolerate the inertial forces of transportation very poorly. Children with a suspected spinal injury should be appropriately immobilised.

Occasionally, in time-critical situations such as trauma or an acute abdominal emergency, this process may not be fully completed before packing and transport. Decisions to transfer in these circumstances should be taken only by senior personnel.

Inadequate resuscitation or missed illnesses (and injuries) may result in instability during transfer and may adversely affect the child's outcome.

Equipment preparation

All equipment must be tested and have adequate power reserves. Supplies of drugs and fluids should be more than adequate for the whole of the intended journey. The essential items of paediatric transport equipment are shown in Box 23.3.

Box 23.3 Paediatric transport equipment

Airway
- Induction drugs
- Oropharyngeal airways: sizes 000, 00, 0, 1, 2, 3 and 4
- Tracheal tubes: sizes 3.5–8.0 mm cuffed (in 0.5 mm steps) and 2.5–6.0 mm uncuffed
- Tracheal tube stylets
- Laryngeal masks: sizes 1.0–5.0
- Laryngoscope handles ×2:
  - straight paediatric blades
  - curved blades
- Magill forceps
- Portable suction unit
- Yankauer suckers: paediatric and adult
- Soft suction catheters: sizes 6, 8, 10 and 12
- Humidity moisture exchange (HME) unit
- Needle cricothyroidotomy set

Breathing
- Oxygen masks with reservoir
- Self-inflating bags (with reservoir): sizes 500 and 1600 ml
- Portable ventilator
- Face masks:
  - infant – circular 0, 01, 1 and 2
  - child – anatomical 2 and 3
  - adult – anatomical 4 and 5
- Catheter mount and connectors
- Ayre's T-piece or Waters' circuit (Mapleson F and C, respectively), as appropriate for child's size

Circulation
- Electrocardiogram monitor + defibrillator (with paediatric pads)
- Invasive and non-invasive (oscillometric) blood pressure monitor (with appropriate-sized cuffs)
- Pulse oximeter (with infant- and child-sized probes)
- End-tidal CO_2 monitor

Usually the four monitors above will be combined within one monitoring device, which will also include temperature and pressure channels

- Intravenous access requirements:
  - intravenous cannulae (as available): 18–25 gauge
  - intraosseous infusion needles: 16–18 gauge
  - graduated burette
  - intravenous giving sets
  - syringes: 1–50 ml
  - three-way taps, Luer-locking T-extensions, etc.
  - intravenous drip monitoring device/syringe pumps
  - central (or umbilical for newborns) and arterial line sets

Fluids
- Plasma-Lyte 148, Hartmann's solution or Ringer's lactate
- 0.9% sodium chloride
- 0.45% sodium chloride and 5% glucose
- 10% glucose

Drugs
- Adrenaline 1:10 000
- Adrenaline 1:1000

Box 23.3 *(Continued)*

- Atropine 600 micrograms/ml or 1 mg/ml
- Sodium bicarbonate 4.2% or 8.4%
- Dopamine 200 mg/5 ml
- Lidocaine 1%
- Amiodarone
- Calcium gluconate 10%
- Furosemide 20 mg/ml
- Mannitol 10% or 20% + 2.7% sodium chloride
- Antibiotics: broad-spectrum antibiotics as per local protocols
- Morphine, benzodiazepine and paralysing agent, made up as infusions

Miscellaneous
- Battery-operated suction device
- Nasogastric tubes: sizes 6, 8 and 10
- Chest drain set
- Stick test for glucose
- Sharps disposal box

Particular care should be taken with supplies of oxygen, inotropes, sedative drugs and batteries for portable electronic equipment. An example oxygen calculation is shown below:

Calculate the amount of oxygen required for the journey using the following:

$$\text{Number of cylinders} = \frac{2 \times \text{Duration of journey} \times \text{Flow (l/min)}}{\text{Cylinder capacity (litres)}}$$

For example, if oxygen is provided at 10 l/min for a journey intended to take 120 minutes, this would need four size E cylinders, each containing 600 litres. This allows for at least twice as much oxygen as the estimated journey time requires. Always take more than one cylinder in case of leakage or failure

A member of the team should be allocated the task of ensuring that all documentation including case notes, investigations, radiographs, reports and a transfer form, accompany the child. The team should carry a mobile phone together with contact names and numbers to enable direct communication with both the receiving and base units. In addition, all personnel need appropriate clothing, food if the journey is long and enough money to enable them to get home independently if needed.

Personnel preparation

The number and nature of staff accompanying children during transport will depend on their transfer category. All staff must practice within their competences. Whatever the category of the child, all personnel should be familiar with the relevant transfer procedures and the equipment that is to be used, as well as the details of the child's clinical condition. The team should be covered by accident insurance with adequate provision for personal injury or death sustained during the transfer.

Packaging

All lines and drains must be secured to the child, the child must be secured to the trolley and the trolley must be secured to the transport vehicle. This is especially important in neonatal transfers using a transport system that typically weighs over 100 kg. In an ambulance, all equipment fastenings should be CEN compliant. When changing oxygen supply (either from hospital to trolley cylinder or to ambulance supply) always conduct a 'tug test' to ensure the oxygen pipe is securely in the valve. This is done by one firm pull on the pipe to check it does not disconnect. Chest drains should be secured and unclamped, with consideration to whether underwater seal devices need to be replaced by an appropriate flutter valve system. A special kit should be prepared to enable chest drain insertion or replacement en route if necessary. The child should be adequately covered to prevent heat loss. Care must be taken to ensure that coverings are arranged to permit ready access to the child, lines and drains during transfer.

Transportation

Mode of transport

The choice of transport needs to take into account several factors.

Road ambulances are by far the most common means of transport. They have a low overall cost and rapid mobilisation time, and are not generally affected by weather conditions. They also give rise to less physiological disturbance. Air transfer may be preferred for journeys of more than 2.5 hours or if road access is difficult. The speed of the journey itself has to be balanced against organisational delays and also the need for inter-vehicle transfer at the start and end of the journey. Staff undertaking air transfers should have received specific training with regard to safety and flight physiology. They should not undertake such transfers without supervised experience.

Factors affecting mode of transfer

- Nature of illness
- Urgency of transfer
- Mobilisation time
- Geographical factors
- Weather
- Traffic conditions
- Cost

Care during transport

Destabilisation may occur during transportation and may arise from the effects of the transport environment on the vulnerable physiology of the child. Careful preparation can minimise the deleterious effects of inertial forces, such as tipping, acceleration and deceleration, as well as changes in temperature and barometric pressure.

The standard of care and the level of monitoring carried out before transfer needs to be continued, as far as possible, during the transfer. Monitoring should include:

- Oxygen saturation
- Electrocardiogram (ECG) and heart rate
- Regular non-invasive or continuous blood pressure
- End-tidal CO_2 in all intubated children and neonates
- Core and ambulance temperature

The child should be well covered and kept warm during the transfer.

Road speed decisions depend on clinical urgency. Although blue lights and sirens may be appropriate in order to get through heavy traffic, excessive speed is very rarely indicated. It is a risk to the child, the transfer team and the general public, and should be the exception rather than the rule.

With adequate preparation, the transportation phase is usually incident-free. However, untoward events do occur. Should this be the case, the child needs to be reassessed using the ABCDE approach and appropriate corrective measures then instituted. If the transport team need to release their seatbelts, the ambulance must stop first at a safe place. If a major deterioration occurs, transfer to the nearest hospital for further stabilisation and support may be appropriate. The benefits of intervention should always be weighed against the risks of delaying arrival at the receiving hospital with its better facilities. Following any untoward events, communication with the receiving unit is important. This should follow the systematic summary described earlier.

Handover

At the end of the transfer, direct contact with the receiving team must be established. A succinct, systematic summary of the child and transfer should be provided *before* transferring the child on to the local bed/cot. It must be accompanied by a written record of the child's history, vital signs, therapy and significant clinical events during transfer. All the other documents that have been taken with the child should also be handed over. Once verbal handover has been completed, the child may be moved with monitoring and ventilator equipment from the transport trolley to the receiving unit's cot or bed. The team can then retrieve all of their equipment and personnel and make their way back to their home unit. Standard documentation with shared proformas may aid this process and ensure all relevant information is handed over, as well as equipment retrieved.

23.3 Summary

This chapter has described the need for paying meticulous attention to the initial assessment and resuscitation. A useful checklist prior to transporting a child is shown in Box 23.4.

Box 23.4 Checklist prior to transporting a child

1. Is the airway secure and protected and is ventilation satisfactory? (Substantiated by blood gases, pulse oximetry and capnography if possible and tug test performed)
2. Is the spine appropriately immobilised?
3. Is there sufficient oxygen (and air) available for the journey?
4. Is appropriate vascular access secure and will the pumps in use during transport work by battery?
5. Have adequate fluids been given prior to transport?
6. Is the child receiving adequate sedation, analgesia and, if used, paralysis?
7. Are fractured limbs appropriately splinted and immobilised?
8. Are appropriate monitors in use?
9. Will the child/baby be sufficiently warm during the journey – ambulance heater, head coverings for child, etc.?
10. Is documentation available? Include:
    - Child's name
    - Age and date of birth
    - Known or estimated weight
    - Clinical notes
    - Observation charts, including neurological charts
    - Time and route of all drugs given
    - Fluid charts
    - Ventilator records
    - Results of investigations, including blood, urine, x-rays and scans
    - Names and contacts of medical and nursing staff involved in referral, receipt and during transport
    - Family/guardian names and contact numbers
11. Is the necessary resuscitation equipment available?
12. Is appropriate treatment available for managing anticipated emergencies, e.g. rising ICP?
13. Has the case been discussed with the receiving team directly?
14. Has the receiving unit been advised of an estimated time of arrival?
15. Have plans been discussed with the parents, including issues of consent?

PART 6
Appendices

Acid–base balance and blood gas interpretation

Learning outcomes

After reading this appendix, you will be able to:

- Describe the approach to acid–base balance in the seriously ill or injured child
- Interpret a blood gas analysis

A.1 Introduction

Acid–base problems may be respiratory or metabolic in origin, or a combination of the two. Impairments to respiration and metabolism usually lead to an accumulation of acid, although respiratory and metabolic alkaloses are sometimes also encountered.

Respiratory. When alveolar ventilation is inadequate, either due to inadequate breathing or inadequate artificial ventilation, carbon dioxide (CO_2) accumulates, and blood PCO_2 rises. The CO_2 combines with water to form carbonic acid, which contributes to an acid (low) pH.

Hence this is called a respiratory acidosis. The treatment is to lower the CO_2 by treating the respiratory problem, or adjusting the ventilator settings, to increase alveolar ventilation.

A respiratory alkalosis will occur with acute hyperventilation and excessive alveolar ventilation such that additional CO_2 is expired, leading to a decrease in PCO_2. This may be observed in acute asthma or with excessive artificial ventilation.

Metabolic. Impairment of normal metabolism may occur, for example in shock when a reduced supply of oxygenated blood reduces oxidative metabolism. In this case lactic acid forms, and it is this that contributes to an acid pH, which is described as a metabolic acidosis. In a pure metabolic acidosis, the PCO_2 is normal or may be low.

A metabolic alkalosis will occur with an intracellular shift of hydrogen ions; a loss of hydrogen ions from the body via the gastrointestinal tract or the kidneys; or the administration of exogenous bicarbonate. It will only persist when the excretion of bicarbonate by the kidneys is impaired, such as with hypochloraemia or hypokalaemia.

The terms acidosis and acidaemia are sometimes loosely used interchangeably. However, acidaemia and alkalaemia represent acidity of the blood that is outside the normal range. The terms acidosis and alkalosis refer to the underlying processes that lead to the acidaemia/alkalaemia, if severe enough to drive the pH or [H⁺] out of the normal range. For example, diabetic ketoacidosis (DKA) starts gradually and the acidaemia only occurs after it has been progressing for a period of time long enough to change the pH/[H⁺] significantly. The DKA still exists early on, yet the pH remains

---

Advanced Paediatric Life Support: A Practical Approach to Emergencies, Seventh Edition. Edited by Stephanie Smith.
© 2023 John Wiley & Sons Ltd. Published 2023 by John Wiley & Sons Ltd.

within the 'normal range' as various buffers in the blood act to inhibit pH changes. In DKA and all other acid–base abnormalities, it is important to identify and treat the underlying process, which is the driver of the pH/[H⁺] change, not simply attempt to normalise the pH/[H⁺].

Alterations in the acid–base status causing acidaemia or alkalaemia can also have significant effects on the body's physiology (Table A.1).

Table A.1 Effects of changes in acid–base status on physiology	
Acidaemia	**Alkalaemia**
Right shift of the oxyhaemoglobin dissociation curve	Left shift of the oxyhaemoglobin dissociation curve
Increased pulmonary vascular resistance	Decreased pulmonary vascular resistance
Decreased response to catecholamines	Decreased cerebral blood flow
Increased risk of ventricular arrhythmias	
Myocardial dysfunction	

Blood gases. The measurement of blood gases allows for the direct analysis of the pH/[H⁺], PCO_2, PO_2, a calculated value of bicarbonate (HCO_3^-) and a derived value for the base excess (BE). It will usually include an oxygen saturation value that may be directly measured or calculated, plus measurements of lactate, glucose and other electrolyte concentrations. These values can then be used to augment the comprehensive ABCDE assessment in terms of the effectiveness of ventilation, oxygenation, circulation and perfusion.

Normal ranges for the blood gas values in air, dependent on the sample type, are given in Table A.2.

Table A.2 Normal blood gas values			
	Arterial	**Venous**	**Capillary**
pH	7.35–7.45	7.33–7.44	7.35–7.45
PCO_2	4.6–6.0 kPa	5.0–6.4 kPa	4.6–6.0 kPa
PO_2	More than 10.6 kPa	5.3 kPa	Variable kPa
HCO_3^-	22–28 mmol/l	22–28 mmol/l	22–28 mmol/l
Base excess (BE)	+2/–2 mmol/l	+2/–2 mmol/l	+2/–2 mmol/l
Oxygen saturation	More than 95%	72–75%	Variable %

A.2   Hydrogen ion concentration, acidity and pH

Many chemical reactions in our cells are rate dependent on the appropriate temperature and acidity. The concentration of many chemicals in the blood is measured in millimoles (mmol: thousandth of a mole). For example, a sodium concentration [Na⁺] may be expressed as 140 mmol/l. Acidity is determined by hydrogen ions, whose concentration [H⁺] is very much lower in the blood and is expressed in nanomoles (nmol: thousand-**millionth** of a mole).

Acidity could be simply expressed as a value of the hydrogen ion concentration in nanomoles. Indeed, it has been argued that blood acidity could and should be expressed directly as the hydrogen ion concentration in nanomoles; however, it remains the case that pH is far more widely used.

Because of the enormous variation in hydrogen ion concentrations that may be encountered in general (Table A.3), the pH scale was devised. In the pH scale, [H⁺] is expressed as the negative logarithm of [H⁺]. The lower the pH, the greater the acidity; quite small differences in the numerical pH reflect large differences in hydrogen ion concentration (Figure A.1 and Table A.3). A whole integer change in pH reflects a 10-fold change in [H⁺], so that [H⁺] is 10 nmol at pH 8, 100 nmol at pH 7 and 1000 nmol at pH 6.

Table A.3 The pH scale		
Concentration of hydrogen ions compared with distilled water	**Approx. pH**	**Examples of solutions of this pH**
10 000 000	pH = 0	Battery acid
100 000	pH = 2	Vinegar
1000	pH = 4	Tomato juice, acid rain
1	pH = 7	'Pure' water at 25°C
0.01	pH = 9	Baking soda
0.0001	pH = 11	Ammonia solution
0.0000001	pH = 14	Liquid drain cleaner

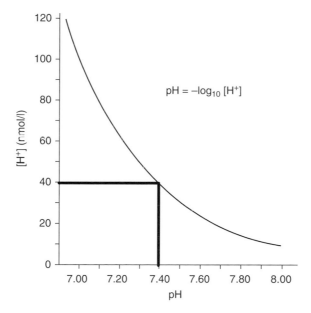

Figure A.1 Relationship between hydrogen ion concentration [H⁺] and pH. As can be seen a pH of 7.4 relates to a hydrogen ion concentration of 40 nmol/l (0.000040 mmol/l)

Thus at a normal blood pH of 7.4, [H⁺] is 40 nmol/l, whereas at pH 7.0 it is 100 nmol/l. Although the concentrations of hydrogen ions may vary widely in proportionate terms, their absolute concentrations in nanomoles are very low compared with other ions in millimoles. Thus, we control the absolute concentration of hydrogen ions much more precisely than sodium ions (measured in millimoles). On the other hand, we may survive a 2.5x increase in [H⁺] from 40 to 100 nmol/l, whereas we would not survive a 2.5x increase in [Na⁺] from say 140 to 350 mmol/l.

Strictly speaking, we should refer to hydrogen ion activity, not concentration, as ions may interact with each other and reduce their effective concentration. However, at the low levels found in the body (Table A.4), this is not a significant consideration.

Table A.4 pH in different parts of the body

Site	pH	Hydrogen ion concentration (mmol/l)	Hydrogen ion concentration (nmol/l)
Stomach, maximum acidity	0.8	150	150 000 000
Urine, maximum acidity	4.5	0.03	30 000
Plasma:			
Severe acidosis	7.0	0.0001	100
Normal	7.4	0.00004	40
Severe alkalosis	7.7	0.00002	20

A.3 Carbonic acid reaction

The chemical relationship between CO_2 and water (the 'carbonic acid reaction') shown in equation 1 is important. It shows how CO_2 can be carried in the blood, as HCO_3^-, and be released in the lungs to allow ventilation to remove this end product of cellular respiration.

$$CO_2 + H_2O \rightleftharpoons H_2CO_3 \rightleftharpoons H^+ + HCO_3^-$$
Equation 1

CO_2 and H_2O can combine to form H_2CO_3 (carbonic acid), which in turn can dissociate into H^+ and HCO_3^-. The [H^+] will depend on the ratio between the PCO_2 and the bicarbonate concentration [HCO_3^-], and this is expressed in equation 2, where K is the dissociation constant:

$$\left[H^+\right] = K \times \left([CO_2] / [HCO_3^-]\right)$$
Equation 2

which can then be expressed logarithmically as the Henderson–Hasselbalch equation:

$$pH = pK + \log\left([HCO_3^-] / PCO_2\right)$$
Equation 3

(The pK is approximately 6.1.)

Importantly, pH is thus dependant on the ratio between [HCO_3^-] and PCO_2, which are not independent of each other (see equation 3).

As we breathe, we exhale CO_2 produced as a metabolic waste product (the PCO_2 thus being determined by the balance between CO_2 production in the body, and the rate at which we exhale CO_2). The rate at which we exhale CO_2 is directly related to alveolar ventilation. In ventilated patients the PCO_2 is determined by the ventilator strategy, while in spontaneously breathing patients the PCO_2 is determined by their respiratory centre.

One of the major stimuli to breathing is the pH of the cerebrospinal fluid (CSF). If the CSF becomes acidotic, then there is increased respiratory drive to exhale CO_2; if the CSF becomes alkalotic, then the reverse is true. Bicarbonate does not cross the blood–brain barrier but is secreted in the CSF as it is produced in the choroid plexus (CSF bicarbonate levels thus approximate serum levels some hours previously). CO_2 does cross the blood–brain barrier easily, with CSF PCO_2 being essentially equivalent to current serum PCO_2.

The CSF pH is thus affected by the underlying bicarbonate levels and the current PCO_2 (remembering that the pH depends on the ratio between the two, which means that if the bicarbonate levels are low, a low PCO_2 is required for a normal pH and if bicarbonate levels are high, the reverse is true). The consequence of this system is that a rise in PCO_2 in the blood will usually be followed by an increase in ventilatory effort from increased respiratory drive.

Thus short-term control of pH happens via the brain and the respiratory system. However, over the longer term, the kidneys can produce bicarbonate by excreting H^+ ions. If pH levels are persistently low, the kidneys will respond by increased excretion of acid and thus increased production of HCO_3^-, which will tend to compensate for the acidosis. This is a relatively slow process, taking place over several hours or days. On the other hand, ventilatory changes can rapidly alter blood PCO_2. Hence in an acute respiratory illness PCO_2 may be raised with a normal HCO_3^-, whereas in a chronic respiratory illness PCO_2 may be raised alongside a raised, 'compensatory' HCO_3^-.

A.4 Standard bicarbonate

Blood gas analysers measure pH, PCO_2 and PO_2, and use the Henderson–Hasselbalch equation to calculate the HCO_3^- levels; other parameters such as BE are in turn derived. As PCO_2 and HCO_3^- are not independent of each other, the concept of 'standard bicarbonate' has been established. The standard bicarbonate (SBC) is 'what the HCO_3^- would have been if the PCO_2 were normal'. In the past, this was measured by exposing the blood in an analyser to a gas mixture with a PCO_2 of 5.3 kPa (40 mmHg in the units then used). Now it is calculated by blood gas analysers using data from in vitro studies.

SBC and BE have been researched in an attempt to provide some insight into whether abnormalities in acid–base balance are related to respiratory or metabolic factors. If acidosis is related to a respiratory problem, then the SBC will be normal or high, with a base excess; if it is related to a metabolic problem, then the SBC will be low and there will be a base deficit. The reverse is true for alkalosis.

A.5 Stewart's strong ion theory

For many years acid–base balance in the body was seen primarily in terms of the carbonic acid reaction. It is still the case that for many acid–base disturbances, the 'traditional' approach to acid–base balance outlined earlier is of the most practical use, and for the clinician the three measures of pH, PCO_2 and SBC or BE are of the most use.

However, there are some problems with this approach as the carbonic acid system is not the only relationship between pH, anion⁻ and acid in the body, and it is not possible to identify and fully understand the causes of metabolic and respiratory acidosis or alkalosis from the carbonic acid reaction alone. There are other pH and anion relationships, including the phosphate systems and the protein system (where albumin is normally the predominant protein). In addition, $[H^+]$ is affected by factors such as the need for electrical neutrality in the body.

In 1978, Stewart proposed his 'strong ion theory'. According to that proposal, there are six 'dependent' ion concentrations, whose concentrations are determined by concentrations of other ions and molecules. These are $[H^+]$, $[OH^-]$, $[HCO_3^-]$, $[CO_3^-]$, $[HA]$ and $[A^-]$ (weak, or poorly dissociated, acids and ions). The concentration of each of the 'dependent variables' is dependent on three 'independent variables'. The three independent variables that affect the pH in the body are:

- PCO_2 as discussed in the carbonic acid reaction section
- SID, the 'strong ion difference', which is the charge difference between negatively charged ions or anions (e.g. chloride) and positively charged cations (e.g. sodium) in the plasma
- $[A_{TOT}]$, the total concentration of all the non-volatile weak acids in the body (this includes phosphates and proteins, of which albumin is usually the dominant factor)

The important consideration is that the variables that actually control pH are PCO_2, SID and $[A_{TOT}]$. All other variables are dependent on these factors. Thus acidosis or alkalosis is the consequence of a combination of changes in these three parameters. Calculating the effect of the three independent variables is complicated, however, involving six complex simultaneous equations. This is a major shortcoming of the direct clinical application of Stewart's ideas, which have, however, made significant contributions to our understanding of acid–base physiology.

Total weak acids

These non-volatile weak acids are albumin and other plasma proteins, and phosphate. Phosphate levels are usually low. Albumin and other proteins are weak acids; hence albumin infusions may contribute to acidaemia.

Strong ion difference

Stewart pointed out that the acid base–balance is profoundly affected by strong ions (which are ions that exist mostly in ionic form, rather than in combined form as molecules). One over-riding principle is that electrical neutrality has to be maintained in a system. The strong ions in the extracellular fluid include the positively charged ions, or cations, Na^+, K^+, Ca^{2+} and Mg^{2+}, and the negatively charged ions, or anions, Alb^-, $Phos^{2-}$, $Lact^-$ and Cl^-.

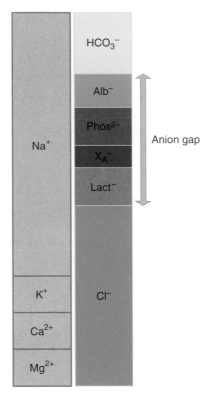

Figure A.2 Ions and their charges in extracellular fluid
X_A^-, unmeasured weak acids

As can be seen in Figure A.2, Na^+ and Cl^- make up the majority of the cations and anions, respectively, and changes in their concentrations (and ratios) will be expected to have the most impact on the $[HCO_3^-]$, while changes in Ca^{2+}, Mg^{2+} or phosphate will have little effect. Under normal circumstances, lactate concentration would also be very low, with minimal effect, although this will change as levels rise. The H^+ concentration is so tiny that in electrical terms it is irrelevant to this balance. HCO_3^- is, in fact, an electrical buffer (not just a 'biochemical' one) and its function is to 'flex up and down' to accommodate other electrolyte changes (and charges). Hence the value of HCO_3^- depends on all the other (metabolic) values in the figure, that is, HCO_3^- is a dependent variable, dependent on metabolic values. The $[HCO_3^-]$ in this context is largely dependent on the need to maintain electrical neutrality.

Hyperchloraemic acidosis

The consequence of this concept is that an increase in $[Cl^-]$ relative to $[Na^+]$ would have the effect of decreasing the $[HCO_3^-]$ and thus create an acidosis. As an example, an infusion of 0.9% saline

(154 mmol/l of both Na^+ and Cl^- in a ratio of 1:1) would increase the ratio of $[Cl^-]$ relative to $[Na^+]$ (as the normal ratio $[Na^+]:[Cl^-]$ in the extracellular fluid is less than 0.8) and create an acidosis. Similarly, an infusion of a weak acid such as albumin would result in a decrease in $[HCO_3^-]$ and create an acidosis.

Conversely, an increase in $[Na^+]$ relative to $[Cl^-]$ would have the effect of increasing $[HCO_3^-]$ and thus create alkalosis. A typical example is what happens when children are given loop diuretics. The diuretic therapy increases Cl^- losses relative to Na^+ and this will create an increase in $[HCO_3^-]$ with metabolic alkalosis.

The important issue to note is that changes in $[HCO_3^-]$ are not the primary cause of changes in acid–base status of the patient but that this is the consequence of other changes. This is true when considering both metabolic and respiratory acidosis or alkalosis.

Figure A.2 represents the ions and their charges in extracellular fluid. The left hand column contains cations (positive charge) and the right hand column anions (negative charge). **Positive and negative charges must be balanced at all times (electroneutrality).** A change in charge will be balanced by an increase or decrease in HCO_3^- and H^+. The unmeasured weak acids (X_A^-) would include acids such as may be present in ketoacidosis (diabetic, starvation, alcoholic), renal failure (residual acids are normally renally eliminated), poisons (e.g. methanol, ethanol, ethylene glycol, aspirin) or organic acidaemia (including methylmalonic acidaemia, propionic acidaemia, isovaleric acidaemia and maple syrup urine disease).

The anion gap is defined as $(Na^+ + K^+) - (Cl^- + HCO_3^-)$. It incorporates all the other anions and/or cations for which measurements are not usually available (sometimes termed unmeasured anions or cations). Strictly speaking the anion gap should be calculated by the formula $(Alb^- + Phos^{2-} + X_A^- + Lact^-) - (Ca^{2+} + Mg^{2+})$, but since Ca^{2+} and Mg^{2+} concentrations are small and vary minimally, we can ignore these ions and so simplify the anion gap (AG) as meaning simply the remaining anions after removing $(Cl^- + HCO_3^-)$. Hence AG = $(Alb^- + Phos^{2-} + X_A^- + Lact^-)$.

The anion gap

The AG is a useful concept. It is calculated by the formula:

$$AG = \left(Na^+ + K^+\right) - \left(Cl^- + HCO_3^-\right)$$

As can be seen from Figure A.2 (and expanded in Figure A.3), a large component of the normal AG is made up of the albumin. As albumin frequently changes dramatically in acute illness or injury, and this might then mask the severity of an acidotic process, it is sometimes useful to use the corrected anion gap (AG_c) in order to take those changes into account.

$$AG_c = \left(Na^+ + K^+\right) - \left(Cl^- + HCO_3^-\right) + 0.25 \times \left(42 - Alb\right)$$

Albumin is only slightly charged (about a quarter of a unit of charge per molecule) compared with 1 or 2 units of charge for most of the strong ions (e.g. Na^+ and $Phos^{2-}$) so we add a quarter of the albumin deficit to the normal, raw, uncorrected AG.

In Figure A.3 the left column shows normal anion values and a normal AG (grey arrow) in a normal child. The middle column shows results from a child with raised lactic acid and hence an increased AG (longer grey arrow) and a fall in HCO_3^-. In the patient shown in the right column, the high lactate has been offset by the fall in albumin, so the AG is apparently normal, hiding the underlying pathology, a lactic acidosis. This would be highlighted by recalculating the albumin-corrected AG, which would be abnormal.

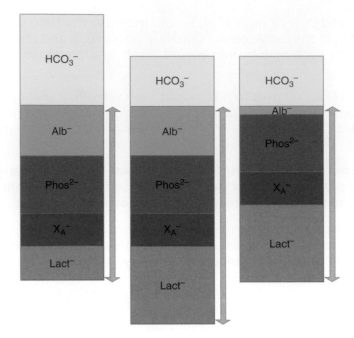

Figure A.3 Expansion of the components of the anion gap

Causes of a raised anion gap
- Lactic acidosis
- Other acids (X_A^-):
  - ketoacidosis (diabetic, starvation, alcoholic)
  - renal failure (residual acids are normally renally eliminated)
  - rhabdomyolysis
  - medications – isoniazid intoxication, salicylate poisoning
  - poisons – methanol, ethanol, ethylene glycol, propylene glycol
  - organic acidaemia: methylmalonic acidaemia, propionic acidaemia, isovaleric acidaemia, maple syrup urine disease

---

A.6 Applying this in practice

Interpretation of a blood gas analysis

Oxygen status: is there hypoxia?

- If the blood gas sample is arterial, is there 'relative' hypoxia in relation to the oxygen being delivered?
  - In air (21% oxygen), the PO_2 should be approximately 13 kPa
  - On 50% oxygen, the PO_2 should be approximately 40 kPa if there is normal gas exchange
- Check the oxygen saturation percentage

Acid–base status: is there acidosis or alkalosis?

- Check the pH:
  - Less than 7.35 – acidosis
  - More than 7.45 – alkalosis

Changes in acid–base homeostasis may be caused by respiratory or metabolic processes or a combination of the two (Figure A.4). In the Henderson–Hasselbalch equation, pH is related to the ratio of the metabolic (HCO_3^-) components to the respiratory (PCO_2) components.

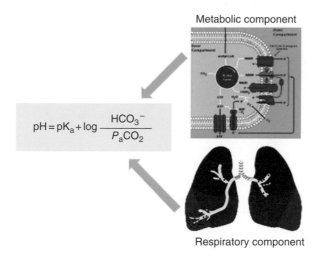

Metabolic component

$$pH = pK_a + \log \frac{HCO_3^-}{P_aCO_2}$$

Respiratory component

Figure A.4 Changes in acid–base homeostasis

What is the cause of the change in acid–base status: is it respiratory or metabolic?

- Check the PCO_2 in relation to the pH
  - pH less than 7.35 and PCO_2 more than 6.0 kPa implies respiratory acidosis
  - pH more than 7.45 and PCO_2 less than 4.6 kPa implies respiratory alkalosis

Primary respiratory abnormalities

Respiratory acidosis

In respiratory failure, there is an increase in PCO_2. If this happens rapidly, there will be a drop in pH (see the Henderson–Hasselbalch equation). However, if this happens gradually, or is persistent, there will be an increase in HCO_3^- production in the kidneys with 'compensation' or correction of the pH (Figure A.5). The SBC will tend to rise as the compensation occurs.

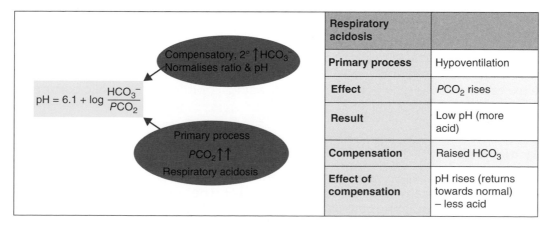

Compensatory, 2° ↑HCO_3^-
Normalises ratio & pH

$$pH = 6.1 + \log \frac{HCO_3^-}{PCO_2}$$

Primary process
PCO_2↑↑
Respiratory acidosis

Respiratory acidosis	
Primary process	Hypoventilation
Effect	PCO_2 rises
Result	Low pH (more acid)
Compensation	Raised HCO_3
Effect of compensation	pH rises (returns towards normal) – less acid

Figure A.5 Primary and compensatory changes in respiratory acidosis. Note the direction of changes in the numerator (HCO_3^-) and denominator (PCO_2) are in the same direction (arrows) – to normalise the ratio

Patient 1

A 3-month-old child with coryza symptoms for 2 days presenting with acute shortness of breath, poor feeding and the following initial assessment:

A Grunting and gasping
B Respiratory rate (RR) 64 breaths/min, SpO_2 90% on 15 litres oxygen, poor air entry throughout, subcostal and intercostal recession
C Heart rate (HR) 194 beats/min, blood pressure (BP) 73/37 mmHg, capillary refill time (CRT) 2–3 seconds, normal peripheries
D V on AVPU
E Looks unwell, no rash, pale; temperature (T) 37.1°C, glucose 5.1

Arterial blood gas:

	Normal values	Patient 1
pH	7.35–7.45	7.18
H^+	45–35	61
PO_2	13	9.5
PCO_2	5	8.1
Standard bicarbonate	24–25	23
Base excess	0±2	0
Saturation	>90	89
Lactate	2	1.8
Glucose	5	5
Na^+	140	134
K^+	4.5	3.5
Cl^-	95–100	102
Albumin	42	32
Urea	<7	4
Creatinine	<90	44

Interpretation:

- There is a relatively low PO_2 and a low saturation in oxygen suggesting significant hypoxia
- The pH is low (acidosis) and the PCO_2 is high with a normal standard bicarbonate and base excess suggesting an acute respiratory acidosis without metabolic compensation

Respiratory alkalosis

A primary increase in ventilation beyond that needed to keep PCO_2 normal drives the PCO_2 down. This reduces the denominator and hence increases pH. The respiratory alkalosis (a fall in PCO_2) moves the carbonic acid equilibrium to reduce HCO_3^- immediately, to a small degree, but over many hours and up to 2 days the HCO_3^- value falls (with a drop in SBC). This reduces the numerator, tending to normalise the ratio of HCO_3^- to PCO_2, thus reducing the impact on pH change and bringing the pH back towards normal (metabolic compensation) (Figure A.6).

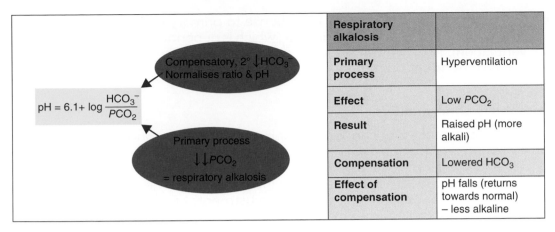

Figure A.6 Primary and compensatory changes in respiratory alkalosis. Note the direction of changes in the numerator (HCO$_3$$^-$) and denominator (PCO$_2$) are in the same direction (arrows) – to normalise the ratio

Patient 2

A 6-year-old child with a family history of atopy presenting to hospital with acute shortness of breath and wheeze and the following initial assessment:

A Able to speak in short phrases
B RR 44 breaths/min, SpO_2 94% on 15 litres oxygen, reduced air entry throughout with some late expiratory wheeze, intercostal recession
C HR 154 beats/min, BP 106/67 mmHg, CRT 1–2 seconds, warm peripherally
D A on AVPU
E No rash, pale; T 36.6°C, glucose 6.4

Arterial blood gas:

	Normal values	Patient 2
pH	7.35–7.45	7.52
H$^+$	45–35	28
PO_2	13	12
PCO_2	5	3.5
Standard bicarbonate	24–25	22
Base excess	0±2	–2
Saturation	>90	93
Lactate	2	2.2
Glucose	5	6
Na$^+$	140	144
K$^+$	4.5	3.0
Cl$^-$	95–100	102
Albumin	42	38
Urea	<7	3
Creatinine	<90	21

Interpretation:

- There is a low normal PO_2 and saturation in oxygen suggesting some hypoxia
- The pH is high (alkalosis) and the PCO_2 is low with a normal standard bicarbonate and base excess suggesting an acute respiratory alkalosis without metabolic compensation

It is important to note that HCO_3^- moves in response to primary changes in PCO_2. Therefore, the value of HCO_3^- is **dependent** on the value of PCO_2, which is dependent on changes in the respiratory system (i.e. ventilation). Next we will see that whilst HCO_3^- represents the metabolic component, paradoxically, it is **dependent** on metabolic issues too!

Primary metabolic abnormalities

A variety of metabolic processes can lead to primary acid–base abnormalities. When using the Henderson–Hasselbalch equation this is indicated by change in HCO_3^-. A reduction in HCO_3^- reduces the numerator and therefore reduces pH (see Figure A.2). An increase in HCO_3^- has the opposite effect. In a spontaneously breathing patient with intact feedback mechanisms, primary metabolic changes can be partially or fully compensated by adjustments of alveolar ventilation and therefore PCO_2. When HCO_3^- is decreased (metabolic acidosis), a resulting drop in pH can be moved back towards normal by increasing ventilation and reducing PCO_2. During a primary metabolic alkalosis (increased HCO_3^-) ventilation slows down, PCO_2 rises and pH is moved back towards normal.

It is important to note that HCO_3^- is only useful as a 'marker' as it is not in itself part of the underlying cause. It is an entirely **dependent** variable – its value changes in response to other (causative) metabolic processes. This provides some explanation of why the administration of sodium bicarbonate may not be helpful in the context of metabolic acidosis. The low bicarbonate is not actually the cause of the problem, it is merely a consequence of the problem and the focus needs to be on what is creating the situation.

Bicarbonate can be calculated from the Henderson–Hasselbalch equation, but it can also be calculated from the SID and $[A_{TOT}]$, where:

$$\left[HCO_3^-\right] = SID - \left[A_{TOT}\right] \qquad \text{Equation 4}$$

SID is the difference between the positive strong ions and the negative strong ions (a strong ion is one that exists mostly in the ionic rather than the associated, un-ionised form). Thus:

$$SID = \left(\left[Na^+\right] + \left[K^+\right] + \left[Ca^{2+}\right] + \left[Mg^{2+}\right]\right) - \left(\left[Cl^-\right] + \left[Lact^-\right]\right) \qquad \text{Equation 5}$$

As $[K^+]$ + $[Ca^{2+}]$ + $[Mg^{2+}]$ are always small numbers that do not vary much, this formula can be simplified to:

$$SID = \left[Na^+\right] - \left(\left[Cl^-\right] + \left[Lact^-\right]\right) \qquad \text{Equation 6}$$

and

$$\left[A_{TOT}\right] = \left(Alb^- + Phos^{2-} + X_A^-\right) \qquad \text{Equation 7}$$

Thus:

$$pH = pK + \log\left\{Na^+ - \left(Cl^- + Lact^- + Alb^- + Phos^{2-} + X_A^-\right)\right\} / PCO_2 \qquad \text{Equation 8}$$

Thus, from a metabolic perspective anything that increases the numerator in the formula (or increases the HCO_3^-) will increase the pH. This would include an increase in sodium or a drop in chloride, albumin or weak acids. Conversely a fall in sodium, or an increase in chloride, albumin or weak acids, would drop the pH.

Quantifying the aetiology of the metabolic acidosis

A metabolic acidosis produces a fall in HCO_3^-. This is mirrored by a fall in BE, that is, it becomes more negative (to put it another way, the base deficit increases). BE is the amount of acid or base that needs to be added to a blood sample in order to return the pH to 7.40 at a temperature of 37°C at a PCO_2 of 5.3 kPa (this is calculated using the standard bicarbonate as mentioned earlier).

Base excess eliminates any respiratory contributions and allows us to quantify the metabolic components of the acid–base abnormality. Both HCO_3^- and BE are useful indicators of the magnitude of the problem and run in parallel.

Each of the numerator components contributes to the overall BE on its own. We can identify and quantify the effects of the contributions of each of the numerator components to the overall net BE (and overall acid–base balance) by using some simple rules. Note that the total BE is the sum of BE changes arising from each component in the numerator:

- BE change due to sodium and chloride relationship $= (Na^+ - Cl^-) - 38$
- BE change due to the lactate present $= 2 - \text{lactate}$
- BE change due to albumin $= 0.25 \times (42 - \text{albumin})$
- BE change due to other acids (X_A^-) $= \text{Total BE} - \text{sum of the others}$

Patient 3

A 3-year-old child post-surgery needing administration of a significant volume of 0.9% saline and the following initial assessment:

A Patent
B RR 42 breaths/min, SpO_2 99% in air, good air entry, no respiratory distress
C HR 139 beats/min, BP 76/43 mmHg, CRT 2–3 seconds, cool peripheries
D A on AVPU, pupils equal and reactive
E No rash, pale; T 35.6°C, glucose 4.9

Arterial blood gas:

	Normal values	Patient 3
pH	7.35–7.45	7.28
H^+	45–35	52.5
PO_2	13	13
PCO_2	5	3.3
Standard bicarbonate	24–25	17.8
Base excess	0±2	–6.7
Saturation	>90	99
Lactate	2	1.5
Glucose	5	5
Na^+	140	142
K^+	4.5	4.2
Cl^-	95–100	115
Albumin	42	28
Urea	<7	5
Creatinine	<90	90
1. Na – Cl – 38 BE	(Na – Cl – 38) =	–11
2. Lactate BE	2 – lactate =	0.5
3. Albumin BE	0.25 × (42 – Alb) =	3.5
4. Residue (X_A BE)	BE – (1) – (2) – (3) =	0.3

Interpretation:

- There is a normal PO_2
- The pH has fallen (acidosis), the PCO_2 is low and the BE is –6.7 suggesting a metabolic acidosis
- For the metabolic acidosis, using formulae 1, 2, 3 and 4 above, it becomes clear that the main contributor is the hyperchloraemia caused by the saline, which alone would generate a base excess of –11 (formula 1)
- This is offset by the dilution effect on the albumin, which generates a metabolic alkalosis, giving a BE change of +3.5 (formula 3). Lactate contributes minimally as it is normal (formula 2) and residual BE is minimal (formula 4)

Patient 4

A 12-year-old patient in the emergency department with abdominal pain, 1 hour after starting treatment with two 10 ml//kg boluses of saline, and the following initial assessment:

A Patent
B RR 23 breaths/min, SpO_2 100% in 15 l/min face mask oxygen (which is not always kept on the face), good air entry, a deep, sighing respiratory pattern
C HR 125 beats/min, BP 82/47 mmHg, CRT 2–3 seconds, cool hands
D V on AVPU, pupils equal and reactive
E No rash; T 37.3°C, glucose unrecordable

Arterial blood gas:

	Normal values	Patient 4
pH	7.35–7.45	6.799
H^+	45–35	159
PO_2	13	18.3
PCO_2	5	1.68
Standard bicarbonate	24–25	4.3
Base excess	0±2	–35.2
Saturation	>90	96.6
Lactate	2	1
Glucose	5	35
Na^+	140	127
K^+	4.5	3.8
Cl^-	95–100	106
Albumin	42	41
Urea	<7	9.7
Creatinine	<90	98
(1) Na – Cl – 38 BE	(Na – Cl – 38) =	–17
(2) Lactate BE	2 – lactate =	1
(3) Albumin BE	0.25 × (42 – Alb) =	0.25
(4) Residue (X_A BE)	BE – (1) – (2) – (3) =	–19.45

Interpretation:

- There is a high PO_2 as the child is receiving 100% face mask oxygen
- The pH is very low (extreme acidosis), the PCO_2 is low and the BE is –35.2 suggesting a metabolic acidosis
- For the metabolic acidosis, using formulae 1, 2, 3 and 4 above, the BE change is partially due to the hyponatraemia and hyperchloraemia (formula 1) and partially due to other acids (formula 4)
- The other acids here are ketones of DKA – note the glucose of 35
- Note that the low pH stimulates respiration, hence Kussmaul breathing and the low PCO_2, respiratory compensation for the metabolic acidosis
- This is a common scenario, where the DKA itself and the treatment with normal saline produce changes in electrolyte status. The metabolic acidosis (and here profound metabolic acidaemia) is initially due to DKA but, as treatment continues, there is a phase of profound (sodium chloride induced) metabolic acidosis

Patient 5

A sick 1 year old patient in the emergency department with fever, hypotension and confusion and the following initial assessment:

A Patent
B RR 52 breaths/min, SpO_2 93% in 15 l/min face mask oxygen, decreased air entry on the right side of the chest and some intercostal recession
C HR 185 beats/min, BP 49/32 mmHg, CRT over 6 seconds, cold up to the elbows and knees
D V on AVPU, pupils equal and reactive
E Non-specific macular rash; T 39.3°C, glucose 3.1

Arterial blood gas:

	Normal values	Patient 5
pH	7.35–7.45	6.83
H^+	45–35	145.7
PO_2	13	8.6
PCO_2	5	6.8
Standard bicarbonate	24–25	6.7
Base excxess	0±2	–22.9
Saturation	>90	80
Lactate	2	15
Glucose	5	3
Na^+	140	133
K^+	4.5	6.6
Cl^-	95–100	104
Albumin	42	8
Urea	<7	17
Creatinine	<90	204
(1) Na – Cl – 38 BE	(Na – Cl – 38) =	–9
(2) Lactate BE	2 – lactate =	–13
(3) Albumin BE	0.25 × (42 – Alb) =	8.5
(4) Residue (XA BE)	BE – (1) – (2) – (3) =	–9.4

Interpretation:

- There is a low PO_2 despite the child is receiving 100% face mask oxygen, suggesting significant hypoxia
- The pH is very low (extreme acidosis), the PCO_2 is mildly elevated and the BE is –22.9, suggesting a mild respiratory and a significant metabolic acidosis
- For the metabolic acidosis, using formulae 1, 2, 3 and 4 above, the BE changes can be quantified. There is some sodium to chloride (strong ion) imbalance (contributing –9 to BE (formula 1)), a profound lactic acidosis (contributing –13 to total BE (formula 2)), the low albumin produces a metabolic alkalosis (+8.5 contribution to overall BE (formula 3)) and there is acute kidney injury (contributing –9.4 to overall BE (formula 4))
- This is a mixed picture of severe sepsis, possibly associated with a lower respiratory tract infection, with both a respiratory and metabolic acidosis with all components contributing somewhat to the BE calculation. Note that the glucose is also relatively low, which is not uncommon in this clinical presentation

A.7 Summary

This appendix has discussed how, in combination with the ongoing ABCDE assessment and resuscitation, correct interpretation of the various parts of blood gas measurements, including oxygenation, the acid–base status, and also quantifying the components of any metabolic acidosis, can allow for a greater understanding of the underlying cause for deterioration in a child, and may also help to guide the appropriate ongoing treatment.

APPENDIX **B**

Fluid and electrolyte management

Learning outcomes

After reading this appendix, you will be able to:

- Describe the approach to the management of fluid and electrolytes in the seriously ill or injured child
- Describe the approach to the management of the child with diabetic ketoacidosis

B.1   Introduction

At birth, approximately 80% of a child's body weight is water. This percentage falls gradually during childhood, reaching 60% water by adulthood. Total body water is normally distributed between the intracellular (67%), interstitial (25%) and intravascular (8%) spaces, moving from one compartment to another depending on various pressure and osmotic gradients. In illness and injury these fluid shifts may be rapid, with significant clinical consequences.

B.2   Fluid balance

Normally, fluid balance is tightly controlled by thirst, hormonal responses and renal function: the quantities in Table B.1 provide a guideline to appropriate fluid intake. These formulae are based on an assumption of 100 kcal/kg/day of caloric intake, 3 ml/kg/h of urine output and normal stool output.

Table B.1   Fluid requirements in well, normal children

Body weight	Fluid requirement per day (ml/kg)	Fluid requirement per hour (ml/kg)
First 10 kg	100	4
Second 10 kg	50	2
Subsequent kilograms	20	1

Advanced Paediatric Life Support: A Practical Approach to Emergencies, Seventh Edition. Edited by Stephanie Smith.
© 2023 John Wiley & Sons Ltd. Published 2023 by John Wiley & Sons Ltd.

For example:

- A 6 kg infant would require 600 ml/day
- A 14 kg child would require 1000 + 200 = 1200 ml/day
- A 25 kg child would require 1000 + 500 + 100 = 1600 ml/day

In critical illness or injury, some or all of these mechanisms may be profoundly disrupted, and fluid therapy has to be tailored to the needs of the specific child. In the presence of anuria due to acute renal failure, fluid requirements may fall below 30 ml/kg/day, while in high-output diarrhoea requirements may be as high as 400 ml/kg/day.

Fluid intake is required to replace fluid losses and to enable the excretion of various waste products through the urine. Insensible losses (via respiration and sweat) generally amount to between 10 and 30 ml/kg/day. The actual volume of insensible fluid loss is related to the caloric content of the feeds, ambient temperature, humidity of inspired air, presence of pyrexia and quality of the skin. Insensible losses from a child on a ventilator in a cool environment with minimal caloric intake may be minimal. Usually between 0 and 10 ml/kg/day are lost in the stool (this will increase markedly in diarrhoea, where losses in excess of 300 ml/kg/day are not uncommon). Urinary losses are between 1 and 2 ml/kg/h (i.e. approximately 30 ml/kg/day).

Dehydration and shock

Concepts

- Dehydration does not cause death, shock does. Shock may occur with the loss of 20 ml/kg from the intravascular space, while clinical dehydration is only evident after total losses of greater than 25 ml/kg
- As a guide, the child with dehydration and no shock can be assumed to be 5% dehydrated; if shock is present, then 10% dehydration or greater has occurred
- The treatment of shock requires the rapid administration of an intravascular volume of fluid that approximates in electrolyte content to plasma
- The treatment of dehydration requires a gradual replacement of fluids with an electrolyte content that relates to the electrolyte losses, or to the total body electrolyte content
- Pathology from electrolyte changes is related to either extreme levels or rapid rates of change
- Administration of sodium bicarbonate is rarely indicated
- Overhydration is potentially as dangerous as dehydration

The intravascular volume of an infant is c. 80 ml/kg, and of an older child 70 ml/kg. A rapid loss of 25% of this intravascular volume (i.e. 20 ml/kg) will cause shock unless that volume is replaced from the interstitial fluid at a similar rate. Clinical signs of dehydration (Table B.2) are only detectable when the patient is 2.5–5% dehydrated. Five per cent dehydration implies that the body has lost 5 g per 100 g body weight, that is, 50 ml/kg of total fluid (intracellular, interstitial and intravascular). Clearly, shock may occur in the absence of dehydration, dehydration may occur in the absence of shock, or both may occur together – all dependent on the rate of fluid loss and the rate of fluid shifts between the intracellular, interstitial and intravascular spaces.

The priorities of management are to identify shock and treat it effectively and rapidly (see Chapter 5), identify dehydration and institute a treatment programme that will enable effective rehydration over 24–48 hours, identify the presence and aetiology of acid–base problems and correct these where necessary, and identify the presence and aetiology of electrolyte abnormalities and correct these gradually without precipitating complications.

One factor remains unknown at the initiation of therapy, namely the ongoing fluid losses that will occur during therapy. Thus any plan of fluid management represents a starting point, and this will have to be modified in the light of data from constant monitoring.

The critical clinical questions are therefore:

- Is the patient shocked?
- Is the patient dehydrated?
- Does the patient have a significant acid–base abnormality?
- Are there significant electrolyte problems?

Table B.2 Signs and symptoms of dehydration and shock (adapted from NICE, 2009)

No clinically detectable dehydration	Clinical dehydration	Clinical shock
Appears well	Appears to be 'unwell'	Pale, lethargic or mottled
Normal breathing pattern	Normal or tachypnoea	Tachypnoea
Normal heart rate	Normal or tachycardia	Tachycardia
Normal peripheral pulses	Normal peripheral pulses	Weak peripheral pulses
Normal capillary refill time	Normal or mildly prolonged capillary refill time	Prolonged capillary refill time
Normal blood pressure	Normal blood pressure	Hypotension
Normal skin turgor	Reduced skin turgor	
Normal urine output	Decreased urine output	Decreased urine output
Alert and responsive	Altered responsiveness (e.g. irritable, lethargic)	Decreased level of consciousness
Eyes not sunken	Sunken eyes Depressed fontanelle*	
Moist mucous membranes (except after a drink)	Dry mucous membranes (except for 'mouth breathers')	
Warm extremities	Warm extremities	Cold extremities

*Only useful in an infant if still patent and in the absence of disorders such as meningitis.

Shock

The treatment of hypovolaemic shock secondary to intravascular fluid loss (after securing the airway and providing high-flow oxygen) is the rapid administration of crystalloid. The starting volume is 10 ml/kg, and this can be repeated if there is inadequate clinical response (with no evidence of intravascular overload). The fluids used should approximate in electrolyte concentrations to those of serum. Options include Plasma-Lyte 148, Hartmann's solution and 0.9% sodium chloride (Table B.3). The first two fluids are consider 'balanced fluids' but should be used with care in significant renal impairment as they contain potassium, while the risk of giving large volumes of 0.9% sodium chloride is hyperchloraemia leading to metabolic acidosis. The presence of hyper- or hyponatraemia does not affect the choice of fluids during this phase of resuscitation.

In the context of presumed severe sepsis, there is some concern about the use of excessive fluid boluses for resuscitation. It seems reasonable to continue with fluid bolus administration of 10 ml/kg with careful monitoring and assessment of the child's response. After 40 ml/kg total of fluid boluses, inotropic support should be considered.

A child with an underlying cardiac condition may not respond as expected to fluid boluses, and may require earlier initiation of inotropic support, as guided by expert advice

Table B.3 Commonly available crystalloid fluids

Fluid	Na⁺ (mmol/l)	K⁺ (mmol/l)	Cl⁻ (mmol/l)	Energy (kcal/l)	Other
Sodium chloride 0.9%	154	0	154	0	0
Plasma-Lyte 148	140	5	98	0	Magnesium, acetate, gluconate
Hartmann's solution	131	5	111	0	Calcium, lactate
Sodium chloride 0.45%, glucose 5%	77	0	77	200	0
Glucose 5%	0	0	0	200	0
Glucose 10%	0	0	0	400	0

Unless there is evidence of cardiac dysrhythmia or neurological abnormality, electrolyte abnormalities should be corrected gradually.

Once shock has been adequately treated, attention can turn to management of hydration. Frequent reassessment remains necessary as the patient may well become shocked again if the underlying cause of the fluid shifts between the various compartments (e.g. gastroenteritis) is ongoing.

Dehydration

Many clinical signs of dehydration are individually unreliable (Table B.2) and have poor interobserver reproducibility, but taken together they provide a reasonable estimate of total body fluid losses. Weight is the only clinically available objective measure of total body fluid changes and enables an accurate assessment of fluid balance over time. Unfortunately, initial fluid therapy must usually be based on a clinical assessment of hydration because the pre-sickness weight is not often available.

The measured weight loss or percentage dehydration is:

5% dehydration = loss of 5 ml of fluid per 100 g body weight, or 50 ml/kg

10% dehydrated = loss of 10 ml of fluid per 100 g body weight, or 100 ml/kg

Management of dehydration consists of the administration of calculated daily maintenance fluids in addition to calculated replacement fluids over a 24-hour period. Therapy should be monitored at 3–4-hourly intervals using weight as an objective measure if possible, to ensure that the patient is gaining weight at an appropriate rate. If the calculated fluid administration rate is too slow or too fast, then the rate should be modified appropriately. See Table B.3 for the commonly available crystalloid fluids.

When the gut is functioning, oral rehydration using standard solutions is preferred (the World Health Organization (WHO) formulation provides 75 mmol sodium, 20 mmol potassium, 65 mmol chloride, 10 mmol citrate and 75 mmol glucose per litre; the formulations recommended in the UK have lower sodium concentrations of 50–60 mmol/l). This fluid should be administered frequently in small volumes (a cup and spoon works very well for this process). Generally, normal feeds should be administered in addition to the rehydration fluid, particularly if the infant is breastfed.

When there is excessive vomiting or there are signs of a damaged bowel, fluid therapy should be given intravenously. Unless there is bowel damage, attempt an early and gradual introduction of oral rehydration therapy during intravenous fluid therapy. If tolerated, stop intravenous fluids and complete rehydration with oral rehydration therapy.

Example
A 6 kg child is clinically shocked and 10% dehydrated as a result of gastroenteritis

Initial therapy
Two 10 ml/kg boluses for shock = 6 × 10 × 2 = 120 ml of Plasma-Lyte 154 given as a rapid intravenous bolus

Estimated fluid therapy over the next 24 hours
100 ml/kg for 10% dehydration = 100 × 6 = 600 ml
100 ml/kg for daily maintenance fluid = 100 × 6 = 600 ml
Rehydration + maintenance = 1200 ml
Therefore start with an infusion of 1200/24 = 50 ml/h

Application of fluid therapy
Reassess clinical status and weight at 4–6 hours, and if satisfactory continue. If the child is losing weight increase the fluid rate, and if the weight gain is excessive decrease the fluid rate. Start giving more of the maintenance fluid as oral feeds if the child is tolerating the fluids

Fluid overload and overhydration

In the same way that fluid losses may cause shock, dehydration or both, excessive fluid administration can cause intravascular fluid overload, overhydration or both.

In the patient with nephrotic syndrome, fluid has leaked out of the intravascular space and into the tissues because of a low serum albumin. Such children may be grossly overhydrated, with diffuse severe oedema. However, many patients with nephrotic syndrome have a contracted intravascular space, and attempts to diurese these patients without first expanding the intravascular space with albumin may result in shock.

By contrast, the patient with myocardial dysfunction may have an intravascular compartment that is grossly overfilled. The clinical signs of intravascular overload may be present, and yet the patient (particularly if they have been on diuretics) may actually be total body fluid depleted and may appear dehydrated.

Children with renal impairment may present with a combination of intravascular and total body fluid overload. Administration of further fluid can worsen fluid overload leading to pulmonary oedema.

> The treatment of fluid overload can be complex and the non-specialist should seek expert advice

Electrolyte abnormalities

Table B.4 shows the normal electrolyte requirements.

Table B.4	Water, electrolyte and energy requirements in well, normal children				
Body weight	Water (ml/kg/day)	Sodium (mmol/kg/day)	Potassium (mmol/kg/day)	Energy (kcal/day)	Protein (g/day)
First 10 kg	100	2–4	1.5–2.5	110	3
Second 10 kg	50	1–2	0.5–1.5	75	1.5
Subsequent kilograms	20	0.5–1	0.2–0.7	30	0.75

Sodium

Both low and high sodium levels are potentially dangerous. Severe hypernatraemia may be associated with brain damage, because brain tissue shrinks as a result of intracellular dehydration and blood vessels may tear or become clotted. Too rapid correction of hypernatraemia may lead to cerebral oedema and convulsions. Similarly, rapid correction of hyponatraemia may also be associated with demyelination and permanent brain injury.

The electrolyte losses during dehydration depend on the reason for dehydration. In gastroenteritis, sodium losses in diarrhoea stool range from approximately 50 mmol/l (rotavirus) to approximately 80 mmol/l (cholera and enteropathogenic *Escherichia coli*). In renal dysfunction, sodium losses may be minimal (diabetes insipidus) or high (renal tubular dysfunction).

Hypernatraemia

Hypernatraemia in the dehydrated patient may be the end result of excessive loss of water (e.g. diabetes insipidus, diarrhoea), excessive intake of sodium (e.g. iatrogenic poisoning, non-accidental injury) or a combination of both (e.g. children with gastroenteritis given excessive sodium in the rehydration fluid).

The electrolyte content of the replacement solution depends on the cause of the dehydration. Previously, 0.45% sodium chloride, containing 77 mmol/L sodium chloride, was considered a safe starting solution for intravenous rehydration. This was based largely on the electrolyte content of stool in diarrhoea. By contrast, patients with rare renal tubular dysfunction who lose excessive sodium and water through their kidneys may require 0.9% sodium chloride to replace the renal losses of sodium. Measurement of the sodium content of the urine and stool may help direct replacement therapy. More recently, consensus guidelines have recommended starting with an isotonic solution such as Plasma-Lyte 148 (± 5% glucose) or 0.9% sodium chloride with 5% glucose for fluid-deficit replacement and maintenance for hypernatraemic dehydration. This is due to a number of children developing a rapid fall in sodium with hypotonic solutions.

The principles in the treatment of hypernatraemia are:

1. Treat shock first.
2. Calculate the maintenance fluid and estimate the fluid deficit carefully.
3. Aim to lower the serum sodium at a rate of no more than 0.5 mmol/h (12 mmol/24 h).
4. Check other electrolyte levels such as calcium and glucose.
5. Monitor the electrolytes frequently – obtain expert advice if the correction is not improving.
6. Clinically assess hydration and weigh frequently.

Hyponatraemia

Hyponatraemia may be due to excessive water intake or retention, excessive sodium losses, or a combination of both.

If the child is fitting or is encephalopathic from hyponatraemia, partial rapid correction of the serum sodium level will be necessary to stop the fitting or improve conscious level. Administration of 5 ml/kg of 3% sodium chloride solution over 15 minutes will raise the serum sodium by approximately 3 mmol and will usually stop the seizures.

If hyponatraemia is due to excessive water intake or retention, and the patient is not symptomatic, the restriction of fluid intake to 50% of normal estimated requirements may be adequate therapy. If dehydrated and intravenous fluids are required then 0.9% sodium chloride or Plasma-Lyte 148 are appropriate fluids.

The principles in the treatment of hyponatraemia are:

1. Treat the child's seizures with hypertonic 3% sodium chloride (seizure control should happen simultaneously).
2. Calculate the maintenance fluid and estimate the fluid deficit carefully.
3. Aim to raise the serum sodium at a rate of no more than 0.5 mmol/h (12 mmol/24 h).

4. Check other electrolyte levels such as calcium and glucose.
5. Monitor the electrolytes frequently – obtain expert advice if the correction is not improving.
6. Clinically assess hydration and weigh frequently.

Potassium

Unlike sodium, potassium is mainly an intracellular ion and the small quantities measurable in the serum and extracellular fluid represent only a fraction of the total body potassium. The intracellular potassium acts as a large buffer to maintain the serum value within a narrow normal range. Cardiac arrhythmias can occur at values outside this range. Thus hypokalaemia is usually only manifest after significant total body depletion has occurred. Similarly, hyperkalaemia represents significant total body overload, beyond the ability of the kidney to compensate, or massive break down of blood cells resulting in the release of potassium. The causes of hypo- and hyperkalaemia are given in Table B.5.

Table B.5 Causes of hypo- and hyperkalaemia	
Hypokalaemia	**Hyperkalaemia**
Diarrhoea	Renal failure
Alkalosis	Acidosis
Volume depletion	Adrenal insufficiency
Primary hyperaldosteronism	Cell lysis
Diuretic abuse	Excessive potassium intake

Hypokalaemia

Hypokalaemia is rarely an emergency and is usually the result of excessive potassium losses from acute diarrhoeal illnesses. The life-threatening symptoms of severe hypokalaemia (i.e. K⁺ less than 2.5 mmol/l) requiring emergency management are cardiac arrhythmias, paralysis and rhabdomyolysis. Electrocardiogram (ECG) changes with hypokalaemia include wide flat T waves, ST depression, T wave inversion, tall wide P waves, prolonged PR segment, U waves, apparent prolonged QT (fusion of T and U waves) and prolonged QRS.

As total body depletion of potassium will have occurred to cause hypokalaemia, large amounts are required to return the serum potassium to normal. Oral supplementation is the preferred initial route. In cases where this is not suitable, or where there are life-threatening symptoms, intravenous supplements are required. However, strong potassium solutions are highly irritant and can precipitate cardiac arrhythmias, thus the concentration of potassium in intravenous solutions ought not to exceed 40 mmol/l, except when given centrally with close cardiac monitoring. Children with symptomatic hypokalaemia require admission to a critical care setting for an infusion of concentrated potassium through a central venous line.

Children who are alkalotic or who are receiving insulin or salbutamol will have high intracellular potassium stores. The hypokalaemia in these cases is the result of a redistribution of potassium into cells rather than potassium deficiency, and management of the underlying causes is indicated. If hypokalaemia is detected, particularly if it is refractory to treatment, the serum magnesium should be checked and any associated hypomagnesaemia corrected.

Hyperkalaemia

Hyperkalaemia is a dangerous condition. Although the normal range extends up to 5.5 mmol/l, it is rare to get arrhythmias below 7.5 mmol/l. Precise blood taking is critical as a squeezed sample lyses blood cells, raising the potassium level spuriously. The most common cause of hyperkalaemia is renal failure – either acute or chronic. Hyperkalaemia can also result from potassium overload, loss of potassium from cells due to acidosis or cell lysis, or endocrine causes such as hypoaldosteronism and hypoadrenalism.

The immediate treatment of hyperkalaemia is shown schematically in Figure B.1. If there is no immediate threat to the patient's life because of an arrhythmia then a logical sequence of investigation and treatment can be followed. Beta-2 stimulants, such as salbutamol, are the immediate treatment of choice. They rapidly act within 30 minutes by stimulating the cell wall pumping mechanism and promoting cellular potassium uptake. They are easily administered by a nebuliser. The serum potassium will fall by about 1 mmol/l with these dosages.

Hyperkalaemia

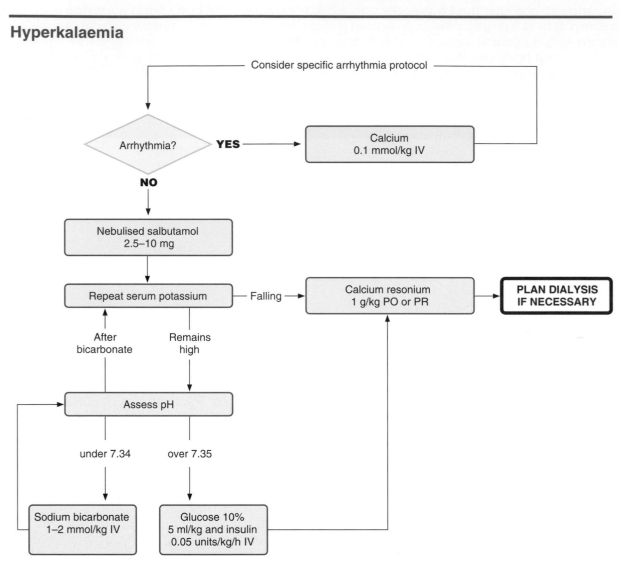

Figure B.1 Management of hyperkalaemia algorithm

Box B.1 summarises the emergency treatment of hyperkalaemia in children.

Sodium bicarbonate is also effective at rapidly promoting intracellular potassium uptake. The effect is much greater in the acidotic patient (in whom the hyperkalaemia is likely to be secondary to the movement of potassium out of the cells). The dosage is the same as that used for treating acidosis, and 1–2 ml/kg of 8.4% NaHCO$_3$ is usually effective. It is important to also check the serum calcium because hyperkalaemia can be accompanied by marked hypocalcaemia, particularly in patients with profound sepsis or renal failure. The use of bicarbonate in these situations can provoke a crisis by lowering the ionised calcium fraction rapidly, precipitating tetany, convulsions or hypotension and arrhythmias, so frequent blood monitoring is required.

Insulin and glucose are the classic treatment for hyperkalaemia. They are not, however, without risk, and the use of salbutamol has reduced the requirement for such therapy. It is easy to precipitate

Box B.1 Summary of emergency management of hyperkalaemia in children

Basics

Definition: K⁺ significantly above upper end of normal for age and/or rising

ABC monitoring: continuous ECG (first signs are tented T waves then loss of P waves,) SaO_2, blood pressure, urine output, weight

Recheck urea and electrolytes urgently – hours may have elapsed since last sample. Sample may have haemolysed

Consider the cause: high K⁺ intake, high production or low output

Stop K⁺ intake	Stop any potassium in diet and in any fluids being infused Stop drugs that can cause hyperkalaemia, e.g. angiotensin-converting enzyme (ACE) inhibitor, angiotension II blockers and β-blockers
Stabilise myocardium	10% calcium gluconate 0.5–1 ml/kg IV over 5 minutes, max 20 ml; give undiluted Give if ECG changes or K⁺ is significantly above upper end of normal for age or is rising. Effect occurs within minutes. Duration of action approximately 1 hour, repeat within 5–10 minutes as necessary
Shift K⁺ into cells	Nebulised salbutamol under 2 years 2.5 mg or over 2 years 5 mg; repeat 2-hourly as necessary. Onset of action within 30 minutes, maximum effect at 60–90 minutes

Advanced

Seek specialist advice

The following strategies can be used depending on the clinical situation:

Shift K⁺ into cells	1. Sodium bicarbonate 1–2 mmol/kg IV over 30 minutes (1 mmol = 1 ml of 8.4% $NaHCO_3$, dilute 1:5 in 5% glucose) 2. Glucose (±insulin): • Peripheral access: 10% glucose 5–10 ml/kg/h • Central access: 20% glucose 2.5–5 ml/kg/h Maintain blood glucose at 10–15 mmol/l. Physiological homeostasis should increase endogenous insulin production. Add insulin after an hour if blood glucose >15 mmol/l Make up a syringe of 50 units insulin in 50 ml 0.9% saline (= 1 unit/ml); commence infusion at 0.05 ml/kg/h Continue to maintain blood glucose at 10–15 mmol/l by adjusting the infusion rate in 0.05 ml/kg/h steps. Can cause severe hypoglycaemia. Measure blood sugar frequently (15 minutes after commencing or increase in dose, then every 30 minutes until stable)
Remove K⁺ from body	Calcium resonium: • By rectum: 250 mg//kg (max 15 g) 6-hourly, repeat if expelled within 30 minutes • By mouth: 250 mg//kg (max 15 g) 6-hourly Limited role for oral route as it is unpalatable. Takes 4 hours for full effect
Dialysis	In specialist environment

hypoglycaemia if monitoring is not adequate. Large volumes of fluid are often used as a medium for the glucose and, particularly in the patient with fluid overload from renal failure, can then be a problem. Many children are quite capable of significantly increasing endogenous insulin production in response to a glucose load, and this endogenous insulin is just as capable of promoting intracellular potassium uptake. It thus makes sense to start treatment with just an intravenous glucose load and then to add insulin as the blood sugar rises.

These treatments are the fastest means of securing a fall in the serum potassium, but all work through a redistribution of potassium into the cells. Thus the problem is merely delayed rather than treated in the patient with potassium overload. The only ways of removing potassium from the body other than by maximising renal excretion with diuretics, are with dialysis or ion exchange resins such as calcium resonium administrated via the gut. Dialysis can only be started when the patient is in an appropriate nephrology or critical care setting, but will be the most effective and rapid means of lowering the potassium.

In an emergency situation, where there is an arrhythmia (heart block or ventricular arrhythmia), the treatment of choice is intravenous calcium. This will stabilise the myocardium temporarily but will have no effect on the serum potassium. Thus the treatments discussed above will still be necessary.

Calcium

Some mention of disorders of calcium metabolism is relevant because both hypo- and hypercalcaemia can produce profound clinical pictures.

Hypocalcaemia

Hypocalcaemia can be a part of any severe illness, particularly septicaemia. Other specific conditions that may give rise to hypocalcaemia are severe rickets, hypoparathyroidism, pancreatitis or rhabdomyolysis, and citrate infusion (in massive blood transfusions). Acute and chronic renal failure can also present with severe hypocalcaemia. In all cases, hypocalcaemia can produce weakness, tetany, convulsions, hypotension and arrhythmias. Treatment is that of the underlying condition. In the emergency situation, however, intravenous calcium can be administered. As most of the listed conditions are associated with a total body depletion of calcium and because the total body pool is so large, acute doses will often only have a transient effect on the serum calcium. Continuous infusions will also often be required, and most appropriately given through a central venous line as calcium is irritant to peripheral veins. In renal failure, high serum phosphate levels may prevent the serum calcium from rising. The use of oral phosphate binders or dialysis may be necessary in these circumstances.

Hypercalcaemia

Hypercalcaemia usually presents as long-standing anorexia, malaise, weight loss, failure to thrive or vomiting. Causes include hyperparathyroidism, hypervitaminosis D or A, idiopathic hypercalcaemia of infancy, malignancy, thiazide diuretic abuse and skeletal disorders. Initial treatment is with volume expansion with sodium chloride and furosemide diuretic. Following this, investigation and specific treatment are indicated.

B.3   Diabetic ketoacidosis

Diabetic ketoacidosis (DKA) is a condition in which a relative or absolute lack of insulin leads to an inability to metabolise glucose. This leads to hyperglycaemia and an osmotic diuresis. Once urine output exceeds the ability of the child to drink, dehydration occurs. In addition, without insulin, fat is used as a source of energy, leading to the production of large quantities of ketones and metabolic acidosis. There is initial compensation for the acidosis by hyperventilation and a respiratory alkalosis but, as the condition progresses, the combination of acidosis, hyperosmolality and dehydration leads to coma. DKA is often the first presentation of diabetes; it can also be a problem in known diabetics who have decompensated through illness, infection or non-adherence to their treatment regimens.

DKA is defined as acidosis and a bicarbonate of less than 15 mmol/l **or** a pH less than 7.3, **and** ketones of greater than 3.0 mmol/l.

- Mild DKA: venous pH 7.2–7.29 or bicarbonate less than 15 mmol/l
- Moderate DKA: venous pH 7.1–7.19 or bicarbonate less than 10 mmol/l
- Severe DKA: venous pH less than 7.1 or serum bicarbonate less than 5 mmol/l

A summary algorithm for DKA management is shown in Figure B.2.

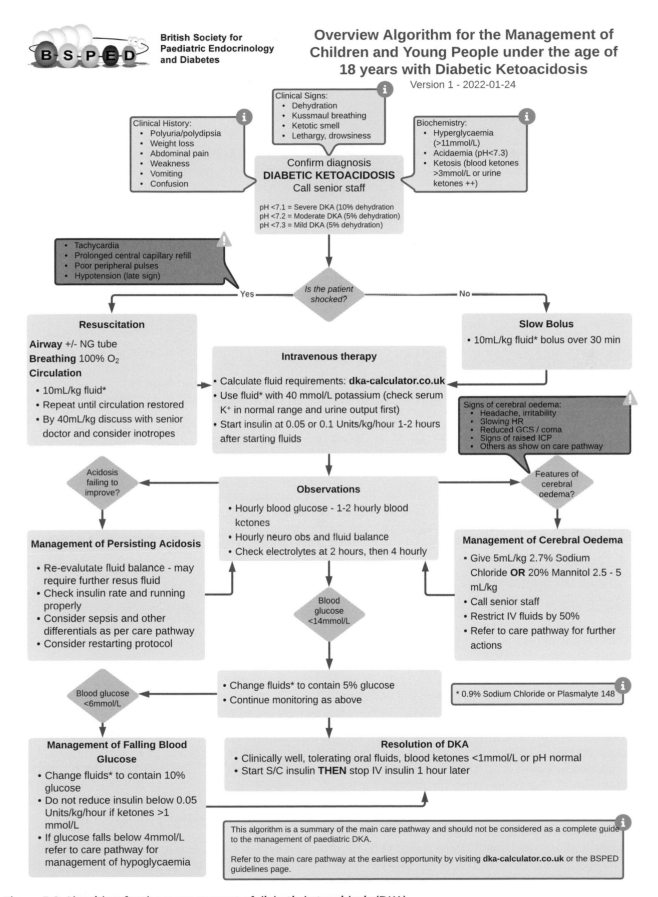

Figure B.2 Algorithm for the management of diabetic ketoacidosis (DKA)
GCS, Glasgow Coma Scale; HR, heart rate; ICP, intracranial pressure; NG, nasogastric

History

The history is usually of weight loss, abdominal pain, vomiting, polyuria and polydipsia, although symptoms may be much less specific in under 5-year-olds who also have an increased tendency to ketoacidosis.

Examination

Children with DKA will be dehydrated. Children with severe DKA are likely to have deep and rapid (Kussmaul) respiration. They may also be drowsy with the smell of ketones on their breath. Salicylate poisoning and uraemia are differential diagnoses that should be excluded. Whilst rare, infection often precipitates decompensation in both new and known diabetics. Fever is not part of DKA. Suspect sepsis in the presence of fever, hypothermia, hypotension and a refractory acidosis or lactic acidosis.

Management of diabetic ketoacidosis

- Assess:
  - Airway
  - Breathing
  - Circulation (including blood pressure)
- Ensure airway patency and insert an oropharyngeal airway if conscious level is reduced
- Give 100% oxygen via a face mask
- Place on a cardiac monitor (observe for peaked T waves from hyperkalaemia)
- Consider placement of a nasogastric tube if reduced conscious level or recurrent vomiting, and leave on open drainage
- Take blood for:
  - Blood gases
  - Urea and electrolytes, creatinine, C-reactive protein
  - Glucose
  - Ketones: near-patient blood ketones (β-hydroxybutyrate) testing should be used.
  - Full blood count (leucocytosis commonly occurs in DKA and is not necessarily a sign of infection)
  - If sufficient blood, send for new diagnosis investigations (HbA1c, thyroid function test, coeliac screen)

Take other investigations only if indicated:

- Chest X-ray
- Blood culture
- Cerebrospinal fluid
- Throat swab
- Urinalysis, culture and sensitivity

The principles of fluid treatment in DKA are:

1. An initial fluid bolus of 10 ml/kg (0.9% sodium chloride or Plasma-Lyte 148) should be given over 30 minutes to all children presenting with DKA. For children in shock, this initial bolus of 10 ml/kg should be given over no more than 15 minutes to reverse signs of shock, after which they should be reassessed and a further bolus of 10 ml/kg may be given as required to restore adequate circulation. If the child remains shocked after 20 ml/kg bolus fluids, contact a paediatric critical care specialist for further advice about managing shock (i.e. more fluid, inotropes/vasopressors).
2. Rehydrate after signs of shock have been reversed with 48 hours of replacement fluid.
3. Calculate fluid requirements:
   - When calculating the fluid requirement for children and young people with DKA, assume a 5% fluid deficit in mild to moderate DKA or a 10% fluid deficit in severe DKA (indicated by a blood pH below 7.1). Replace this deficit over 48 hours
   - Calculate the maintenance fluid requirement for children and young people with DKA using the usual fluid requirements:

Body weight	Fluid requirement per day (ml/kg)
First 10 kg	100
Second 10 kg	50
Subsequent kilograms	20

- For children who are not shocked, the first 10 ml/kg of fluid resuscitation should be subtracted from the calculations for the fluids for the next 48 hours
- For children who are shocked, resuscitation fluid volumes should NOT be subtracted from the fluid volume calculated for the 48-hour replacement
- The total replacement fluid to be given over 48 hours for a non-shocked patient is calculated as follows:

$$\text{Hourly rate} = \left(\{\text{deficit} - \text{initial bolus}\} / 48 \text{ hours}\right) + \text{maintenance per hour}$$

- To avoid excessive amounts of fluid in overweight children, it is recommended that consideration be given to using a maximum weight of 75 kg or 97th centile weight for age (whichever is lower) when calculating both deficit and maintenance requirements
- Urinary losses should not be routinely replaced
4. Replace insulin; start an IV insulin infusion 1–2 hours after beginning intravenous fluid therapy. Use a soluble insulin infusion at a dosage between 0.05 and 0.1 units/kg/h. Unless the child is in severe DKA, it would be usual to start at 0.05 units/kg/h.
5. Return the glucose level to that approaching normal.
6. Avoid hypokalaemia; all fluids should contain 40 mmol/l KCl, as long as the serum potassium is less than 5.5 mmol/l and there is a history of patient passing urine.
7. Avoid rapid changes in corrected sodium/serum osmolarity.
   - The corrected sodium (Na_{corr}) represents the expected serum sodium in the absence of hyperglycaemia:

$$\text{Corrected sodium} (\text{mmol} / \text{l}) = \text{measured sodium} + \frac{(\text{glucose} - 5.6)}{3.5}$$

   - Corrected sodium levels should typically rise as blood glucose levels fall during treatment (expected rise of 5 mmol/l over first 8 hours of treatment). Corrected sodium levels give an indication of the risk of cerebral oedema, with a falling corrected sodium indicating an excess of free water and an increased risk of cerebral oedema
   - Effective osmolality should remain stable during treatment of DKA and can also be calculated and monitored:

$$\text{Effective osmolality} = (2 \times \text{measured sodium}) + \text{glucose}$$

The detailed management of DKA is complex. Advice should be sought from experienced local practitioners and published guidelines.

Complications

All of the complications in Box B.2 require intensive monitoring on a paediatric critical care unit.

Box B.2 Major complications of diabetic ketoacidosis

Cerebral oedema	Most important cause of death and poor neurological outcome. Attempt to avoid by slow normalisation of osmolarity with attention to glucose and sodium levels, and hydration over 48 hours
	Monitor for headache, recurrence of vomiting, irritability, Glasgow Coma Scale score, inappropriate slowing of heart rate and rising blood pressure
	Treat with 3% sodium chloride 3 ml/kg or mannitol infusion (250–500 mg/kg over 20 minutes), and reduce fluids to half the maintenance rate
	Avoid intubation and ventilation if airway is maintained
	Exclude other diagnoses by computed tomography scan; other intracerebral events may occur (thrombosis, haemorrhage, infarction) and present similarly. Treatment of suspected cerebral oedema should not be delayed awaiting imaging
Cardiac arrhythmias	Usually secondary to electrolyte disturbances, particularly potassium
Systemic infections/sepsis	Antibiotics not routinely given unless severe bacterial infection is suspected. Fever, raised lactate and raised inflammatory markers indicate possible infection
Aspiration pneumonia	Avoid by placing a nasogastric tube in a vomiting child with impaired consciousness
Pulmonary oedema	Careful fluid replacement may limit the occurrence of pulmonary oedema
Acute renal failure	Uncommon because of high osmotic urine flow

B.4   Summary

This appendix has described the approach to the management of fluid and electrolytes in the seriously injured or seriously ill child, including specific reference to diabetic ketoacidosis.

Paediatric major trauma

Paediatric major trauma – resuscitation checklist

Age:			
Sex:			
W	**Weight**	**1–12 months: (0.5 x age in months) + 4** **1–5 years: (2 x age in years) + 8** **6–12 years: (3 x age in years) + 7** Adult doses over 40 kg Adapt on arrival if needed	
E	**Energy**	**4 joules/kg** Over 40 kg: 150 joules	
T	**Tube**	**(Age/4) + 4 (0.5 less for cuffed tube)** Over 40 kg: size 7	
F	**Fluids** Crystalloid **Consider MHP**	**10 ml/kg bolus (5 ml/kg blood)** Over 25 kg: 250 ml bolus **Consider MHP/rapid infuser/splinting**	
L	**Lorazepam**	**0.1 mg/kg** (Max 4 mg)	
A	**Adrenaline**	**10 micrograms/kg** Over 50 kg: 10 ml of 1:10 000	
G	**Glucose**	**3 ml/kg glucose 10%** (Max 100 ml)	
TXA Tranexamic acid		**Under 12 years: 15 mg/kg bolus** **Over 12 years: 1 g bolus** Followed by infusion of 2 mg/kg/h over 8 hours (max 125 mg/h)	
Saline 3% Hypertonic saline		**3 ml/kg over 10–20 minutes** Over 40 kg: 250 ml bolus (NUH: 2.7% sodium chloride)	
Calcium gluconate		**0.2 ml/kg 10% over 10 minutes** Over 40 kg: 10 ml 10% over 10 minutes	
Consider analgesia			
Morphine		**0.03–0.1 mg/kg (0.2 mg/kg max)** Over 50 kg: 2–10 mg	
Fentanyl		**0.5–1 microgram/kg** Over 50 kg: 50–100 micrograms	
Ketamine		**0.2–0.5 mg/kg IV (adult: 20–40 mg)** **3 mg/kg intranasal (adult: 100 mg)** **2 mg/kg IM (adult: 100–200 mg)**	
Paracetamol		**15 mg/kg IV infusion** Over 50 kg: 1 g	

The final responsibility of delivery of the correct dose remains that of the physician prescribing and administering the drug.

Paediatric major trauma and analgesia calculations

Please note: All doses can be given via INTRAVENOUS (IV) or INTRAOSSEOUS (IO) route

Age	Birth	1/12	3/12	6/12	1 yr	2 yr	3 yr	4 yr	5 yr	6 yr	7 yr	8 yr	9 yr	10 yr	11 yr	12 yr	14 yr	Adult
Weight (kg)	3.5	4	5	8	10	12	14	16	18	20	23	24	28	30	35	40	50	70
Blood (FFP) 5 ml/kg	17.5 ml	20 ml	25 ml	40 ml	50 ml	60 ml	70 ml	80 ml	90 ml	100 ml	115 ml	120 ml	140 ml	150 ml	175 ml	200 ml	250 ml	250 ml
Tranexamic acid (TXA 15 mg/kg)	52.5 mg	60 mg	75 mg	120 mg	150 mg	180 mg	210 mg	240 mg	270 mg	300 mg	345 mg	360 mg	420 mg	450 mg	525 mg	1 g	1 g	1 g
Hypertonic saline (2.7–3%) 3 ml/kg over 10-20 min >40 kg: 250 ml	10.5 ml	12 ml	15 ml	24 ml	30 ml	36 ml	42 ml	48 ml	54 ml	60 ml	69 ml	72 ml	84 ml	90 ml	105 ml	250 ml	250 ml	250 ml
Calcium gluconate 0.2 ml/kg over 10-20 min >40 kg: 10 ml	0.7 ml	0.8 ml	1 ml	1.6 ml	2 ml	2.4 ml	2.8 ml	3.2 ml	3.6 ml	4 ml	4.6 ml	4.8 ml	5.6 ml	6 ml	7 ml	8 ml	10 ml	10 ml
Morphine 50–100 mcg/kg >40 kg: 2–10 mg	0.175–0.35 mg	0.2–0.4 mg	0.25–0.5 mg	0.4–0.8 mg	0.5–1 mg	0.6–1.2 mg	0.7–1.4 mg	0.8–1.6 mg	0.9–1.8 mg	1–2 mg	1.15–2.3 mg	1.2–2.4 mg	1.4–2.8 mg	1.5–3 mg	1.75–3.5 mg	2–4 mg	2–10 mg	2–10 mg
Fentanyl 0.5–1 mcg/kg >40 kg: 50–100 micrograms	1.75–3.5 mcg	2–4 mcg	2.5–5 mcg	4–8 mcg	5–10 mcg	6–12 mcg	7–14 mcg	8–16 mcg	9–18 mcg	10–20 mcg	11.5–23 mcg	12–24 mcg	14–28 mcg	15–30 mcg	17.5–35 mcg	20–40 mcg	50–100 mcg	50–100 mcg
Paracetamol 15 mg/kg IV infusion >50 kg: 1 g	52.5 mg	60 mg	75 mg	120 mg	150 mg	180 mg	210 mg	240 mg	270 mg	300 mg	345 mg	360 mg	420 mg	450 mg	525 mg	600 mg	1 g	1 g

Safeguarding

Learning outcomes

After reading this appendix, you will be able to:

- Recognise non-accidental injury and neglect as a potential differential diagnosis in the critically ill or injured child
- Describe your approach to a child where physical, sexual and emotional abuse and neglect may be suspected
- Identify your role and that of other agencies within safeguarding

---

D.1   Introduction

The United Nations Convention on the Rights of the Child 1989 provides a set of principles and standards to ensure that, among other things, children are protected. These apply to the practice of children's healthcare for all children and young people up to the age of 18 years.

> **Article 3** provides that any decision or action affecting children either as individuals or as a group should be taken with 'their best interest' as the most important consideration
>
> **Article 9** holds that children have a right not to be separated from their parents or carers unless it is judged to be in their child's best interest
>
> **Article 12** obliges health professionals to seek a child's opinion before taking decisions that affect their future
>
> **Article 19** states that legislative, administrative, social and educational measures should be taken to protect children from all forms of physical and mental violence, injury and abuse (including sexual abuse) and negligent treatment
>
> **Article 37** states that no child shall be subjected to torture or other cruel, inhuman or degrading treatment or punishment

In 2012, World Health Organization (WHO) data showed that 54 581 children died from intentional injuries globally – this is the equivalent of 150 children every day. This appendix focuses on generic principles associated with managing safeguarding concerns in the acute situation including recognition, urgent interventions and referral. Health professionals should seek guidance and legal details plus safeguarding specific to their setting from national sources.

Healthcare workers will come into contact with:

- Children who have suffered NAI or neglect by adults or by other children
- Children who have injured or neglected other children
- Adults who suffered NAI or neglect as children

Advanced Paediatric Life Support: A Practical Approach to Emergencies, Seventh Edition. Edited by Stephanie Smith.
© 2023 John Wiley & Sons Ltd. Published 2023 by John Wiley & Sons Ltd.

- Safeguarding is everyone's responsibility. If you have concerns that a child has suffered non-accidental injury (NAI) or neglect, you have an obligation to refer
- NAI should always be considered as a potential differential diagnosis (it can often be rapidly excluded but if it is not thought about it will be missed)

Present classifications are shown in Box D.1.

Box D.1 Classification of child abuse

Neglect	The persistent failure to meet a child's basic physical and/or psychological needs, likely to result in the serious impairment of the child's health or development. Neglect can occur during pregnancy as a result of maternal substance abuse such as alcohol or drug use. Once a child is born, neglect may involve a parent or carer failing to: • Provide adequate food, clothing and shelter (including exclusion from home or abandonment) • Protect a child from physical and emotional harm or danger • Ensure adequate supervision (including the use of inadequate care givers) • Ensure access to appropriate medical care or treatment It may also include neglect of, or unresponsiveness to, a child's basic emotional needs
Physical abuse	A form of abuse that may involve hitting, shaking, throwing, poisoning, burning or scalding, drowning, suffocating or otherwise causing physical harm to a child. Physical harm may also be caused when a parent or carer fabricates the symptoms of, or deliberately induces, illness in a child
Sexual abuse	Involves forcing or enticing a child or young person to take part in sexual activities, not necessarily involving a high level of violence, whether or not the child is aware of what is happening. The activities may involve physical contact, including assault by penetration (e.g. rape or oral sex) or non-penetrative acts such as masturbation, kissing, rubbing and touching outside of clothing. They may also include non-contact activities, such as involving children in looking at, or in the production of, sexual images, watching sexual activities, encouraging children to behave in sexually inappropriate ways, or grooming a child in preparation for abuse (including via the internet). Sexual abuse is not solely perpetrated by adult males. Women can also commit acts of sexual abuse, as can other children
Emotional abuse	The persistent emotional maltreatment of a child such as to cause severe and persistent adverse effects on the child's emotional development. It may involve conveying to a child that they are worthless or unloved, inadequate or valued only insofar as they meet the needs of another person. It may include not giving the child opportunities to express their views, deliberately silencing them or 'making fun' of what they say or how they communicate. It may feature age or developmentally inappropriate expectations being imposed on children. These may include interactions that are beyond a child's developmental capability, as well as overprotection and limitation of exploration and learning, or preventing the child participating in normal social interaction. It may involve seeing or hearing the ill treatment of another. It may involve serious bullying (including cyber bullying), causing children frequently to feel frightened or in danger, or the exploitation or corruption of children. Some level of emotional abuse is involved in all types of maltreatment of a child, although it may occur alone

Susceptibility to abuse

Concerns over safeguarding or child protection must be considered in the differential diagnosis of all children who have suffered injury or who have unexplained illness. Child abuse/ill treatment occurs in all social classes. However, the possible features of parenting known to be associated with abuse or neglect include:

- Where the relationship between the parent and child does not appear loving and caring
- Where one or both parents have been abused themselves as children
- Parents who are young, single, unsupportive or substitutive
- Parents with learning difficulties
- Parents who have a poor or unstable relationship
- Situations where there is domestic violence or drug or alcohol dependence
- Parents who have mental illness or personality disorders

Factors in the child that make them vulnerable to abuse or neglect include:

- Prematurity
- Separation and impaired bonding in the neonatal period
- Physical disability
- Learning difficulties
- Behavioural problems
- Challenging temperament or personality
- Soiling and wetting past developmental age
- Neurodiversity
- Screaming or crying interminably and inconsolably

D.2 Recognition of child abuse and/or neglect

As highlighted, abuse should always be considered as a potential differential diagnosis. It can often be rapidly excluded but if it is not thought about it will be missed. In emergency paediatrics consider the following key areas:

A/B	Asphyxial event: suffocation, hanging
A/B	Rib cage and long bone fractures
A/B	Drowning
C	Ruptured abdominal viscus
D	Subdural haemorrhage
D	Cervical spine injury
E	Burns
E	Poisoning and other induced illness (e.g. septicaemia)

The following sections list presentations where you may have a higher index of suspicion.

Presentations of physical abuse

- Bruising inappropriate to developmental stage; any bruising in a non-mobile infant
- Cuts and bruises – imprints of hands, sticks, whips, belts, bites, etc. may be present
- Burns and scalds – 'glove and stocking' appearance for scalds, implement imprints for contact burns
- Cold injury – hypothermia, frostbite
- Suffocation
- Internal damage, such as rupture of the bowel
- Head injuries – fractures or intracranial injury. These may present as an acute life-threatening event with breathing difficulty or apnoea, or with raised intracranial pressure including symptoms or signs of poor feeding, vomiting, drowsiness and seizures
- Fractured ribs and spinal injuries
- Fractures of long bones – single fracture with multiple bruises, multiple fractures in different stages of healing, possibly with no bruises or soft tissue injury, or metaphyseal or epiphyseal injuries (often multiple)
- Poisoning – drugs or household substances

Presentations of sexual abuse

- Disclosure by child
- Disclosure by witness
- Suspicion by third party because of the behaviour of the child, especially changes in behaviour. These include insecurity; fear of men; sleep disorders; mood changes, tantrums and aggression at home; anxiety, despair, withdrawal and secretiveness; poor peer relationships; lying, stealing or arson; school failure; eating disorders like anorexia and compulsive overeating; running away and truancy; suicide attempts, self-poisoning, self-mutilation and abuse of drugs, solvents and alcohol; unexplained acquisition of money; and sexualised behaviour and promiscuity
- Symptoms such as a sore bottom, vaginal discharge, bleeding per vagina in a prepubertal child, bleeding per rectum or inflamed penis that the care-giver believes is due to sexual abuse
- Symptoms as above and/or signs (e.g. unexplained perineal tear and/or bruising, torn hymen or perineal warts), but the doctor is the first person to suspect abuse
- Faecal soiling or relapse of enuresis
- Sexually transmitted disease
- Pregnancy where the girl refuses to name the putative father or even indicate the category (e.g. boyfriend, casual acquaintance)
- Sexual intercourse with a child younger than 13 years is unlawful and therefore pregnancy in such a child means the child has been maltreated
- Female genital mutilation (FGM)

Presentations of neglect

- It may be difficult to distinguish between neglect and material poverty. However, care should be taken to balance recognition of the constraints on the parents' or carers' ability to meet their children's needs for food, clothing and shelter with an appreciation of how people in similar circumstances have been able to meet those needs
- A child's clothing or footwear is consistently inappropriate (e.g. for the weather or the child's size)
- A child is persistently smelly and dirty, especially if seen at times of the day when it is unlikely that they would have had an opportunity to become dirty or smelly (e.g. early morning)
- Repeated observation or reports of the home environment being of a poor standard of hygiene that affects a child's health
- The home environment is unsuitable for the child's stage of development and impacts on the child's safety or well-being
- Poor/inadequate supervision which may lead/has led to injury
- Child abandonment
- Non-organic failure to thrive
- Severe and persistent infestations, such as scabies or head lice
- Repeated non-attendances at appointments that are necessary for the child's health and well-being
- Parents or carers fail to administer essential prescribed treatment for their child
- Parents or carers fail to seek medical advice for their child to the extent that the child's health and well-being is compromised

Other presentations to consider

There are also some other pointers to be aware of during history taking and examination:

- There is delay in seeking medical help or medical help is not sought at all
- The story of the 'accident' is vague, is lacking in detail and may vary with each telling and from person to person. Innocent accidents tend to have vivid accounts that ring true
- The account of the accident is not compatible with the injury observed
- The injury is not compatible with the child's level of development or of the level of development of another child alleged to have caused the injury

- The parents' affect is abnormal. Note anything that appears abnormal to you in this regard
- The parents' behaviour gives cause for concern. They may become hostile, rebut accusations that have not been made or leave before the consultant arrives
- The child's appearance and interaction with the parents is abnormal. The child may look sad, withdrawn or frightened. There may be visible evidence of failure to thrive. Full-blown frozen watchfulness is a late stage and results from repetitive physical and emotional abuse over a period of time

D.3 Assessment

The assessment of all children should follow the standard ABCDE procedure and full medical assessment approach.

Consent for examination is mandatory in all cases unless a serious life-threatening injury is suspected. This needs to be given by an adult with parental responsibility or the child if competent. Social care may need to get a court order if appropriate consent is not available or has been refused. This is also an aspect that will be subject to national laws, policies and procedures and you should familiarise yourself with those relevant to your practice using national guidance.

Details of medical assessment

History

A full history should be taken as in any medical assessment. There are some specific issues to consider if child abuse and/or neglect are on your list of differential diagnoses.

- Full details of the history of the incident(s) should be obtained from the child and the caregivers. If social workers and police officers have previously talked to the child, then taking this history from them may be appropriate, especially for alleged sexual offences. Frequent repetition of the details can be very disturbing to the child and can jeopardise evidence
- In history related to the gastrointestinal tract remember to ask about soiling, constipation, rectal pain and rectal bleeding
- In history related to the urogenital system remember to ask about wetting, vaginal bleeding, vaginal discharge and, when appropriate, menarche, cycle, sanitary protection and previous sexual intercourse
- Personal history must start with pregnancy, birth, the neonatal period and subsequent developmental milestones. Then obtain details of immunisations, drug history (including alcohol and street drugs) and allergies. Information on the child's performance at nursery or school should include social factors
- Enquiries are made about previous illnesses and injuries, with dates of attendance at hospital or the surgery of the family doctor. Past records should be obtained and relevant information should be extracted
- The traditional family history should include details of the birth parents, all co-habitees and any other people who regularly care for the child, such as relatives and childminders
- Parental illness should be discussed, particularly psychiatric illness
- The presence of domestic abuse should be explored
- Then the names, ages and medical histories of all siblings and half-siblings are obtained. Any miscarriages, stillbirths or deaths of siblings are discussed sensitively
- Familial illnesses that are particularly important are inherited skin or blood disorders

Remember to remain objective and show professional sensitivity. Document who is present and their relationship to the child. Use open questions and avoid leading questions. Full contemporaneous notes are essential. If the child has been video-interviewed you may be able to obtain the transcript of this prior to examination to avoid unnecessary repetition.

Examination

Ensure an appropriate chaperone is present. The general examination starts while the history is being taken. During that time the doctor observes the affect of the child, the relationships between the child, mother, father and others present, and any behavioural problems. If the child is reluctant to be examined, then playing with toys or the doctor's stethoscope often breaks the ice. No child should be examined against his or her will as this constitutes an assault. Examination under anaesthesia is rarely required.

General examination

- Full head-to-toe examination
- Plot growth on growth chart including head circumference in younger children
- Comment on general level of hygiene, clothing, etc.
- Document any injuries on a body map
- Comment on developmental level and interaction with carers

Sexual abuse examination

- This should be undertaken by a doctor with the necessary specialist competences
- If there has been acute assault, then forensic examination taking forensic swabs will be needed and will require a forensic medical examiner for this to occur in a sexual assault resource centre (SARC)
- Consider post-coital contraception and/or screening and treatment for sexually transmitted infections

---

Investigations

The investigations are dependent on the initial presentation and injuries.

Young babies presenting with concerns about physical abuse all need:

- Full blood count and clotting
- Neuro-imaging
- Fundoscopy
- Imaging in line with *The Radiological Investigation of Suspected Physical Abuse in a Child* (RCR/SCoR, 2018) endorsed by the Royal College of Paediatrics and Child Health (RCPCH)

Blood investigations to exclude differential diagnosis will also depend on clinical presentation and may include:

- Blood cultures
- Metabolic investigations
- Renal and bone profile
- Extended clotting studies

D.4   Initial management

Medical treatment is the priority, especially if the child has serious or life-threatening injuries. At the end of the medical assessment the diagnosis may be clear. More often, there is a differential diagnosis that includes abuse.

For paediatric trauma, ask the following questions:

- Does the story of the mechanism fit with the injury pattern seen? (e.g. a 'fall down the stairs' with bruising on the abdomen)
- Do the injuries fit with what is reasonable for this child's developmental age? (e.g. a 1-month-old baby who 'rolled off the bed')
- Could the parents or carers have done anything in advance to prevent the accident happening? (e.g. a burn injury in an unsupervised toddler)
- Could the parents or carers have done anything after the accident to improve medical care? (e.g. an injury that has not had prompt care)

When the diagnosis or differential diagnosis is one of child abuse, then the decisions to be made about management are the following:

- Does the child need admission for treatment of the injuries?
- Will the child be safe if returned home?
- If the child needs protection from an abuser who is in their own home, how can this be done?
- What support/protection is needed for the rest of the family, including siblings?

D.5   Child in need/safeguarding

Where there are concerns regarding safeguarding or child protection, discussion must take place among the professionals involved (medical/social/police) who have information about the family, to balance the probabilities of abuse having occurred. Approaches to this will vary from country to country, but in all cases should include a decision about whether it may be necessary to arrange for the child to be taken to a place of safety.

If abuse and neglect are likely then a multiagency assessment involving social care, health and police will be required. As a separate, parallel process, police will consider whether criminal investigation is appropriate or necessary; in many cases a full criminal investigation will not take place. The approach to this will vary according to national laws, policies and procedures.

All safeguarding work is based on cooperation between families, social workers, police officers, healthcare workers and educationalists. This multiagency approach is to ensure that all aspects of the care of the family are considered when decisions are being made. Certain decisions in management must be made by a professional, for example only a doctor can decide on the treatment required for a fracture and only a police officer can initiate criminal investigations. However, whenever possible, unilateral decisions are avoided in the best interests of the child and the family.

Because of the complexity of interaction between these agencies, communication is a crucial element.

Doctors may be concerned about sharing information with other professionals because of the ethical consideration of confidentiality. In the UK, the General Medical Council (2018) gave the following advice:

> Ask for consent to share information unless there is a compelling reason for not doing so. Information can be shared without consent if it is justified in the public interest or required by law. Do not delay disclosing information to obtain consent if that might put children or young people at risk of significant harm.

Advice on consent will vary between countries and you should be aware of your own national guidance and advice.

D.6   Medicolegal aspects

Healthcare professionals must be familiar with the medicolegal aspects of their work. These may vary according to the jurisdiction where the clinician practices. Court orders may enable the following:

- Emergency protection
- Child assessment
- Residence
- Police protection
- Consent to examination

In some cases where there is involvement of either a criminal or family court, healthcare professionals may be required to write statements and/or present evidence.

D.7   Summary

This appendix has stressed that safeguarding is everyone's responsibility. Abuse or neglect should always be considered as a potential differential diagnosis and as a health professional you have an obligation to refer any concerns to a statutory agency.

Advance decisions and end of life

Learning outcomes

After reading this appendix, you will be able to:

- Recognise and act on advance decision making, understanding when limitations of treatment and intervention may be appropriate
- Identify the function of care plans to help guide appropriate, individualised management of the child and family
- Describe the purpose of recognising the possibility of end of life and be able to communicate this effectively with families to ensure appropriate management
- Recognise the importance of continued care and comfort at the end of life
- Identify important factors when dealing with the death of a child
- Describe your approach to the death of a child
- Identify your role and that of other agencies

E.1   Introduction

The purpose of the Advanced Paediatric Life Support (APLS) programme is to bring a structured approach and simple guidelines to the emergency management of seriously ill and injured children. While these should always be the default, it is equally important to recognise that they are guidelines and that there may be times when some adaption and individualisation of these guidelines may be necessary.

The numbers of children with life-limiting conditions and complex needs are increasing. Best practice ensures that an advance care plan (ACP) is recorded for these children. The plan should document anticipated interventions that may offer benefit to the child and therefore should be considered. It should also record recommendations to reduce or exclude interventions that offer no benefit or are seen to be excessively burdensome purely to sustain life at all costs.

Advanced Paediatric Life Support: A Practical Approach to Emergencies, Seventh Edition. Edited by Stephanie Smith.
© 2023 John Wiley & Sons Ltd. Published 2023 by John Wiley & Sons Ltd.

E.2   Advance care planning

An ACP (sometimes alternatively referred to as an anticipatory care plan) is a summary document completed to communicate the wishes of a child or young person (and their family) who has a chronic, complex or life-limiting condition (incorporating professional views and experience of what would or would not be beneficial).

The plan may set out an agreed plan of care to be followed when a child or young person's condition deteriorates, including specific resuscitation plans and end of life plans.

ACPs are advisory and the recommendations that are recorded are not binding. They must be interpreted by the clinicians involved in the context of the clinical scenario.

Referencing the child's 'normal/baseline' status

Many of these children have complex backgrounds and abnormal physiology. A good care plan should describe their normal or baseline status to help assess any deterioration or deviation requiring intervention.

For example, the presence of dystonia and posturing in a child with cerebral palsy (or other neurological impairment) may represent their baseline (and not necessarily an acute neurological deterioration). Likewise, however, if this has deteriorated it is important to recognise it and act accordingly.

Specific management plans

The child may have individualised management care plans which are varied depending on the clinical situation. These should have been written to capture previous experience of managing the child and input from specialists. For example, recommendation of specific antibiotics based on the likely organisms/sensitivities specific to the child, or a specific seizure protocol based on knowledge of the child's condition or individual experience of what works (or indeed does not work) for that child.

Resuscitation

Many ACPs detail decisions on the appropriate management of acute deteriorations and on what level of intervention would be appropriate for this child and their family.

This may or may not include limitations in the form of a modified resuscitation plan or a 'do not attempt cardiopulmonary resuscitation' (DNACPR).

It is important to note that a limitation of treatment refers to specific interventions, more accurately representing a 'reorientation' of care. It does not indicate limitation or withdrawal of care.

End of life

An ACP may indicate priorities of care towards the end of life, including preferences of place of care at the end of life and after death. Advance care planning assists professionals who are not familiar with the child's care to direct clinical management in accordance with those wishes wherever possible and to aid further discussion and decision making if necessary.

Whilst it can be difficult to recognise that end of life is imminent, it is important to communicate this to the child/family, such that important decisions can be made and appropriate care can be given (such as focused symptom control).

For example, a family may indicate that they wish their child to receive active treatment if conditions are reversible. However, if a deterioration represents the end of life, they may prefer transfer to a hospice. In which case this must be recognised, communicated to the family and then actioned (if possible and stable enough for transfer), all whilst continuing optimal symptom control. The presence of an advance care plan makes this discussion considerably easier.

Local differences

Different ACPs exist nationally and familiarisation with your local format is recommended. It is important to recognise that careful and often difficult decision making will have been applied to an ACP and it should be respected even if it deviates from the normal APLS approach.

One example of an ACP in the UK is the 'child and young persons advance care plan' (CYPACP) (Figure E.1). Information can be found on the website www.cypacp.uk (last accessed January 2023).

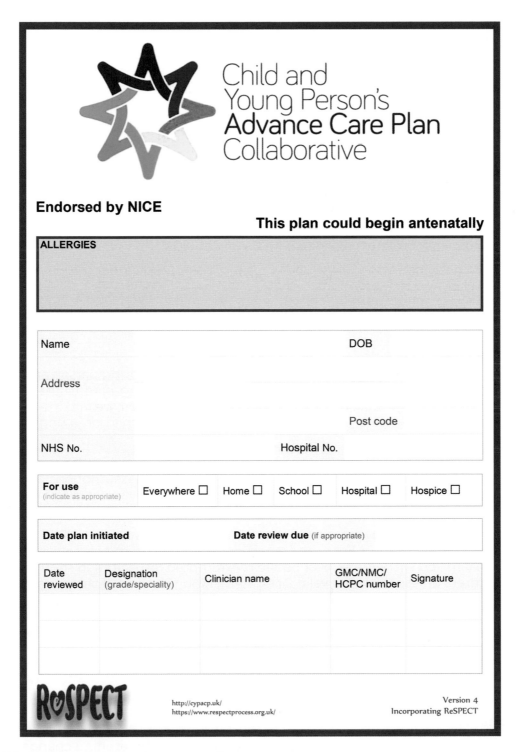

Figure E.1 Child and young person's advance care plan
CYPACP, https://www.nnuh.nhs.uk/publication/child-and-young-persons-advance-care-plan-collaborative-formerly-known-resuscitation-plan-for-children-respect-form (last accessed March 2023)

Legality

Advance care plans are not legally binding and the child/parents are entitled to change their mind at any point. This does not detract from the importance of such documents, but highlights the wishes and preferences around treatment and care. As they are not a legal document they do not need to be signed by parents.

Advance care conversations and documentation of decisions should be considered within the ethical, legal and clinical frameworks that guide clinicians working with children and young people.

When differing opinions emerge in the type of medical intervention that represents a child's best interests, parents and clinicians should work together to resolve the disagreement, with the child's welfare being paramount. Parents and clinicians have a moral and legal duty to protect children from significant harm. If local resolution is not possible, it may be appropriate to consult a clinical ethics committee and consider mediation. The Royal College of Paediatrics and Child Health (RCPCH) have published guidance on both conflict resolution and withholding and withdrawal of life-sustaining treatment, which can be found on the RCPCH website (www.rcpch.ac.uk; last accessed January 2023).

E.3   Resuscitation decisions

Parents and clinicians are required to act in the child's best interests when making decisions on behalf of or with a person under the age of 18 years. This is described in the General Medical Council (GMC) ethical guidance for doctors working with 0–18-year-olds.

An assessment of best interests will include what is clinically indicated in a particular case. The following should also be considered:

- The views of the child or young person, so far as they can express them, including any previously expressed preferences
- The views of parents
- The views of others close to the child or young person
- The cultural, religious or other beliefs and values of the child or young person and their parents
- The views of other healthcare professionals involved in providing care to the child or young person, and of any other professionals who have an interest in their welfare
- Which choice, if there is more than one, will least restrict the child or young person's future options

This list is not exhaustive. The weight attached to each point will depend on the circumstances, and any other relevant information should be considered. Unjustified assumptions about a child or young person's best interests should not be made based on irrelevant or discriminatory factors, such as their behaviour, appearance or disability.

Whatever the prognosis and advance decisions that may be in place, the child's comfort should always be a primary consideration. Every attempt should be made to minimise distress and to fulfil the child and the families' wishes wherever possible. Attempted resuscitation should be the default action for all children, unless there is a valid DNACPR decision in place. If there is any doubt about the validity of a DNACPR decision, then resuscitation should be initiated. However, it is important to make it clear to families that if the most senior clinician present believes that resuscitation is unlikely to restart the heart or breathing then cardiopulmonary resuscitation (CPR) would be futile and should not be continued. If the ACP (or alternative document) states that the child should not be resuscitated or that a modified resuscitation plan is detailed then this should be followed (if the child/parents/family still agree with this and it is felt to be in the child's best interest).

DNACPR decisions

Clinicians should adhere to a valid DNACPR in the event of a life-threatening change in the child's clinical condition, unless this is a potentially reversible cause such as choking or anaphylaxis. It is worth noting that on occasions even reversible causes are included, in these circumstances this should be detailed clearly. The recorded DNACPR decision should, therefore, be considered in context.

In hospital, a clinical emergency call (e.g. a 2222 medical emergency call) will not usually be made, and no active interventions (e.g. ventilation and chest compressions) will be made to assist the child's failing respiratory or circulatory function.

In the pre-hospital environment, ambulance control and the general practitioner (GP) (and other professionals as appropriate – schools, respite centres, etc.) should be made aware of the existence (and the contents) of an ACP.

A valid DNACPR decision:

- Reflects the agreed wishes of the child (where appropriate), those with parental responsibility for the child and the healthcare professionals caring for the child
- Is clearly recorded, signed and dated in the DNACPR section of the ACP
- Falls within the time period specified for review (if this is not the case, then a decision needs to be made if this is still appropriate or not between the clinicians and those with parental responsibility)

The DNACPR applies only to CPR. Other types of resuscitation may be described in care plans and can be considered independently of CPR decisions.

It is worth noting that CPR may be interpreted in different ways and thus when creating an ACP it is worth specifying EXACTLY what is meant. Unless specified it would be reasonable to assume that DNACPR applies to both ventilation (bag and mask) and cardiac compressions (including cardiac drugs such as adrenaline). If the resuscitation plan includes ventilation efforts but not cardiac compressions this should be specified (see later section).

Exclusions from and suspension of DNACPR decisions

A DNACPR decision does not apply to immediately remediable and acutely life-threatening clinical emergencies such as choking and anaphylaxis (unless otherwise specified). Appropriate emergency interventions should be attempted, which may include CPR. Wherever possible, the lead consultant should be contacted as a matter of urgency for ongoing management advice.

A valid DNACPR decision may be temporarily suspended, for example around the time of specific interventions such as anaesthesia or surgery that have an associated increased risk of cardiorespiratory arrest. If such procedures are planned, then any advance decisions should be reviewed and whatever decision is made should be documented and communicated accordingly.

Modified resuscitation

As explained, whilst a DNACPR indicates that there should be no attempt made to resuscitate a child in the event of a cardiorespiratory arrest it does not indicate the level of intervention that has been agreed to be appropriate for that child.

The ACP (or alternative document) may give more specific details on which interventions are deemed appropriate/acceptable. These decisions have been made considering the burdens of interventions and the benefits achieved by their actions. An example may be that a family wish for reversible conditions such as an acute pneumonia to be treated by admission to hospital, administration of intravenous antibiotics and oxygen if necessary. However, any intervention above this may be agreed to be too burdensome and thus not appropriate. The advantage of a good quality ACP is that it communicates these prior decisions so that clinicians can follow them, ensuring that an individually appropriate level of intervention is given to that child.

E.4 End of life

This is not meant to be a complete guide to end of life; it is advisable to seek specialist advice should this be needed.

Recognising end of life

Recognising end of life is often difficult, especially in paediatrics.

However, some potential indicators that a child may be in the later stages of life may include:

- Reduced level of consciousness
- Abnormal breathing (apnoeas, Cheyne–Stokes)
- Peripheral shutdown (cold extremities)

Additionally, it is often stated that many families (and professionals) instinctively recognise the considerable deterioration in these children and have a 'gut feeling' that they are at the end of their life. This should not be ignored but communicated carefully with the family. However, we also need to recognise that it is not always possible to accurately predict death and that parallel planning is of vital importance, ensuring one has prepared for the possibility that a child survives despite expectations.

Place of care

It should be recognised that the duration of the end of life stage can be variable (and not always predictable). This should be communicated with the family (and considered, when deciding on management). In particular, when deciding upon place of care for the dying patient.

Where possible, attempts should be made to follow families' wishes. If it is recognised that a patient is not stable enough for transfer this should be communicated to the family and alternative plans should be made (perhaps to a quieter side room if possible).

Symptom control at end of life

As already stated, if available, the ACP should be consulted to see if there is any patient-specific guidance on this.

It is worth considering some of the main symptoms that are likely/possible at the end of life and targeting treatment towards these (including anticipatory prescribing, such that medications are available at short notice for troublesome symptoms). The main symptoms to consider are pain, agitation, nausea and vomiting, secretions and breathlessness and rarely, but importantly, the possibility of catastrophic haemorrhage.

Further information regarding appropriate doses and means of administration (e.g. syringe drivers) can be found in the Association for Paediatric Palliative Medicine (APPM) *Master Formulary* (available at www.appm.org.uk; last accessed January 2023).

Catastrophic haemorrhage

It should be noted that at the end of life this is managed very differently to a major haemorrhage described in the trauma section of this manual. Whilst direct pressure to bleeding sites and topical tranexamic acid and adrenaline can help, if bleeding is catastrophic, priority is given to ensuring a calm, reassuring environment for the child and family. Dark towels (to reduce the visual impact of a large bleed) and anxiolytic medications can be very helpful if available quickly.

Other issues at end of life

Hydration and nutrition

A child should always be encouraged to eat and drink as they wish, if they are able. If, however they are not able, burdens versus benefits of continuing hydration and nutrition should be considered.

Implantable cardioverter defibrillator

Consider if the child has an implantable cardioverter defibrillator (or pacemaker) and ensure that this is deactivated.

Portable ventilators

Children may be on portable ventilators, which may need to be removed at the end of life.

Prioritise comfort and benefit of any intervention

Review which interventions are of benefit to the child, including blood tests, antibiotics, blood glucose monitoring, observations and oxygen.

Consider which of the child's regular medications may still be of benefit, and discontinue non-essential medications. The route of administration may also need to be considered or changed.

Consider and address any issues relating to skin and mouth care.

Spirituality/religion

Ask the child and family if spirituality or religion is important and whether their beliefs affect the care they would like. Consider chaplain support if appropriate.

Family and friends

Honest and open communication around the time of end of life may enable family and friends to be informed and visit where possible.

E.5   When a child dies

Even with the best preventative measures in place and the use of the most effective resuscitation methods, children will still unfortunately die from serious illness and severe injury. When a death occurs, medical and nursing staff must be able to deal effectively with the child's family and the legal requirements of death as well as cope with their own emotional reactions. Sympathetic and sensitive support of the family at such times can help the grief process and adjustment to loss.

The principles in dealing with a family that has experienced a sudden child death are shown in Box E.1.

Box E.1 Principles in dealing with a family

- Be kind, caring and compassionate
- Use the deceased child's name and ask the family how they would like to be addressed (e.g. mum/mummy or by first name)
- Spend as much time as necessary with the family in an unhurried fashion and allow them to spend as much time with their child as they need
- Offer information regarding the death as the family requires
- Offer support for when the family leaves hospital

Parental presence during resuscitation is increasingly common and has been shown to help in the grieving process; this should occur through a combined decision between the healthcare team and the parents/carers. If parents are present during resuscitation, a member of staff should be available exclusively to support them. If the presence of parents is impeding the progress of the resuscitation, they should sensitively be asked to leave.

There may be suspicious circumstances around the death, evidence of abuse or concerns regarding the family; however this must not influence our approach as healthcare staff to the family, our responsibility is to flag this under local safeguarding arrangements. The response when a child dies unexpectedly should include a multiagency discussion to ensure an appropriate planned response. In some circumstances, the police may decide to undertake an immediate criminal investigation with which medical staff will need to cooperate.

Dealing with the family

Breaking the news

Informing parents that their child has died is a difficult task and is usually undertaken by a senior and experienced staff member. Before speaking to the parents ensure they are in a private, comfortable environment and that you know the name of the child. Sometimes a bigger family circle may be important and should be respected.

A direct and sympathetic approach is best, avoiding euphemisms and clichés. If it is appropriate and you feel comfortable doing it, you may show sympathy by holding the parent's hand or putting an arm around them. The parents may wish to ask questions about the cause of death and what they should do now. The parents will often want to know what happened and what treatments were instituted. If you are asked about the cause of death answer as simply and honestly as you can, making it clear that some answers are not yet available.

Caring for the parents

Provide the family with a private room in which they can be alone with their child for as long as they wish. Encourage the family to touch and hold the child. Offer to stay with the family; however, if they wish to be left alone, assure them you will be nearby if they wish to speak to you. In cases where there have been child protection concerns or in a sudden unexpected death, it will be necessary for the parents to be accompanied by a professional when they are with the child.

Accept the family's distress as natural and support them in this by acknowledging their feelings. Be prepared for a variety of responses: there is no 'correct' way to grieve and each person will have a different reaction. Be sensitive to and respectful toward varying cultural norms and rituals surrounding death. Facilitate contact with other family members and friends as required. Even very young children may be included in the grief process right from the start; assist the family in feeling comfortable with this.

Each institution will have its own bereavement support programme: ensure that you are familiar with local resources and that the family is offered ongoing support and medical advice. For example, in Wales as part of the procedural response to unexplained death in childhood, a locally established charity 2 Wish (www.2wish.org.uk; last accessed January 2023) offers immediate support to anyone affected by the sudden and unexpected death of a child or young person aged 25 and under. Remember that if a child dies, most parents/families do not know what will happen or how the procedures work. It is advisable to give them guidance.

Post-death procedures

Every jurisdiction will have specific legal requirements that need to be adhered to. It is usually necessary for the coroner, the police or another statutory authority to be informed of the death. The requirements for a police or coronial investigation, an autopsy and an inquest will vary from case to case.

An overview of the *Child Death Review – Statutory and Operational Guidance (England)* (HM Government, 2018) document is given here.

The death of a child is a devastating loss that profoundly affects bereaved parents as well as siblings, grandparents, extended family, friends and others who were involved in caring for the child. Families experiencing such a tragedy need to be met and supported with empathy and compassion. They need clear and sensitive communication. They also need to understand what happened to their child, and want to know that people will learn from what happened. The process of systematically and expertly reviewing all children's deaths is grounded in deep respect for the rights of children and their families, with the intention of preventing future child deaths.

Figure E.2 sets out the main stages of the child death review process.

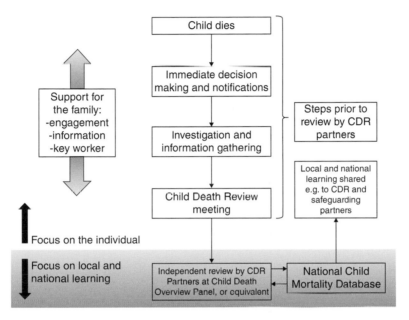

Figure E.2 Chart illustrating the full process of a child death review (CDR)

Immediate decision making and notifications

A number of decisions need to be made by professionals in the hours immediately following the death of a child. These include:

- How best to support the family
- Whether the death meets the criteria for a joint agency response
- Whether a Medical Certificate of Cause of Death (MCCD) can be issued following discussion with the local medical examiner, or whether a referral to the coroner is required
- Whether the death meets the criteria for a serious incident investigation

A number of notifications must also be made, to the child's GP and other professionals, to the Child Health Information System, the relevant Child Death Overview Panel (CDOP).

Investigation and information gathering

After immediate decisions and notifications have been made, a number of investigations may then follow. These include:

- Coronial investigation
- Multiagency response
- Serious incident investigation

Postmortem examinations may be required in a number of cases. Which investigations are necessary will vary depending on the circumstances of the individual case. They may run in parallel, and timeframes will vary greatly from case to case.

Child death review meeting

Although investigations following the death of a child will vary, every child's death should be discussed at a child death review meeting. This is the final multiprofessional meeting involving the individuals who were directly involved in the case. The nature of this meeting will vary according to the circumstances of the child's death and the practitioners involved. It would, for example, take the form of a final case discussion following a Joint Agency Response to a SUDC (sudden unexpected death in children), or a hospital-based mortality meeting following a death on a neonatal unit. It has common aims and principles in all cases.

Child Death Overview Panel

The Child Death Overview Panel (CDOP) is a multiagency panel for a defined geographical area, whose role is to review the death of all children normally resident in that area, and also, where appropriate, the deaths of non-resident children, in order to learn lessons for the prevention of future child deaths. It provides independent scrutiny of each child's death from a multiagency perspective. As such, it differs from the child death review meeting in two essential aspects: (i) the information reviewed is made anonymous; and (ii) the CDOP is made up of senior professionals who have had no involvement in the cases under discussion.

CDOPs are required to report specified data on child death reviews to the relevant UK Departments of Health. In England they also submit data on all child deaths directly to the National Child Mortality Database.

Support for the family

Supporting and engaging the family who have lost a child is of prime importance throughout the whole child death review process.

Recognising the complexity of the process, and the state of total shock that bereavement can bring, families should be given a single, named point of contact who they can turn to for information on the processes following their child's death, and who can signpost them to sources of support.

Specific situations

Guidance in the *Child Death Review* is also included for a number of specific situations, including:

- Deaths of UK-resident children overseas
- Children and young people with learning disabilities
- Deaths of children and young people in adult healthcare settings such as adult intensive care units
- Suicide and self-harm
- Inpatient mental health settings
- Deaths in custody

In addition to the CDOP guidelines, a customised checklist is invaluable for ensuring that procedures or information are not forgotten. Box E.2 gives an outline of such a list although local hospital/organisational guidelines should be followed if they are different (for example many hospices have significantly different procedures for expected deaths). In all cases of sudden unexpected death in the UK there are local procedures for reporting to, and investigation by, a multiagency team led by the designated doctor for unexpected deaths.

Box E.2 Checklist for post-death procedure in the emergency department

The child
- Full and thorough examination
- Assess core temperature
- Wrap child in clean warm clothes for parents to see and hold (if consistent with forensic requirements)
- Samples or swabs if agreed as mandatory in local protocol

The parents
- Explain that the child (use name) has died
- Gently get as full a history as possible
- Ask if they would like a religious leader present and whether there are any important religious practices to be carried out (although these may not always be possible)
- Ask if they want any close relative to be contacted or extended family to be present
- Encourage the parents to see and hold the child
- Let them know if postmortem examination needs to be carried out and ensure they understand all that they wish to know about the procedure and have their written consent where appropriate. Explain the full process of a postmortem and what will be done with the dead child. Remember that sometimes a postmortem might not include the whole body, but may be limited to specific regions, depending on pre-mortem illness, etc.
- Let them know that the police and coroner are always informed of sudden unexpected deaths and will need to ask a few simple questions of the carers
- Explain options open to the family following death (perhaps the opportunity of transfer of the body to a children's hospice, or even home)
- Ask what address the family will be going to on leaving the hospital
- Arrange transport from the hospital to home and, if alone, make sure they are accompanied on the journey and not left alone at home
- Be gentle, unhurried, calm and careful
- Do not guess at the diagnosis

Details to be obtained
- Child's and parents' names
- Child's date of birth
- Address at which death occurred
- Time of arrival in department
- Time last seen alive
- Usual address if different from above

Inform
- GP – advise of child's death and give the address to which the parents will be going from hospital
- Health visitor
- Social worker
- Any relative as requested by the family
- Coroner – who will need to know the full name and address and date of birth of the child, time of arrival, place of death, brief recent history and any suspicious circumstances

Please also refer to any ACP in place as this may also give guidance on appropriate management of the child and family after death. It should be noted that there are certain circumstances in which care plans cannot be followed exactly. For instance, it may be that these wishes stated that a child should be buried within 24 hours after death in line with religious beliefs. Although in certain circumstances (e.g. in sudden unexpected deaths, which require a postmortem) this may not be possible. The reasons for this need to be communicated sensitively and sympathetically.

E.6 Take care of the staff/'debrief'

The death of a child is extremely distressing for all involved. This is equally true for sudden and unexpected deaths as for those with life-limiting conditions where death itself was not unexpected.

There is increasing recognition in the importance of a debrief following a distressing situation such as this (https://www.paediatricfoam.com/2017/01/hot-debrief/; last accessed January 2023). They serve several purposes including analysis of team performance, education and emotional support. Learning can be made through things that went well and things that did not go so well, and can be used to improve future performance.

Two terms are often used with a 'hot' debrief relating to a meeting immediately after the event and a 'cold' debrief sometime after. There is value in both of these and they should not be seen as an 'either/or'.

Useful guidance on some important issues to address in these debriefs include those listed in Box E.3.

Box E.3 Issues to consider in the debrief

Where
Use a quiet area, ensuring you will not be disturbed

How
- Try to handover bleeps to ensure you are not disturbed
- Treat everyone as equals, all team members' opinions are valued and encourage participation from everyone
- Identify the leader/chair of the debrief – this does not need to be the leader of the resuscitation itself
- Set out structure of the debrief – informal and no blame
- One suggestion is to initially run through the facts of the events
- After the facts are established – invite **thoughts**/emotions of the events
- What were people's reactions – how did people **feel** afterwards (and now), is there anything anyone is struggling with?

What
- Human factors
- Team process
- Clinical learning points
- Remember to focus on processes not outcome. A child may still die following a perfectly executed resuscitation
- Try to focus on some key points (what is important to the group)
- Consider a framework to this process:
  - what happened?
  - what needs to change?

What next?
- Establish an action plan
- If another 'cold' debrief is necessary:
  - who will organise this
  - get contacts for everyone
- Ensure everyone is able to either continue their shift or get home
- Ways people can access further support:
  - supervisor
  - local counselling/psychology/chaplain services
  - British Medical Association's counselling service for doctors
  - local charity organisations (e.g. www.2wish.org.uk)
- Feedback on the debrief itself

It should be reiterated that staff may be vulnerable following such an event and a good debrief should not assign 'blame' or force people to contribute if they do not want/are unable to. It may be appropriate to approach staff individually at a later time in private.

It should be recognised that these debriefs are equally important in situations where the child survives. These are often still distressing and staff may be in need of support. Additionally, even in survival, there are often many learning points to be gained including examples of good practice.

E.7 Summary

This appendix has explored some of the possible challenges of managing children with complex medical needs and life-limiting conditions. These situations need to be recognised and individualised plans swiftly identified and acted upon.

General approach to poisoning and envenomation

Learning outcomes

After reading this appendix, you will be able to:

- Describe the approach to the management of poisoning in children
- Describe the approach to the management of envenomation in children
- Describe the approach to the management of button battery and strong magnet ingestion

F.1 Poisoning: introduction

Deaths from ingested poisons are uncommon in children (globally in 2012 there were 35 205 – only 4.7% of the number of deaths caused by 'injury'). They are due to therapeutic (especially tricyclic antidepressants) or 'recreational' drugs, household products and, rarely, plants. Infrequently, groups of children may be exposed to inhalational toxins such as chlorine gases in the event of accidents (or occasionally deliberate attempts to cause harm).

In some parts of the world, poisoning with agricultural products such as organophosphates and carbamates may also be a significant problem, and in others children ingest corrosives from time to time and end up with severe oesophageal burns and complications.

Most poisoning episodes in childhood and adolescence are of low lethality and little or no treatment is required. This appendix will not address the milder cases but will enable the student to develop an approach to the seriously ill poisoned child, with additional advice on the management of specific poisons.

Incidence

There has been a steady decline in the number of childhood deaths from poisonings globally from 52 149 in 2000 to 35 205 in 2012 (World Health Organization data). The selective introduction of child-resistant containers, together with other measures, has reduced the number of poisonings and hospital attendances. It should be remembered, however, that 20% of children under the age of 5 years are capable of opening child-resistant containers.

Advanced Paediatric Life Support: A Practical Approach to Emergencies, Seventh Edition. Edited by Stephanie Smith.
© 2023 John Wiley & Sons Ltd. Published 2023 by John Wiley & Sons Ltd.

The decrease in deaths from the inhalation of toxic fumes may be related to the gradual effect of legislation in some countries on the banning of toxic substances in furnishing items. The continued substantial death rate from carbon monoxide poisoning is disappointing but may be related to the fact that although smoke alarms are more readily found in dwellings, they are often non-functional. The decline in mortality from drug poisoning may be due both to more effective treatment and possibly to the more widespread use of less toxic antidepressant drugs.

Accidental poisoning

This is usually a problem of the young child or toddler, with a mean age of presentation of 2.5 years. Accidental poisoning usually occurs when the child is unsupervised, and there is an increased incidence in poisoning following recent disruption in households, such as a new baby, moving house or where there is maternal depression.

Intentional overdose

Suicide or parasuicide attempts are usually made by young people in their teens; however, sometimes they may be as young as 8 or 9 years old. These children or adolescents should undergo psychiatric and social assessment.

Drug abuse

Alcohol and solvent abuse are among the commonest forms of drug abuse in children.

Iatrogenic drugs

The commonest offender is diphenoxylate with atropine (Lomotil). This combination is toxic to some children at therapeutic doses. The most frequently fatal drug is digoxin.

Deliberate poisoning

Rarely, symptoms are induced in children by adults via the administration of drugs. A history of poisoning will often not be given at presentation.

F.2   Primary assessment and resuscitation in poisoning

- Respiratory rate: the rate may be increased in poisoning from amphetamines, ecstasy, salicylates, ethylene glycol and methanol
- Acidotic sighing respirations: this may suggest metabolic acidosis from salicylates or ethylene glycol poisoning as a cause for the coma
- Heart rate: tachycardia is caused by amphetamines, ecstasy, β-agonists, phenothiazines, theophylline and tricyclic antidepressants (TCAs); bradycardia is caused by β-blockers, digoxin and organophosphates
- Blood pressure: hypotension is commonly seen in serious poisoning; hypertension is caused by ecstasy and monoamine oxidase inhibitors
- If heart rate is above 200 beats/min in an infant or above 150 beats/min in a child, or if the rhythm is abnormal, perform cardiac monitoring. QRS prolongation and ventricular tachycardia are seen in TCA poisoning
- Depression of conscious level suggests poisoning with opiates, sedatives (such as benzodiazepines), antihistamines and hypoglycaemic agents
- Pupillary size and reaction should be noted. Very small pupils suggest opiate or organophosphate poisoning; large pupils suggest amphetamines, atropine and TCAs

- Note the child's posture. Hypertonia is seen in amphetamine, ecstasy, theophylline and TCA poisoning
- The presence of convulsive movements should be sought. Convulsions are associated with any drug that causes hypoglycaemia (ethanol) and with TCA poisoning
- A fever suggests poisoning with ecstasy, cocaine or salicylates
- Hypothermia suggests poisoning with barbiturates or ethanol

Airway

- A patent airway is the first requisite. If the airway is not patent it should be opened and maintained with an airway manoeuvre and the child ventilated by bag–valve–mask oxygenation. An airway adjunct can be used. The airway should then be secured by intubation with experienced senior help
- Management of the airway may be particularly challenging in situations such as: corrosive ingestion; patients with cardiac arrhythmia related to medication such as TCAs; or in patients with profuse respiratory secretions as may occur following organophosphate ingestions
- If the child has an AVPU score of 'P' or 'U', their airway is at risk. It should be maintained by an airway manoeuvre or adjunct and senior help requested to secure it

Breathing

- All children with respiratory abnormalities, shock or a decreased conscious level should receive high-flow oxygen through a face mask with a reservoir as soon as the airway has been demonstrated to be adequate
- A number of agents taken in overdose (particularly narcotics) can produce respiratory depression. Oxygen should be given, but it is important to remember that these patients may have an increasing carbon dioxide level despite a normal oxygen saturation whilst breathing oxygen. Inadequate breathing should be supported using a bag–valve–mask device with oxygen or by intermittent positive pressure ventilation in the intubated patient

Circulation

- A number of poisons can produce shock, by a number of different mechanisms. Hypovolaemia may be caused by gastrointestinal bleeding from iron poisoning or there may be vasodilatation from barbiturates. Shock should be treated with a fluid bolus, as usual. If possible, inotropes should be avoided in poisoning cases as the combination of toxic substance producing shock and an inotrope may be proarrhythmogenic
- Cardiac dysrhythmias can be expected in TCA, digoxin, quinine and antiarrhythmic drug poisoning. Some antiarrhythmic treatments are contraindicated with certain poisons. See later in this chapter for advice on TCA poisoning and contact a poisons centre urgently for other advice
- Gain intravenous or intraosseous access
- Take blood for a full blood count, urea and electrolytes, toxicology, paracetamol and salicylate levels (in patients who have taken an unknown drug), glucose stick test and laboratory test
- Give 3 ml/kg of 10% glucose followed by maintenance glucose infusion to any hypoglycaemic patient
- Give a 10 ml/kg rapid bolus of a balanced crystalloid to any child with signs of shock
- If a child has a tachyarrhythmia and is shocked, up to three synchronous electrical shocks at 1, 2 and 4 joules should be given. If the arrhythmia is broad complex and the synchronous shocks are not activated by the defibrillator then attempt an asynchronous shock. A conscious child should be anaesthetised first if this can be done in a timely manner. A direct current (DC) shock may be dangerous in digoxin poisoning. Antiarrhythmics may be used on advice from a poisons centre

Disability

- Treat convulsions with either diazepam, midazolam or lorazepam
- Give a trial of naloxone in cases where depressed conscious level and small pupils suggest opiate poisoning

> In all cases of serious poisoning, early consultation with a poisons centre is mandatory. Such centres have a wealth of expertise in the management of poisoning and will advise on the individual child's needs

Monitoring

- Electrocardiogram (ECG)
- Blood pressure (use appropriate size of cuff)
- Pulse oximetry
- Core temperature
- Blood glucose
- Urea and electrolytes
- Blood gases (where indicated)

Lethality assessment

At the end of the primary assessment it is important to assess the potential lethality of the overdose. This requires knowledge of the substance that has been taken, the time it was taken and the dosage. This information may be unattainable in the unwitnessed poisoning episode of a toddler or that of an unconscious or uncooperative adolescent. Some clues about the drug ingested may be available from physical signs noted during the primary assessment (Table F.1).

Table F.1 Diagnostic clues from the primary assessment

Signs	Drug
Tachypnoea	Aspirin, carbon monoxide, cyanide, theophylline
Bradypnoea	Barbiturates, ethanol, opiates, sedatives
Metabolic acidosis (sighing respirations)	Carbon monoxide, ethanol, ethylene glycol
Tachycardia	Amphetamines, antidepressants, cocaine, sympathomimetics
Bradycardia	Beta-blockers, clonidine, digoxin
Hypotension	Barbiturates, benzodiazepines, β-blockers, calcium channel blockers, iron, opiates, phenothiazines, phenytoin, tricyclic antidepressants
Hypertension	Amphetamines, cocaine, sympathomimetic agents
Small pupils	Opiates, organophosphate insecticides, phenothiazines
Large pupils	Amphetamines, atropine, cannabis, carbamazepine, cocaine, quinine, tricyclic antidepressants
Convulsions	Carbamazepine, lindane, organophosphate insecticides, phenothiazines, tricyclic antidepressants
Hypothermia	Barbiturates, ethanol, phenothiazines
Hyperthermia	Amphetamines, cocaine, ecstasy, phenothiazines, salicylates

Some investigation results can add clues to the diagnosis of an unknown poison (Table F.2).

Table F.2   Clues to the diagnosis of an unknown poison

Poison	Metabolic acidosis	An enlarged anion gap [(Na + K) – (HCO$_3$ – Cl)] of more than 18	Hypokalaemia	Hyperkalaemia
Beta-agonists			✓	
Carbon monoxide	✓			
Digoxin				✓
Ecstasy	✓			
Ethanol		✓		
Ethylene glycol	✓	✓		
Iron	✓	✓		
Methanol	✓	✓		
Salicylates	✓	✓		
Theophylline			✓	
Tricyclic antidepressants	✓			

The risks of a particular overdose can be assessed once all the information has been gathered. Complex or life-threatening cases should be discussed with a poisons centre. The poisons centre will require the following information:

- Age and weight of the child
- Time since exposure
- Substance taken
- Amount taken together with any description or labelling
- Child's condition

If the nature of the overdose is unknown then a high potential lethality should be assumed.

Many childhood poisoning incidents have zero lethality and no treatment is required.

F.3   Emergency treatment in poisoning

Drug elimination

Many children have taken a trivial overdose or an overdose of a non-poisonous substance. If the overdose episode is assessed as having a low lethality, then no treatment is required.

If the drug overdose is assessed as having a potentially high lethality or its exact nature is unknown, then measures to minimise blood concentrations of the drug should be undertaken. In general, this means stopping further absorption. Occasionally measures to increase excretion can be employed and in some circumstances specific antidotes may be available. Seek advice from a poisons centre.

There are a number of active elimination techniques such as haemoperfusion and plasmapheresis; their use is infrequent and should be guided by the advice of the poisons centre.

Activated charcoal

Activated charcoal has a surface area of 1000 m²/g and is capable of binding a number of poisonous substances without being systemically absorbed. It is now widely used in cases of poisoning. However, there are some substances that it will not absorb. These include alcohol and iron. Repeated doses of activated charcoal are useful in some types of poisoning because they promote drug reabsorption from the circulation back into the bowel and interrupt enterohepatic cycling. These types include aspirin, barbiturates and theophylline.

It is often difficult to give charcoal to children as it is unpalatable. Flavouring may be necessary but can diminish the charcoal's activity. The charcoal can be given via a nasogastric or lavage tube after a gastric washout. The dose is at least 10 times the estimated dose of poison ingested. Children should usually be given 25–50 g.

Aspirated charcoal causes severe lung damage, so airway protection is especially important in the child who is not fully conscious or in whom the predicted trajectory of the poisoning is likely to result in an at-risk airway.

Emesis

Emesis caused by ipecacuanha is now rarely used although for many years it was routinely given for the management of poisoning incidents in children. The dose schedule is 15 ml with water (10 ml in children of 6 months to 2 years), repeated once after 20 minutes if necessary. It must not be used in the child with a depressed conscious level. Evidence now suggests that unless emesis occurs within 1 hour of ingestion of the poison, little of the poison will be eliminated. Only about 30% is retrieved even within the hour.

Emesis should only be used for those poisons requiring removal that are not bound by charcoal, or in children who are at risk from developing symptoms from the poison they have taken, who present within 1 hour of ingestion and who will not take the charcoal. It should not be used in children who may have ingested corrosive substances.

Gastric lavage

Gastric lavage is rarely required as the benefit rarely outweighs the risk. Advice should be sought from the National Poisons Information Service if a significant quantity of iron or lithium has been ingested within the previous hour.

F.4   Emergency treatment of specific poisons

Iron

Depending on the elapsed time since ingestion, the child with iron poisoning may present with shock, which may be due to gut haemorrhage. If over 20 mg/kg of elemental iron has been taken, toxicity is likely. Over 150 mg/kg may be fatal. Intubation, ventilation and circulatory support are necessary in the severely affected child. Initial symptoms of toxicity are vomiting, diarrhoea and abdominal pain. These may lead on to drowsiness, fits and circulatory collapse.

Whole bowel irrigation can be considered once the airway is secured and circulatory access has been gained. Charcoal is not helpful. Desferrioxamine can be administered orally and left in the stomach, or intravenously and infused at a dose of up to 15 mg/kg/h. This treatment should be given immediately to children with serious symptoms such as shock, coma or fits and to all with a serum iron level (4 hours or more after ingestion) of 3 mg/l and gastrointestinal symptoms, leucocytosis or hyperglycaemia. Note that high levels of iron can itself cause haemolysis, so a haemolysed sample should raise alarm bells.

Radiography of the abdomen can help to show how much iron remains within.

Tricyclic antidepressant poisoning

The toxic effects of these agents result from their inhibition of fast sodium channels in the brain and myocardium – this action is known as 'quinidine-like'. With serious intoxication, the cardiac problems are due to intraventricular conduction delay. This results in QRS prolongation (a QRS of more than four little squares on the ECG paper is predictive of serious effects). TCA poisoning causes anticholinergic effects (tachycardia, dilated pupils, convulsions) and cardiac effects (conduction delay, any arrhythmia). Convulsions should be treated as described in Chapter 6.

In addition, alkalinisation up to an arterial pH of at least 7.45, and preferably 7.5, has been shown to reduce the toxic effects of TCAs on the heart. This can be achieved by hyperventilation (PCO_2 no lower than 3.33 kPa (25 mmHg)) and by infusing sodium bicarbonate (1–2 mmol/kg). Hypotension should be treated with volume expansion, and if an intravenous infusion is necessary, a vasopressor such as noradrenaline is preferable to an inotrope such as dopamine, dobutamine or adrenaline. Glucagon also has an inotropic effect and can be used in this circumstance.

The use of antiarrhythmics should be guided by a poisons centre. Lidocaine and phenytoin may be helpful. Quinidine, procainamide and disopyramide are contraindicated.

Opiates (including methadone)

Following stabilisation of airway, breathing and circulation, the specific antidote is naloxone. An initial bolus dose of 10 micrograms/kg should be given. Naloxone has a short half-life, relapse often occurring after 20 minutes. Larger boluses, or an infusion of 5–20 micrograms/kg/h, may be required.

It is important to normalise carbon dioxide (CO_2) through increased ventilation before the naloxone is given because adverse events such as ventricular arrhythmias, acute pulmonary oedema, asystole or seizures may otherwise occur. This is because the opioid system and the adrenergic system are inter-related. Opioid antagonists and hypercapnia stimulate sympathetic nervous system activity. Therefore, if ventilation is not provided to normalise CO_2 prior to naloxone administration, the sudden rise in adrenaline concentration can cause arrhythmias.

Paracetamol

Significant paracetamol poisoning in childhood is almost always intentional; the accidental ingestion of paediatric paracetamol elixir preparations by the toddler very rarely achieves toxicity. Doses of less than 150 mg/kg will not cause toxicity except in a child with hepatic or renal disease.

Current treatment of paracetamol poisoning may include oral charcoal if presentation occurs within 1 hour of ingestion or is considered to be of high risk. A paracetamol blood level should be taken at 4 hours or later. In liquid ingestions, because of rapid absorption, no oral charcoal should be given. Figure F.1 shows a nomogram indicating the level of blood paracetamol at which acetylcysteine should be given intravenously. A total dose of 300 mg/kg is given over approximately 12–24 hours (depending on the regimen used). Contact a poisons centre for individual details.

Salicylates

Aspirin slows stomach emptying, so gastric lavage can be undertaken up to 4 hours after ingestion. Repeated charcoal doses should be given for children who have ingested sustained-release preparations. The salicylate level can be measured initially at 2 hours. However, repeated measurements are necessary and no reliance should be placed on a single salicylate level. The levels will usually rise significantly over the first 6 hours (longer if an enteric-coated preparation is used). Salicylate poisoning causes a respiratory alkalosis and metabolic acidosis. Arterial blood gas estimation is necessary for managing the child. Alkalinisation of the child improves the excretion of salicylate: 1 mmol/kg of sodium bicarbonate should be infused over 4 hours. Forced diuresis is no longer used.

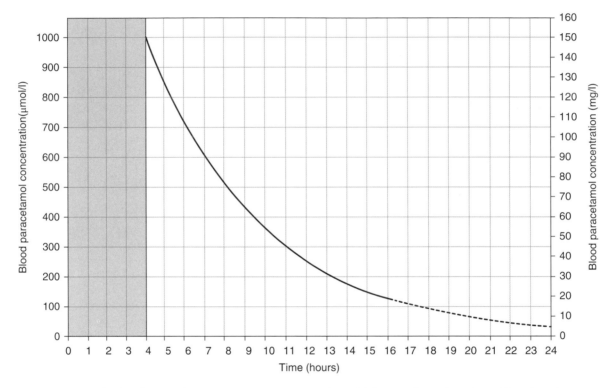

Figure F.1 Nomogram indicating the level of blood paracetamol at which acetylcysteine should be given intravenously
From Daly FS, Fountain JS, Murray L, Graudins A, Buckley NA; Panel of Australian New Zealand Clinical Toxicologists. Guidelines for the management of paracetomol poisoning in Australia and New Zealand: explanation and elaboration. A consensus statement from clinical toxicologists consulting to the Australasian poisons information centres. *Med J Australia* 2008; 188(5): 296–301. © 2008 Reproduced with permission from Medical Journal of Australia

Ethylene glycol

This sweet-tasting substance is available as an antifreeze and de-icer fluid for vehicles. It produces a clinical appearance of inebriation accompanied by metabolic acidosis and causes widespread cellular damage, especially to the kidneys. In unwitnessed ingestions the clue is in metabolic acidosis with an inexplicable anion gap. Activated charcoal is ineffective. Ethanol is a competitive inhibitor of alcohol dehydrogenase and can block metabolism of the ethylene glycol to its poisonous metabolic by-products. An oral loading dose of 2.5 ml/kg of 40% ethanol (the strength of most spirits) should be started. The aim is to have a blood ethanol concentration of 100 mg/dl. Fomepizole may also be used and haemodialysis may be necessary. Co-factors thiamine and pyridoxine are also recommended.

Cocaine

Cocaine poisoning leads to the local accumulation of the neurotransmitters noradrenaline, dopamine, adrenaline and serotonin. The accumulation of noradrenaline and adrenaline leads to tachycardia, which increases myocardial oxygen demand while reducing the time for diastolic coronary perfusion. Vasoconstriction causing hypertension results from the accumulation of neurotransmitters at the peripheral β-adrenergic receptors, and peripheral hydroxytryptamine (5-HT) receptor stimulation causes coronary artery vasospasm. In addition, cocaine stimulates platelet aggregation. Together, these changes can produce what is effectively a coronary event in a child or an adolescent.

Acute coronary syndrome producing chest pain and varying types of cardiac rhythm disturbances is the most frequent complication of cocaine use, and leads to hospitalisation. Cocaine is also a sodium channel inhibitor, similar to a type I antiarrhythmic agent, and so can prolong the QRS duration and impair myocardial contractility. Through the combination of adrenergic and sodium channel effects, cocaine use may cause various tachyarrhythmias including ventricular tachycardia and ventricular fibrillation. Treatment should be guided by a poisons centre.

Initial treatment of the acute coronary syndrome consists of oxygen administration, continuous ECG monitoring and administration of a benzodiazepine (e.g. diazepam or lorazepam), aspirin and heparin. Hyperthermia should be treated with cooling. Beta-adrenergic blockers are contraindicated in the setting of cocaine intoxication. Ventricular tachycardia should be treated with DC shock as antiarrhythmic drugs may cause further proarrhythmic effects. Since cocaine is a sodium channel blocker, administration of sodium bicarbonate in a dose of 0.5–1 mmol/kg should be considered in the treatment of ventricular arrhythmias.

Ecstasy

Most ecstasy tablets contain 30–150 mg of 3,4-methylenedioxymethamphetamine (MDMA). This drug, which has a half-life of around 8 hours, most probably stimulates both the peripheral and the central α- and β-adrenergic receptors. Early deaths are usually due to cardiac dysrhythmias, while deaths after 24 hours occur from a neuroleptic malignant-like syndrome.

Mild adverse effects occur at low doses and include increased muscle tone, agitation, anxiety and tachycardia. A mild elevation of temperature may also occur. At higher doses, hypertonia with hyper-reflexia, tachycardia, tachypnoea and visual disturbance can be seen. In the worst affected children, coma, convulsions and cardiac dysrhythmias can occur. Hyperpyrexia with increased muscle tone can lead to rhabdomyolysis, metabolic acidosis with acute renal failure and disseminated intravascular coagulation.

Activated charcoal should be given to conscious children. Blood pressure and temperature must be monitored. Diazepam can be used to control anxiety – major tranquillisers should not be used because they exacerbate symptoms. If core temperature exceeds 39°C then active cooling should be commenced and the use of dantrolene sodium (2–3 mg/kg over 10–15 minutes) should be considered. Some children may require ventilation.

Organophosphate poisoning

In organophosphate poisoning you will note the following signs and symptoms:

- B: dyspnoea
- D: pinpoint pupils
- E: rhinorrhoea

The treatment is according to the algorithm in Figure F.2. Very large doses of atropine (up to 250 mg) may be required.

Organophosphate poisoning

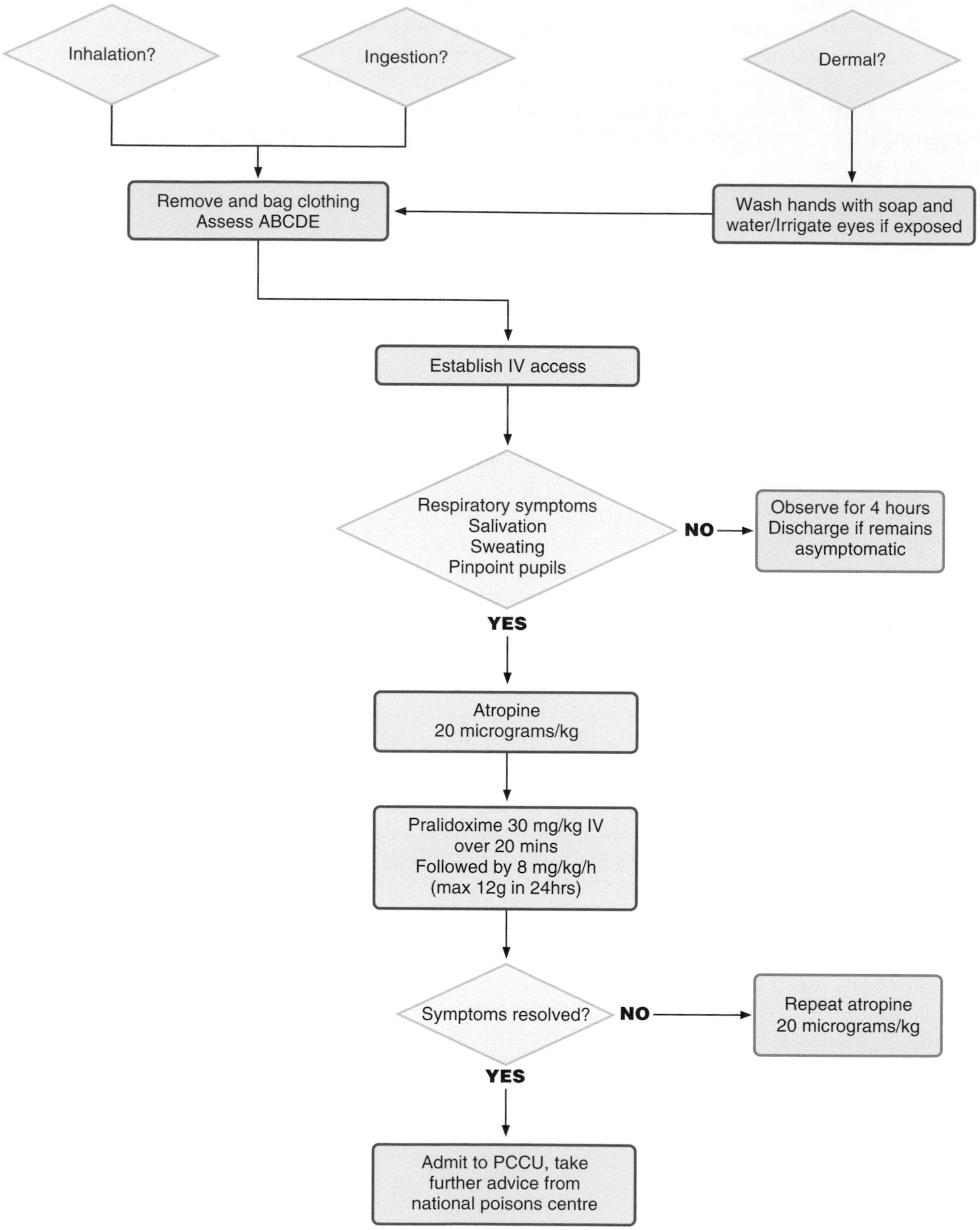

Figure F.2 Management of organophosphate poisoning algorithm
PCCU, paediatric critical care unit

F.5   Envenomation (envenoming): introduction

Envenoming may occur as a result of bites or stings from a wide variety of animals, which includes snakes, spiders, insects (e.g. bees, wasps, ants), ticks, jellyfish and fish. The best management of envenoming is prevention, because once major envenoming occurs, reversal through the use of antidotes (antivenoms) may not resolve all medical problems.

Awareness of risk and avoidance of risky behaviour, plus use of simple clothing such as shoes and long trousers in potential risk areas, may prevent effective bites/stings or reduce the severity of envenoming. Bites and stings by venomous animals are a risk in both rural and large urban centres.

Symptoms of envenoming may be either the direct result of the venom or allergic reactions to the venom, or a combination of both. In all cases the principles of management consist of:

- Removal from danger (particularly important for venomous animals)
- Standard resuscitation practice of managing the airway, breathing and circulation
- Limiting the uptake of venom into the circulation where possible
- Administration of antidote (antivenom) where available and appropriate
- Supportive care to the systems affected by the venom
- Management of pain
- Treatment of sites of local injury

Envenoming is not an inevitable consequence of a venomous bite/sting, as the animal can often control how much venom is injected, penetration through clothing may reduce or prevent venom injection into the skin, and the size of the child will affect the concentration of injected venom and so the potential severity of envenoming. The smaller the child, the higher the potential venom concentration after a bite/sting, with consequently greater potential for severe or lethal envenoming. Even for venomous snakebites in small children, a significant number of bites fail to be effective ('dry' bites) and so do not result in envenoming. However, all snakebites should be initially managed as potentially lethal.

The diagnosis of envenoming is crucial and there are three points that are important to consider:

1. Is there a history of exposure to a bite/sting? Even if not, consider envenoming in a child presenting with unexplained paralysis, myotoxicity, coagulopathy, renal failure, collapse or convulsions.
2. Is there an indication of the type of animal involved? Knowing the type of animal can enable prediction of potential risks and targeted therapy. It may help determine if the animal is actually venomous (e.g. in parts of Queensland, Australia, python bites are a common but non-venomous cause of snakebites).
3. Is there evidence of envenoming or allergic reaction to the bite/sting? This is the key question in determining both emergency and ongoing management.

Determining if envenoming is present may be simple (e.g. the child who screams and then collapses after swimming in areas with box jellyfish, who has numerous adherent jellyfish tentacles – a likely box jellyfish sting with severe envenoming) or complicated (e.g. the child who is bitten by a snake but initially appears well). Considering the setting, history, examination and laboratory findings may all be vital. For snakebites in particular, laboratory testing for coagulopathy (international normalised ratio (INR), activated partial thromboplastin time, D-dimer) and myolysis (creatine kinase) are essential in determining the degree of envenoming, in conjunction with examination looking for paralytic features.

Laboratory tests, conversely, are not important in determining if envenoming is present or the extent of envenoming for spider and tick bites, insect stings (except massive multiple stings) or marine stings.

F.6 Resuscitation and support in envenomation (envenoming)

Danger

A venomous animal can injure multiple humans (although honey bees can sting only once), including first responders (e.g. a box jellyfish in shallow water at a beach, or a cornered snake), so it is important to avoid further bites/stings. In general, attempting to catch or kill the animal entails risks that exceed the benefits, but there are exceptions (e.g. it is important to locate and carefully remove all attached ticks in cases of tick paralysis).

Airway

The airway may be threatened for a number of reasons, including depressed level of consciousness, bulbar palsy, paralysis and swelling of tissues around the airway. The airway must be assessed frequently. Clearance of secretions from the pharynx is the most common problem. Children who require intubation for reasons other than a depressed level of consciousness require anaesthesia for intubation. **It is extremely important to note that a totally paralysed child may be fully conscious**.

Breathing

Many venoms cause paralysis, and children affected by these venoms require ventilatory support. The support must be provided prior to respiratory arrest. As a child may be paralysed but fully awake, anaesthesia for intubation is essential. Severe muscle spasm or seizures may occur following some types of envenoming, and these children will require ventilatory support. Also, secretions may contribute to respiratory distress and ventilatory support may prevent the accumulation of secretions.

Circulation

Shock may occur for a variety of reasons including cardiac arrhythmia, bleeding secondary to coagulopathy and massive leakage of fluid into tissues damaged by cytotoxic venoms. Adequate vascular access must be secured with fluid resuscitation appropriate to the clinical situation. Beware fluid overload in children and avoid cannulation/sampling from subclavian, jugular and femoral veins if a coagulopathy is a possibility (snakebites). Some venoms are associated with the development of renal and/or electrolyte problems; fluid and electrolyte therapy must be adapted to the specific venom.

Disability

Assess the child's conscious level, remembering that failure to respond may be a consequence of paralysis and not of the level of consciousness. Look specifically for local neurological problems such as ptosis, ophthalmoplegia and/or bulbar palsy.

Exposure

Full exposure may be required to identify the site of a bite, and in the case of stings it is also important to examine areas of the body covered by hair. The search of cryptic areas such as the scalp and in and behind the ears is particularly important for tick envenoming.

F.7   Specific envenomation (envenoming) issues

Limiting uptake of venom (snakes, funnel web spiders, blue ringed octopus)

Where possible, the rate of uptake of venom into the circulation should be limited. If the bite or sting has affected a limb, it may be possible to slow the rate of absorption of venom from the bite/sting by the application of pressure bandaging and immobilisation (PBI) first aid. PBI is based on limiting lymph transport of the venom, using a broad bandage firmly applied over the bite site, then over the rest of the bitten limb and over the top of clothing, followed by immobilisation of the limb using a splint. To be effective, the limb must be immobilised and the child prevented from moving or walking. The bandage should be as firm as for a sprain, but not so tight as to act as a tourniquet. Crepe bandage has traditionally been recommended, but recent evidence suggests an elasticised bandage is easier to apply effectively and therefore may be preferred. Once applied, PBI should only be discontinued once the child is in a hospital able to treat envenoming with the appropriate antivenom.

Pressure bandaging and immobilisation is inappropriate for red back spider and tick bites and stonefish and jellyfish stings.

Inactivating venom locally (jellyfish and fish)

Box jellyfish stings are potentially lethal, so inactivating unfired stinging cells on tentacles adherent to the skin is vital. Flooding the tentacles with vinegar is recommended. The application of a cold pack is also recommended by some authorities. For other jellyfish stings and fish/stingray stings, the use of hot water (a shower or immersion at 45°C) is recommended, but ensure the water is not so hot as to cause thermal injury.

Local bite/sting trauma

Stingrays can cause significant local trauma, including the laceration of nerves, tendons and blood vessels, and can penetrate the abdomen or chest wall, including direct injury to the heart. Stingray venom can cause local tissue damage/necrosis. It is therefore important to carefully wash and, where appropriate, debride a stingray wound and control excessive bleeding. For stings penetrating near the heart, incautious removal of the sting may result in lethal injury.

Venom sprayed or spat into the eyes may cause intense pain, temporary blindness and corneal injury, but is not likely to cause envenoming. Urgent irrigation of the eyes is required, then examination of the cornea and appropriate treatment given if there is a corneal injury.

All bites/stings have the potential to introduce tetanus or other infections. Tetanus immune status should be ensured, but not until after any acute envenoming coagulopathy (snakebite cases) has fully resolved. Antibiotics should only be used if there is acute infection, not as routine prophylaxis.

Antidotes (antivenom)

Antivenom consists of immunoglobulin G (IgG) antibodies (or fractions thereof) raised in animals against selected venoms. Each antivenom is specific for a particular species or group of animals only. Antivenoms can cause both early (rash, febrile, anaphylactic) and late (serum sickness) adverse reactions. Antivenoms will only bind to their target venoms, not other venoms, and may neutralise venom action but cannot reverse damage caused by venom. It is therefore crucial: (i) that the correct antivenom is used; (ii) that antivenom is only used when clearly indicated; and (iii) that everything is to hand to treat an acute adverse reaction, before antivenom is infused.

Indications for antivenom vary depending on the type of animal/antivenom involved:

- For Australian snakebites antivenom is indicated if there is evidence of significant systemic envenoming, including coagulopathy, myolysis, paralysis, renal damage and collapse/convulsions, but excludes children who have only general symptoms (headache, vomiting, abdominal pain) without evidence of the foregoing problems

- For funnel web spider bites any evidence of systemic envenoming is an indication to give antivenom
- For red back spider bites the use of antivenom is more controversial, but most experts would consider it if there is intractable regional envenoming or any degree of systemic envenoming
- For stonefish stings any significant local pain is an indication to use antivenom
- For box jellyfish stings the role and indications for antivenom are currently unclear, but it should be used in any child with life-threatening envenoming

The choice of antivenom will be determined by the type of venomous animal involved. For snakes there are five different 'specific' antivenoms plus a polyvalent antivenom covering all five types of snake. Currently, the specific antivenoms are polyvalent but the doses are specific for the species indicated. For lower volume specific antivenoms (brown snake and tiger snake in particular), it is preferable to use the correct specific antivenom rather than the polyvalent product, for safety and cost reasons. A snake venom detection test is available to help choose the appropriate specific antivenom, but should be used in conjunction with diagnostic algorithms. Snake venom detection is not a screening test for snakebites and a negative result does not exclude snakebite.

Antivenom should be given as soon as indicated, by the intravenous route. The intramuscular route has traditionally been used for red back spider and stonefish antivenoms, and is anecdotally effective, but the intravenous route is more likely to give a rapid, effective response. For all other antivenoms, the intravenous route is mandatory. The dose is based on quantity of venom injected, not the size of the child. Therefore, there is no paediatric dosing and children receive the same dose as adults. Intravenous antivenom is usually infused as a dilute solution in 0.9% sodium chloride or similar, but the degree of dilution should be carefully adjusted in children to avoid volume overload.

The use of premedication prior to giving antivenom is no longer accepted practice, but adrenaline must **always** be immediately available before giving antivenom.

Drugs

In addition to antivenom (where available and appropriate), there are a number of problems that may require symptomatic therapy.

Analgesia

Pain may be a major feature of envenoming and adequate analgesia is critical. For painful marine stings, hot water (45°C, but avoid thermal injury) may be effective. Antivenom can be the most effective treatment for pain caused by stonefish stings, red back spider bites and possibly box jellyfish stings. If these treatments are not appropriate or insufficient in cases with severe pain, then consider intravenous opioids titrated to effect or regional nerve block (for marine fish stings).

Sedation

Bites and stings may be associated with extreme anxiety. Reassurance and supportive care is the basis of therapy, but sedation and anxiolysis may be helpful, particularly if a child requires transportation. However, be cautious sedating children with potential for developing neurotoxic paralysis.

Coagulation factor therapy

Antivenom can neutralise venom components attacking the haemostasis system if given early enough, but cannot replace consumed clotting factors. In cases with consumptive coagulopathy (defibrination, venom-induced consumptive coagulopathy) following snakebite, it may take many hours for key clotting factors to return to 'safe' levels. If there is also significant active bleeding, then, once appropriate antivenom has been given, clotting factor replacement therapy (fresh frozen plasma, cryoprecipitate) should be considered.

Monitoring

Many cases of bites/stings by potentially dangerous animals – including snakes, funnel web spiders, box jellyfish and blue ringed octopuses – may result in either no or only minor envenoming, not requiring antivenom. (There is no antivenom available for the blue ringed octopus anyway.) These cases of 'dry' or minor bites/stings require an adequate period of observation, including recurrent examination and blood testing (snakebites only) to ensure late developing envenoming is not missed.

- For snakebites monitoring should be for at least 12 hours if there is no evidence of envenoming or if only minor envenoming is present. In remote areas it might be wise to monitor the child for longer before sending them home. Blood tests should be performed on presentation, 1 hour after PBI is removed and at 6 and 12 hours post bite
- For suspected funnel web spider bites (= 'big black spider' bite) monitor for at least 4 hours post bite; in significant funnel web spider bites envenoming develops within 4 hours
- For red back spider bites only symptomatic children require hospital assessment
- For marine envenoming the requirement for hospital monitoring is determined by the type of bite/sting and symptomatology. Severe or life-threatening envenoming generally occurs very early after exposure, within the first hour or less, and always within the first 4 hours. The exception is stingray wounds to the trunk, which may seem initially alright but should always be fully assessed and observed for a longer period

Table F.3 contains a summary of the major types of venomous animals, with clinical effects of envenomation, first aid and primary treatments.

Table F.3 Major types of venomous animals injuring humans with a summary of clinical effects, first aid and treatment

Type of animal	Major clinical effects	First aid	Prime treatment
Venomous snakes			
Brown snake	Coagulopathy (defibrination), renal damage, paralysis (rare)	PBI	Brown snake AV, 1–2 vials IV
Tiger snake, rough scaled snake	Coagulopathy (defibrination), paralysis, myolysis, renal damage	PBI	Tiger snake AV, 1–2 vials IV
Copperheads	Paralysis	PBI	Tiger snake AV, 1–2 vials IV
Broad headed, pale headed and Stephen's banded snakes	Coagulopathy (defibrination)	PBI	Tiger snake AV, 1–2 vials IV
Red bellied and blue bellied black snakes	Myolysis, coagulopathy (anticoagulant)	PBI	Tiger snake AV, 1–2 vials IV
Mulga and Collett's snakes	Myolysis, coagulopathy (anticoagulant)	PBI	Black snake or polyvalent AV, 1 vial IV
Taipan	Coagulopathy (defibrination), paralysis, myolysis, renal damage	PBI	Taipan or polyvalent AV, 1 vial IV

(Continued)

Table F.3   *(Continued)*

Type of animal	Major clinical effects	First aid	Prime treatment
Death adder	Paralysis	PBI	Death adder or polyvalent AV, 1 vial IV
Arthropods			
Funnel web spider	Neuroexcitatory envenoming, catecholamine storm effects, pulmonary oedema	PBI	Funnel web spider AV, 2–4+ vials IV
Red back spider	Neuroexcitatory envenoming, pain, sweating, hypertension, nausea	No first aid is effective	Red back spider AV, 2 vials IV or IM
Paralysis tick	Progressive flaccid paralysis (ascending)	No specific first aid; respiratory support	Respiratory support, remove all ticks
Bee, wasp and ant stings	Anaphylaxis in susceptible individuals	PBI, cardiorespiratory resuscitation, EpiPen®	Adrenaline, cardiorespiratory support
Marine			
Box jellyfish sting	Local pain, skin damage, cardiorespiratory collapse (rare, severe cases only)	Flood tentacles with vinegar before removing, cardiorespiratory support (if indicated)	Supportive and symptomatic care, box jellyfish AV IV in selected cases
Irukandji syndrome	Neuroexcitatory envenoming, catecholamine storm effects, intense pain in limbs and back, hypertension, sweating, rash	Flood sting area with vinegar, supportive care	Opioid analgesia, supportive care, consider magnesium sulphate infusion
Other jellyfish stings	Local pain, erythema	Hot water shower or immersion of stung area (45°C, but avoid thermal injury)	Hot water shower or immersion of stung area (45°C, but avoid thermal injury)
Stonefish sting	Local pain	Hot water shower or immersion of stung area (45°C, but avoid thermal injury)	Hot water shower or immersion of stung area (45°C, but avoid thermal injury), stonefish AV IV or IM
Other fish stings	Local pain	Hot water shower or immersion of stung area (45°C, but avoid thermal injury)	Hot water shower or immersion of stung area (45°C, but avoid thermal injury)
Stingray sting	Local pain, local trauma, potential necrosis	Hot water shower or immersion of stung area (45°C, but avoid thermal injury), staunch active bleeding, supportive care	Hot water shower or immersion of stung area (45°C, but avoid thermal injury), supportive care, manage open wound
Blue ringed octopus bite	Rapid flaccid paralysis, collapse	PBI, respiratory support if paralysis develops	Cardiorespiratory support

AV, antivenom; IM, intramuscular; IV, intravenous; PBI, pressure bandaging and immobilisation.

For all cases of envenoming seek **urgent expert advice** from your National Poisons Centre

F.8   Button battery ingestion

Any child who has ingested or is suspected of ingesting a button battery is a **time critical emergency**. Ingestion of button batteries can kill even if the child is asymptomatic. It is also important to suspect button battery ingestion in any presumed 'coin' or other foreign body ingestion.

Button battery ingestion affects all age groups, although most cases involve children under the age of 6 years who mistake the battery for a sweet, or older people with confusion or poor vision who mistake the battery for a pill. Older children, young people and adults may ingest batteries as a means of self-harming (Box F.1). There may be no history of foreign body ingestion (20–40% patients).

Box F.1   Safeguarding and mental health

- For all children of any age it is important to investigate circumstances around the ingestion of a button battery
- Any potentially vulnerable children or young people must be referred to the local safeguarding team
- Consider the possibility of attempted suicide in the older child or adolescent who will need a full CAMHS (Child and Adolescent Mental Health Services) assessment in addition to medical management

Children at greatest risk are:

- Those younger than 6 years of age
- Ingested battery over 20 mm diameter, which is more likely to become lodged in the oesophagus, and have been found to be responsible for more fatal or serious ingestions (Litovitz et al., 2010)
- Multiple batteries ingested or co-ingestion with strong magnets

Consider the possibility of battery ingestion in those with:

- Acute airway obstruction (stridor), drooling, wheezing or other noisy breathing
- Vomiting, abdominal pain or diarrhoea
- Chest pain or discomfort
- Difficulty swallowing
- Decreased appetite or refusal to eat, or coughing, choking or gagging with eating or drinking

In severe cases, there may be severe abdominal pain, bloody stools, irritability, fever and haemorrhage with subsequent stricture or fistula formation, even after removal of the battery.

Early use of a metal detector may help to confirm the presence of an ingested button battery.

Pathophysiology

- Disk or button batteries are small, coin-shaped batteries used within watches, calculators, hearing aids and many children's toys
- The batteries can contain several different metals (such as mercury, silver and lithium) along with sodium or potassium hydroxide to facilitate the chemical reaction
- Severe tissue damage is caused by sodium hydroxide (caustic soda) as a result of the electric current discharged from the battery, **not** battery leakage
- Even apparently discharged ('flat') batteries can still have this effect
- Injury is likely to have started within minutes of mucosal contact with burns, ulceration and perforation being seen within 2–4 hours of an ingestion becoming lodged in the oesophagus (or rarely the stomach)
- Sodium hydroxide causes tissue burns, often in the oesophagus, which can then cause necrosis, perforation, stricture and fistulae between the oesophagus and aorta or trachea. Several children have died from haemorrhage via aorto-oesophogeal fistulae – in one case 18 days after battery removal

- Oesophageal perforation and fistulae may be delayed for up to 28 days after removal of a button battery. Oesophageal strictures may not manifest for weeks to months after ingestion of a button battery and symptoms may develop after it has been passed in stool
- Passage of a button battery to the stomach alone cannot be used as a criterion that the child is free from a potentially catastrophic underlying injury, and passage through the gastrointestinal (GI) tract can take up to 2 weeks with prolonged transit time increasing the likelihood of symptoms
- Co-ingestion with a magnet may increase the chance of injury due to attraction across the bowel wall

Investigation

- Urgent chest X-ray: anteroposterior and lateral (including the neck)
- Abdominal X-ray

Important radiological characteristics suggestive of a button battery include:

- Radiopaque foreign body
- The halo effect/double rim
- Step-off on a lateral X-ray

Beware that the step-off may not be seen if the battery is thin or if the lateral film is not precisely perpendicular to the plane of the battery.

Management

Oesophageal location

- **Batteries lodged in the oesophagus or airway should be removed immediately irrespective of the presence or absence of symptoms.** If there is active GI bleeding within 28 days of removal of a button battery, assume the present of an aortoenteric fistula and summon the appropriate expertise
- Urgent anaesthetic, ENT and/or surgical teams must be contacted for immediate removal (Figure F.3)

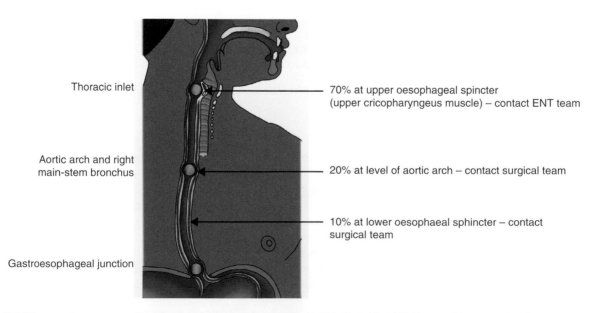

Thoracic inlet — 70% at upper oesophageal spincter (upper cricopharyngeus muscle) – contact ENT team

Aortic arch and right main-stem bronchus — 20% at level of aortic arch – contact surgical team

10% at lower oesophaeal sphincter – contact surgical team

Gastroesophageal junction

Figure F.3 The most common sites for button batteries to become lodged in children and young people

- Active bleeding and/or clinically instability – obtain urgent intravenous or intraosseous access and activate local major haemorrhage protocols
- There is experimental evidence to suggest that early administration of honey or sucralfate reduces acute alkali injury of the oesophagus by coating the battery and reducing hydroxide generation
- If clinically stable, consider the administration of sucralfate suspension whilst awaiting endoscopy in children over the age of 12 months if:
  - Honey has not been given in the pre-hospital setting
  - Provided it is immediately available
  - The child can swallow
  - It is less than 12 hours since ingestion
- Endoscopic removal is recommended so that the extent of mucosal damage can also be visualised and can help determine the requirement for oesophageal rest and further investigations. **This procedure should be completed within 2 hours of ingestion**
- All patients should be observed until the resolution of symptoms but if there is endoscopic evidence of oesophageal injury they are at risk of developing vascular injury (e.g. aortoenteric fistula) so further imaging (computed tomography or magnetic resonance imaging) after battery removal should be considered. Refer for ongoing specialist management as appropriate

Gastric location or beyond

- If the child is less than 5 years of age AND the button battery is ≥20 mm, they should have endoscopic assessment of any oesophageal injury and/or removal of the battery within 24–48 hours
- If the child is more than 5 years of age with any size button battery OR 5 years or younger and the button battery is less than 20 mm, consider outpatient observation only
- For any button battery over 20 mm the child will require a repeat X-ray in 48 hours
- The child needs a repeat X-ray after 10–14 days if the button battery fails to pass in the stool OR for any button battery over 20 mm
- At any point the child will require endoscopic removal if GI symptoms develop or if the battery has not passed through the stomach by the time of the repeat X-ray

Discharge

All patients should be observed in hospital until there is complete resolution of symptoms.

Parents should be advised to return to the emergency department for further urgent assessment if they have:

- Difficulty in breathing
- Features of intestinal obstruction (e.g. persistent vomiting, distended tender abdomen)
- Haematemesis or melaena
- Abdominal pain/gastritis
- Parental concern about a change in their child's eating patterns, such as refusing food or fluids

These symptoms may develop after the battery has passed through the intestine and should warrant a full medical review and discussion with the regional paediatric gastroenterology and/or surgical team.

F.9 Strong magnet ingestion

A symptomatic child or young person who has ingested a rare earth magnet requires urgent discussion with a tertiary paediatric surgical team. **The presence of symptoms with a history of rare earth magnet ingestion is highly likely to require surgical intervention.** Perforation and fistula formation are the most likely surgical findings.

The ingestion of a single rare earth magnet is unlikely to cause significant harm; however, if multiple magnets are ingested, or if a magnet is swallowed along with a metal object, significant GI injury can occur. Magnets can attract each other across layers of bowel to cause ischaemia and pressure necrosis of the gut with serious complications.

Consider the possibility of rare earth magnet ingestion in children with:

- Stridor, wheezing or other noisy breathing
- Drooling, difficulty swallowing, coughing, choking or gagging when eating or drinking
- Vomiting
- Chest pain or discomfort
- Abdominal pain
- Decreased appetite or refusal to eat

Abdominal symptoms may not manifest for weeks after the ingestion of magnets but intestinal injury can occur early, within 8–24 hours following ingestion, despite the child often remaining well.

Pathophysiology

- Neodymium magnets (also known as NdFeB, NIB, neo-magnet or super strong rare-earth magnets) have become easy to purchase and are promoted as 'adult desk toys' or 'stress relievers'
- Neodymium is a rare earth element that is used alongside iron and boron in the production of newly engineered powerful magnets. They are between five and 10 times stronger than ceramic magnets
- Anecdotal evidence from across the UK has identified that the incidence of magnet ingestion is increasing, especially in older children who may have been attempting to mimic tongue and cheek piercings, as well as permanent dental work leading to accidental ingestion
- As they are often brightly coloured and can be of a variety of shapes, they are also attractive to younger children and can be accidentally swallowed with ease
- Injuries seen include ulceration, necrosis, perforation, rupture, stricture, fistula, haemorrhage, mediastinitis, gastric outlet or bowel obstruction, volvulus, sepsis and death
- Surgical intervention is indicated when endoscopic removal is not indicated or is not possible because of the location, the number of magnets or where several bowel loops are attached to each other

Unlike most other 'foreign body' ingestions, the passage of rare earth magnets into the stomach must not be considered to be an indication that a child is free from any potentially catastrophic underlying injury. **The progression of the magnet/magnets through the GI tract is crucial to determining whether surgical intervention is required.** See Box F.2 for risk factors for complications.

Box F.2 Risk factors for complications following ingestion rare earth magnets

- Those who have co-ingested a magnet with a button battery
- Those who have ingested multiple magnets or a magnet and another metal object
- Children and young people with developmental, behavioural or psychiatric problems
- Delayed presentation (more than 12 hours after presentation)

Investigation

> **Do not use metal detectors for the assessment of children with suspected rare earth magnet ingestion**

- Chest X-ray
- Abdominal X-ray (with the child lying down, ideally anteroposterior)

X-rays are used to assess both the position of any magnets and the number of magnets. In the case of a single magnet being identified on an abdominal X-ray, further imaging may be needed to confirm that only one magnet has been ingested.

Pitfalls in radiological interpretation include:

- A neodymium magnet appears like a ball-bearing on an X-ray, be careful to not misdiagnose it as a metal ball
- Misdiagnosis of multiple magnets as solitary magnet ingestion can lead to a delay in diagnosis and subsequent complications

Management

- Symptomatic children, signs of deterioration and the ingestion of two or more rare earth magnets should be discussed with a specialist regional paediatric surgical centre
- Admission under the care of a local surgical team may be appropriate after discussion with the regional paediatric centre for close observation, repeat imaging and, in the event of any deterioration, intervention locally or transfer
- Children in the following categories should be considered suitable for discharge:
  - Single magnet ingestion
  - Accidental ingestion
  - No co-morbidities
  - Tolerating oral intake
  - Presenting within 24 hours of ingestion
  - Care-giver able to provide close observation (there is no need to examine the child's faeces)
- All children who are being discharged with rare earth magnet ingestion require at least one follow-up image to confirm magnet progression
- If the child becomes symptomatic before the repeat radiograph, urgent surgical review will be required
- If a single magnet is ingested, it can be expected to be passed spontaneously if the magnet is not too large

F.10 Summary

This appendix has described the standard approach to the management of envenomation and poisoning of various types.

Resuscitation of the baby at birth

Learning outcomes

After reading this appendix, you will be able to:

- Describe the approach to the resuscitation of the baby at birth and how this differs from the resuscitation of older children

---

G.1   Introduction

The resuscitation of babies at birth is different from the resuscitation of all other age groups as it usually supports the process of transition from intra- to extrauterine life, rather than the recovery of a child with serious illness or injury. Knowledge of the physiology of normal transition and how interruption to transition leading to hypoxia is essential in understanding the process outlined in the algorithm for resuscitating newborn babies (Figure G.1). The majority of babies will establish normal respiration and circulation without help. A tiny minority will not, and will require intervention.

As some babies are born unexpectedly out of hospital, or in a non-maternity setting within a hospital, or are unwell as a result of peripartum circumstances, it is important that clinicians working in any unit that receive neonates have an understanding of the differences between resuscitating older children and a newborn. Ideally, someone trained in newborn resuscitation should be present at all deliveries. It is advisable that all those who attend deliveries regularly should have been on courses such as the newborn life support (NLS) course organised by Resuscitation Council UK, European Resuscitation Council courses or the Neonatal Resuscitation Program organised by the American Academy of Pediatrics.

G.2   Normal physiology

Successful transition at birth involves moving from a fetal state, where the lungs are fluid filled and respiratory exchange occurs through the placenta, to that of a newborn baby whose air-filled lungs have successfully taken over that function. Preparation for this in a pregnancy progressing without incident is thought to begin in advance of labour, with detectable cellular changes occurring that may subsequently prime the lung tissues for reabsorption of the intra-alveolar fluid.

Advanced Paediatric Life Support: A Practical Approach to Emergencies, Seventh Edition. Edited by Stephanie Smith.
© 2023 John Wiley & Sons Ltd. Published 2023 by John Wiley & Sons Ltd.

Newborn life support

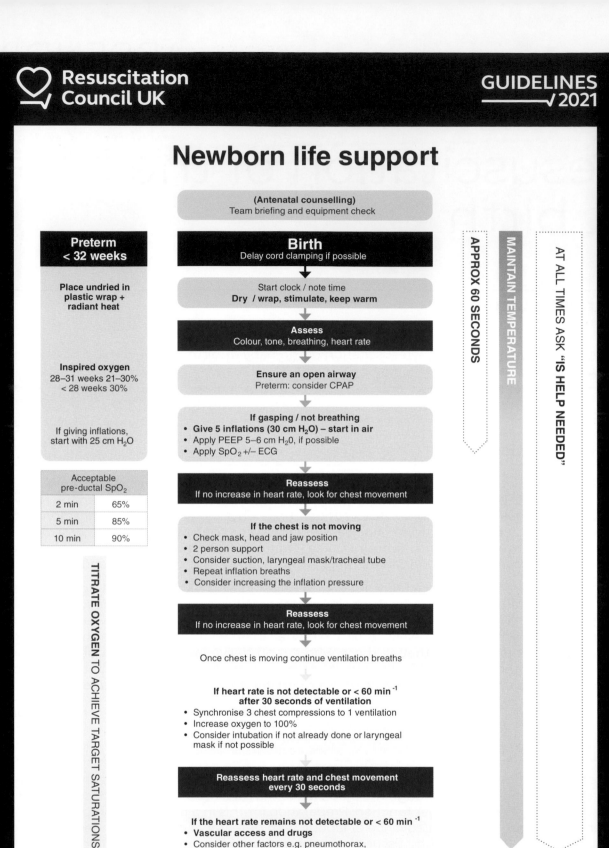

(Antenatal counselling)
Team briefing and equipment check

Birth
Delay cord clamping if possible

Start clock / note time
Dry / wrap, stimulate, keep warm

Assess
Colour, tone, breathing, heart rate

Ensure an open airway
Preterm: consider CPAP

If gasping / not breathing
- **Give 5 inflations (30 cm H_2O) – start in air**
- Apply PEEP 5–6 cm H_2O, if possible
- Apply SpO_2 +/– ECG

Reassess
If no increase in heart rate, look for chest movement

If the chest is not moving
- Check mask, head and jaw position
- 2 person support
- Consider suction, laryngeal mask/tracheal tube
- Repeat inflation breaths
- Consider increasing the inflation pressure

Reassess
If no increase in heart rate, look for chest movement

Once chest is moving continue ventilation breaths

**If heart rate is not detectable or < 60 min^{-1}
after 30 seconds of ventilation**
- Synchronise 3 chest compressions to 1 ventilation
- Increase oxygen to 100%
- Consider intubation if not already done or laryngeal mask if not possible

**Reassess heart rate and chest movement
every 30 seconds**

If the heart rate remains not detectable or < 60 min^{-1}
- **Vascular access and drugs**
- Consider other factors e.g. pneumothorax, hypovolaemia, congenital abormality

Update parents and debrief team
Complete records

Preterm < 32 weeks

Place undried in plastic wrap + radiant heat

Inspired oxygen
28–31 weeks 21–30%
< 28 weeks 30%

If giving inflations, start with 25 cm H_2O

Acceptable pre-ductal SpO_2	
2 min	65%
5 min	85%
10 min	90%

TITRATE OXYGEN TO ACHIEVE TARGET SATURATIONS

APPROX 60 SECONDS

MAINTAIN TEMPERATURE

AT ALL TIMES ASK "IS HELP NEEDED"

Figure G.1 Newborn resuscitation algorithm
Resuscitation Council UK 2021: https://www.resus.org.uk/sites/default/files/2021-05/Newborn%20Life%20Support%20 Algorithm%202021.pdf (last accessed March 2023)
CPAP, continuous positive airway pressure; ECG, electrocardiogram; PEEP, positive end-expiratory pressure

Airway/Breathing

After delivery, a healthy full-term baby usually takes their first breath within 60–90 seconds. Several factors drive this first breath to occur: exposure to the relative cold of the extrauterine environment; the physical stimulus of delivery; and the fact that even an uncomplicated vaginal delivery involves a degree of exposure to hypoxia. In a term baby, approximately 100 ml of fluid is cleared from the airways and alveoli, initially into the interstitial pulmonary tissue, and then later into the lymphatic and capillary systems. During vaginal delivery around 35 ml of fluid from the uppermost airways will be displaced by physical forces experienced by the baby during passage through the birth canal.

The respiratory pattern in newborn mammals has specifically evolved to facilitate replacement of the fluid in the lungs with air during the first few breaths. Animal studies show that at initiation of breathing, the inspiratory phase is longer than the expiratory phase (expiratory braking): expiration occurs against a partially closed glottis, heard as either crying or sometimes a grunting sound, creating increased pressure in the airways and driving the fluid into the lung tissue. In a healthy baby, the first spontaneous breaths may generate a negative inspiratory pressure of between –30 and –90 cmH$_2$O. This pressure is 10–15 times greater than that needed for later breathing but is necessary to overcome the resistance from the viscosity of the fluid filling the airways, the surface tension of the fluid-filled lungs, and the elastic recoil and resistance of the chest wall, lungs and airways. These powerful chest movements also aid displacement of fluid from the airways into the interstitial tissue of the lung. As long as the functional residual capacity (FRC) is successfully established, then the fluid displaced into the lung interstitial tissues will subsequently be cleared via the lymphatic system into the circulation.

If this process fails, and the fluid is not cleared from the interstitial tissue or leaks back into the alveolar spaces, then respiratory compromise will be seen with increased respiratory rate and effort of breathing.

Circulation

Neonatal circulatory adaptation commences at the same time as the pulmonary changes. Lung inflation and alveolar distension releases vasomotor compounds that reduce the pulmonary vascular resistance as well as increasing oxygenation. Evidence shows that as pulmonary vascular resistance falls during establishment of the FRC, pulmonary blood flow increases and consequently venous return to the left atrium increases. This leads to improved left ventricular filling and an increased stroke volume.

If the umbilical cord is clamped prior to the first breath, reduced venous return from the placenta to the right side of the heart results in an immediate decrease in heart size and a bradycardia as the pulmonary vascular resistance drops. There is then a return to its original size and recovery of the heart rate as long as the baby has successfully started to breath. The increase in size subsequently seen is likely due to the increased volume of blood returning to the left side of the heart from the expanded pulmonary circulation that occurs once the lungs are aerated. The loss of the low-resistance placental circulation results in increased systemic resistance and a spike in blood pressure. Immediate cord clamping is associated with a bradycardia that is avoided if cord clamping is deferred, particularly until after the first breath is taken (Figure G.2).

Circulatory adaptation proceeds with closure of the foramen ovale due to pressure changes as the pulmonary venous return to the left atrium increases and finishes with functional, then permanent, closure of the ductus arteriosus over the following days.

For these reasons, after a baby is born, the drying, thermal care and initial assessment starts with the cord intact. If assessment shows the baby is well, good thermal care should continue and the cord should remain unclamped for at least 60 seconds (preferably until the baby has taken their first breaths). If assessment demonstrates compromise warranting immediate resuscitation, then the cord can be clamped and cut to allow the baby to be taken to the resuscitative platform.

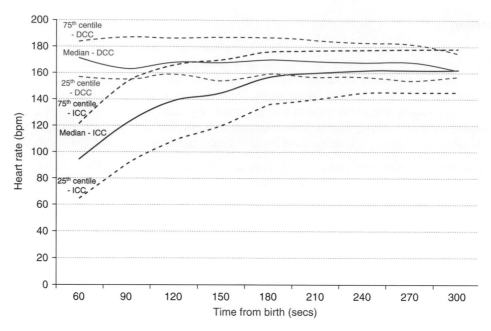

Figure G.2 Heart rates for babies who received immediate umbilical cord clamping (ICC) versus those who had their cord clamped after their first breath (deferred cord clamping (DCC))

G.3 Pathophysiology

The approach to resuscitating newborn humans evolved from observation of the pathophysiology of induced, acute, fetal hypoxia during pioneering mammal-based research in the early 1960s. The results of these experiments, which followed the physiology of newborn animals during acute, total, prolonged asphyxia and subsequent resuscitation, are summarised in Figure G.3.

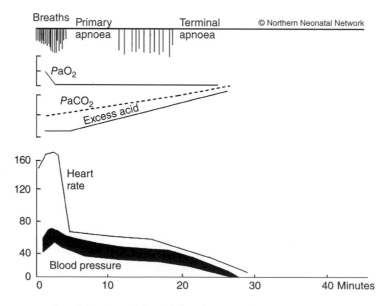

Figure G.3 Response of a mammalian fetus to total, sustained asphyxia starting at time 0
Reproduced with permission from Northern Neonatal Network

When the placental oxygen supply is interrupted or severely reduced, the fetus will initiate respiratory movements (i.e. attempt to breathe) in response to hypoxia. These breathing efforts fail to provide an alternative oxygen supply as the fetus is still in the womb surrounded by amniotic fluid: consequently the baby will become unconscious. If hypoxia continues, the higher respiratory centre in the brain becomes inactive and unable to continue to drive respiratory movements. The breathing therefore stops, usually within 2–3 minutes. This cessation of breathing is known as **primary apnoea** (Figure G.4).

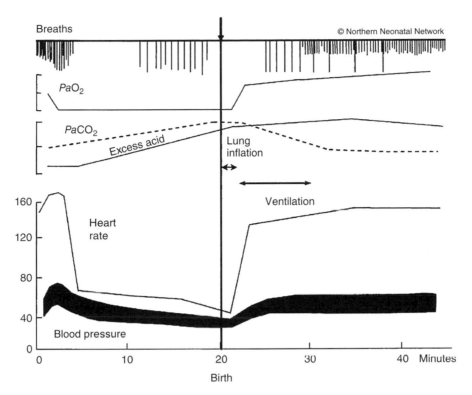

Figure G.4 Effects of lung inflation and a brief period of ventilation on a baby born in early terminal apnoea but before failure of the circulation
Reproduced with permission from Northern Neonatal Network

At the onset of hypoxia, a marked bradycardia will occur quickly. Intense peripheral vasoconstriction helps to maintain blood pressure with diversion of blood away from non-vital organs. The reduced heart rate also allows a longer ventricular filling time, and thus an increased stroke volume, which also helps maintain blood pressure.

As hypoxia continues, primary apnoea is broken: loss of descending neural inhibition by the higher respiratory centre allows primitive spinal centres to initiate forceful, gasping breaths. These deep, irregular gasps are easily distinguishable from normal breaths as they only occur 6–12 times per minute and involve all accessory muscles in a maximal, 'whole body' inspiratory effort. If this fails to draw air into the lungs and hypoxia continues, even this reflexive activity ceases and **terminal apnoea** begins. Without intervention, no further innate respiratory effort will occur. The time taken for such activity to cease is longer in the newly born baby than at any other time in life, taking up to 30 minutes.

The circulation is almost always maintained until **after** all respiratory activity ceases. This resilience is a feature of all newborn mammals at term and is largely due to the reserves of glycogen in the heart permitting prolonged, anaerobic generation of energy in the cardiomyocytes. Resuscitation is therefore relatively uncomplicated if undertaken before all respiratory activity has stopped. Once the lungs are aerated, oxygen will be carried to the heart and then to the brain provided the circulation is still functional (Figure G.4). Recovery will then be rapid. Most babies who have **not** progressed to terminal apnoea will resuscitate themselves if their airway is open. Once gasping ceases, however, the circulation starts to fail and resuscitation becomes more difficult. Support for the circulation is then required in addition to support for the breathing (Figure G.5).

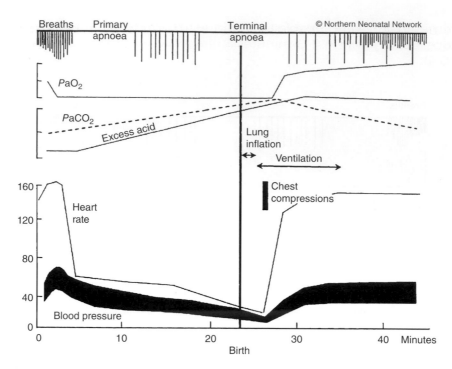

Figure G.5 Response of a baby born in terminal apnoea. In this case lung inflation is not sufficient because the circulation is already failing. However, lung inflation delivers air to the lungs and then a brief period of chest compressions delivers oxygenated blood to the heart, which then responds

Reproduced with permission from Northern Neonatal Network

G.4 Equipment

For many newborn babies, especially those born outside the delivery room, the need for resuscitation cannot be predicted. It is therefore useful to plan for such an eventuality. Equipment that may be required to resuscitate a newborn baby is listed in Box G.1.

Box G.1 Equipment required to resuscitate a newborn baby

- A flat surface
- Radiant heat source
- Dry towels
- Plastic bag for preterm babies
- Suitable hats
- Suction with catheters of at least 12 French gauge
- Face masks
- Bag–valve–mask or T-piece resuscitator with pressure-limiting device
- Source of air and/or oxygen
- Laryngeal mask size 1 (such as laryngeal mask airway or i-gel®)
- Laryngoscopes with straight blades, 0 and 1
- Nasogastric tubes
- Cord clamp
- Scissors
- Tracheal tubes sizes 2.5–4.0 mm
- Umbilical catheterisation equipment
- Adhesive tape
- Disposable gloves
- Monitoring saturations/ECG
- Stethoscope

Most babies can be resuscitated if there is access to a few pieces of key equipment: a firm, flat surface; means to provide warmth; a way to deliver air or oxygen to the lungs in a controlled fashion to displace the fluid present in the airways at delivery if the baby does not breath itself (ranging from using mouth-to-mouth to equipment-based techniques); and guidance from someone who is familiar with the process of newborn resuscitation (either as part of the resuscitation team or by telephone at the time of need).

G.5   Strategy for assessing and resuscitating a baby at birth

Resuscitation is likely to be rapidly successful if commenced before the baby has progressed beyond the point at which the circulation has started to fail. Babies in primary apnoea can usually resuscitate themselves if they have a clear airway. Unfortunately, it is not possible during the initial assessment to distinguish reliably whether an apnoeic, newborn baby is in primary or terminal apnoea. A structured approach that will work in either situation must therefore be applied to **all** apnoeic babies. The structured approach is outlined here. In reality the first four steps (up to and including assessment) are completed simultaneously. After this, appropriate intervention can begin following an ABCDE approach.

- Call/shout for help
- Start the clock or note the time
- Dry and wrap the baby in warmed dry towels. Maintain the baby's temperature
- Assess the situation
- Airway
- Breathing
- Chest compressions
- (Drugs/vascular access)

Call for help

Ask for help if you expect or encounter any difficulty or if the delivery is outside the labour suite. Where a pre-alert is received in hospital, convene the team for briefing and allocate roles.

Start the clock

Start the clock, if available, or note the time of birth.

At birth

There is no need to rush to clamp the cord at delivery. It should be left unclamped while the following steps are completed. Dry the baby quickly and effectively. Remove the wet towel and wrap the baby in a fresh, dry, warm towel. (For very small or significantly preterm babies it is better to place the wet baby in a food-grade plastic bag – and under a radiant heater as soon as possible.) Put a hat on **all** babies regardless of gestation. Assess the baby during and after drying: decide whether any intervention is needed. If your assessment suggests that the baby is in need of resuscitation, clamp and cut the cord. Otherwise wait for at least 60 seconds from the complete delivery of the baby (or, if safe, until the baby has started to breathe) before clamping the cord.

If the baby is assessed as needing assistance/resuscitation then this becomes the priority. If the equipment and skills are available resuscitation can be started whilst the baby is still attached to the placenta by a functioning umbilical cord. However, more commonly the cord needs to be clamped and cut in order to deliver assistance/resuscitation.

Keep the baby warm

The normal temperature range for a newborn baby is 36.5–37.5°C. For each 1°C decrease in admission temperature below this range in pre-term, low birthweight newborn babies there is an associated increase in baseline mortality of 28%. In environments likely to receive sick babies or infants the room temperatures should be kept as close as possible to the recommended minimum for term babies (23–25°C) and if a preterm baby is known to be about to deliver the environment should be warmed to at least 26°C if possible. Where delivery or admission of a newborn baby is imminent **outside** these environments, anticipation and active management of room temperature to achieve this baseline as quickly as possible is required: eliminate any draughts from the room (close window and doors where possible) and heat the room to above 23°C (term babies) or above 25°C (preterm babies).

Once delivered, dry the baby immediately and then wrap in a warm, dry towel. In addition to increased mortality risk, a cold baby has an increased rate of oxygen consumption and is more likely to become hypoglycaemic and acidotic. If this is not addressed at the beginning of resuscitation it is often forgotten. Most heat loss at delivery is caused by the baby being wet (evaporation) and in a draught (convection). Babies also have a large surface area to weight ratio, exacerbating heat loss. An overhead heater or external heat source should be used as well if available, but drying effectively and wrapping the baby in a warm, dry towel with the head covered by a hat are the most effective interventions to avoid hypothermia. A naked dry baby can still become hypothermic despite a warm room or the use of a radiant heater, especially if there is a draught.

In **all** babies, the head represents a significant part of the baby's surface area (see Section G.10) so attention to providing a hat is invaluable in maintaining normothermia.

Out of hospital. Babies of all gestations born outside the normal delivery environment may benefit from placement in a food-grade polyethylene bag or wrap *after* drying and then swaddling. Alternatively, well newborn babies of more than 30 weeks' gestation who are breathing may be dried, have a hat put on and be nursed with skin-to-skin contact (or kangaroo parent care) with a cover over any remaining exposed skin to maintain their temperature whilst they are transferred. Ensure the baby remains positioned in a way that maintains airway patency.

Assessment of the newborn baby

During and immediately after drying and wrapping the baby, make a full assessment:

A/B	Breathing	Regular, gasp, none
C	Heart rate	Fast (more than 100 beats/min), slow (60–100 beats/min), very slow/absent (less than 60 beats/min)
D	Tone	Well flexed, reduced tone, floppy
E	Colour	Pink/pale/blue

Unlike resuscitation at other ages, **all** four items are assessed in parallel and a rapid ABCDE assessment helps decide on the need for resuscitation. Once resuscitative measures are started, regular reassessment should assess their effect.

This is different to the linear hierarchy of assessment and treatment used at other ages. In the newborn baby, heart rate and breathing provide the most useful information and are the **only** items that need regularly reassessing during resuscitation to assess effectiveness of intervention. At the initial assessment, however, taking note of the baby's tone can also be informative: a very floppy baby is likely to be unconscious, suggesting that the baby may have been subject to hypoxia.

Colour is a potentially useful indicator of status. Normal babies are born 'blue' and become 'pink' in the first minutes of life. A baby who is pale ('shut down') due to intense peripheral vasoconstriction is more likely to be acidotic: this sort of appearance suggests significant cardiovascular response to peripartum compromise.

Breathing movements and colour can be determined by observation during drying; tone can be evaluated whilst in the act of drying the baby. Heart rate is determined by auscultation of the heart using a stethoscope which can be done during the drying by a second person or immediately afterwards if the responder is on their own.

Breathing

Most well, term babies will take their first breath 60–90 seconds after delivery and establish spontaneous, regular breathing sufficient to maintain the heart rate ≥100 beats/min within 3 minutes of birth. If there is no breathing (apnoea), gasping or irregular, ineffective breathing that persists after drying, intervention is required.

Heart rate

In the first couple of minutes, auscultating at the cardiac apex is the best method to assess the heart rate. Palpating peripheral pulses is not practical and is not recommended. Palpation of the umbilical pulse can only be relied upon if the palpable rate is ≥100 beats/min. A rate less than this should be checked by auscultation. It may not be possible to feel a cord pulse when there **is** a heart rate that can be detected by auscultation.

In delivery suites, saturation monitors are used by neonatal intensive care unit (NICU) teams when resuscitation is required at term, or when preterm babies have been delivered. However, applying a saturation monitor should not interrupt the process of resuscitation. It is also good practice to correlate the probe reading (heart rate), once good detection signal strength is achieved, with the auscultated heart rate. An electrocardiogram (ECG), if available, can give a rapid, accurate and continuous heart rate reading during newborn resuscitation, but the use of ECG must also not delay the delivery of resuscitative care. In low-resource or non-specialist settings (especially if the only saturation monitor probe available is designed to fit a larger child or adult), the use of a stethoscope is recommended to allow resuscitation to proceed without delay.

The probe for the saturation monitor must be applied to the **right** (not left) hand or wrist in order to accurately reflect the preductal saturations (which are most likely to reflect the oxygenation of blood being distributed to the coronary arteries and cerebral circulation). A correctly applied pulse oximeter can give an accurate reading of heart rate and saturations within 60–90 seconds of application. Oxygen saturation levels in healthy babies in the first few minutes of life may be considerably lower than at other times (Table G.1). Attempting to judge oxygenation by assessing colour of the skin or mucous membranes is not reliable, but it is still worth noting the baby's colour at birth as well as whether, when and how it changes later in the resuscitation. Very pale babies who remain pale and bradycardic after resuscitation may be hypovolaemic as well as acidotic. Similarly, tone immediately at birth should be assessed, and changes noted as resuscitation progresses.

Table G.1 Oxygen saturation levels in babies in the first few minutes of life

Time from birth	Acceptable preductal SpO$_2$ levels
2 minutes	65%
5 minutes	85%
10 minutes	90%

An accurate and prompt initial assessment of heart rate is vital because an increase in the heart rate will be the first sign of success during resuscitation.

Outcome of the initial assessment

Initial assessment will categorise the baby into one of the three following groups.

1. **Vigorous breathing or crying; good tone; heart rate ≥100 beats/min.** These are healthy babies. They should be dried and kept warm, with a hat on, and the umbilical cord clamped after 60 seconds. They can be given to their mothers and nursed skin-to-skin if this is appropriate and the baby can be protected from drafts by covering. The baby will remain warm through skin-to-skin contact under a cover and may also be put to the breast at this stage.

2. **Irregular or inadequate breathing or apnoea; normal or reduced tone; heart rate less than 100 beats/min.** If gentle stimulation (drying will be an adequate stimulus in this situation) does not induce effective breathing, consider whether the cord needs to be clamped and cut to allow resuscitation to commence. After drying and wrapping are completed, the airway should be opened. Most of these babies will improve with inflation of the lungs using a mask and the heart rate should be used to assess the effect of this intervention. Some babies in this group will then require a period of ventilation by mask until they recover respiratory drive and are able to breathe for themselves.

3. **Breathing inadequately, gasping or apnoeic; globally floppy; heart rate very slow (less than 60 beats/min) or absent and colour blue or pale (pale often suggests poor perfusion).** Ensure good thermal care and begin intervention as per the algorithm (see Figure G.1).

Whether an apnoeic baby is in primary or terminal apnoea (see Figure G.2), the initial management is the same although it will be quickly apparent that in this case deferred cord clamping (DCC) is not appropriate. Cord milking ('stripping') has sometimes been advocated as an alternative to DCC in babies who are in need of immediate assistance. This can be done in babies more than 28 weeks' gestation but is not recommended below this as there is some evidence it is associated with harm (cerebral intraventricular haemorrhage).

Dry and wrap the baby, assessing as you go, and then commence resuscitation. Open the airway and then inflate the lungs using five 2–3-second inflation breaths. A reassessment of heart rate response and chest rise with mask inflation directs further resuscitation. After assessment, resuscitation follows the broad categories of the structured approach seen in the algorithm (see Figure G.1):

- Airway
- Breathing
- Circulation
- Drugs, used in a few selected cases

G.6 Resuscitation of the newborn baby

Airway

To achieve an open airway, the baby should be positioned with the head in the neutral position (Figure G.6) (see Chapter 17).

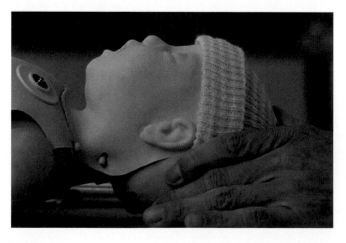

Figure G.6 Neutral position in babies
Children's Health Queensland / CC BY 4.0

A newborn baby's head has a large, often moulded, occiput that tends to cause the neck to flex when the baby is supine on a flat surface. A 2 cm folded towel placed under the neck and shoulders (Figure G.7) may help to maintain the airway in a neutral position and a jaw thrust may be needed

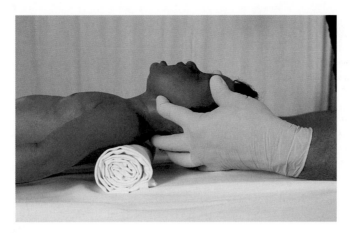

Figure G.7 Neutral position in babies with towel
Children's Health Queensland / CC BY 4.0

to bring the tongue forward and to open the airway, especially if the baby is floppy. However, over-extension may also collapse the newborn baby's pharyngeal airway, leading to obstruction. If using a towel under the shoulders, care must be exercised to avoid such overextension of the neck.

Most secretions found in and around the oropharynx at birth are thin and rarely cause airway obstruction. Priority should be given in **all** babies to the application of a well-fitting mask and inflating the lungs once airway position and control is established, even those born through meconium.

If, during resuscitation, there is concern that there might be an airway obstruction (e.g. if the heart rate is poor and the chest does not move with appropriately applied mask ventilation), then airway opening options including a two-person jaw thrust (Figure G.8), insertion of a laryngeal mask, or suction of the oropharynx under direct vision using a laryngoscope should be considered. Any obvious material obstructing the airway should be removed by gentle suction with a large-bore suction catheter. Deep pharyngeal suction without direct visualisation should not be performed as it may cause extensive soft tissue injury, vagal nerve-induced bradycardia and laryngospasm. Suction, if it is used, should not exceed –20.0 kPa (–150 mmHg).

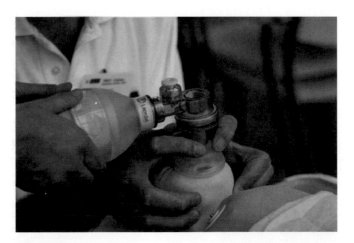

Figure G.8 Two-person jaw thrust
Children's Health Queensland / CC BY 4.0

A two-person jaw thrust or a laryngeal mask airway are used in preference to oropharyngeal airways as these can occasionally worsen airway obstruction in smaller babies. Oropharyngeal airways can sometimes be useful in the context of a difficult airway.

Meconium aspiration

Meconium-stained liquor (light green tinge) is relatively common and occurs in up to 10% of births. Meconium aspiration is a **rare** event, when it happens the aspiration usually occurs in utero as the fetus approaches term. It requires intrauterine fetal compromise severe enough to have caused both the reflexive passage of meconium and the onset of gasping respiratory movements for meconium to be aspirated.

That meconium has been inhaled *before* delivery means that the previously widely advocated and used combined obstetric–neonatal strategy of suctioning the airways after delivery has not been shown to be of use. No difference in incidence of meconium aspiration syndrome has been shown in the most obtunded of babies who were subjected to tracheal intubation followed by suction and those who were not intubated. All that these procedures do is delay the application of appropriate resuscitative measures to the baby in need in a timely fashion. Thus, when faced with a baby who has been born through meconium-stained liquor, and who needs assistance, lung aeration should be the priority, **not** clearance of meconium.

In the context of a baby delivered through meconium who needs resuscitation, start with the standard NLS algorithm; only suction under direct vision if you fail to get chest movement with inflation breaths delivered for the correct length of time (five breaths, each 2–3 seconds long) with the head in the correct (neutral) position.

From the perspective of effective resuscitation, the only type of meconium that may cause an immediate issue is that which is thick and viscid and which has the potential to block the airway. If suction under direct vision is required, a suitable wide-bore catheter or Yankauer sucker should be used. Routine tracheal intubation is not recommended for babies born through meconium, although if very thick meconium blocks the airway then using a meconium aspirator attached to a tracheal tube can be helpful, if the team present have the required skills. A small proportion of babies born through thick meconium will need more advanced intensive care management on a neonatal unit.

Breathing (inflation breaths and ventilation)

The first five breaths in term babies should be 'inflation' breaths in order to replace lung fluid in the alveoli with air. These should be 2–3-second sustained breaths ideally delivered using a T-piece resuscitator with a continuous gas supply, a pressure-limited device (e.g. Neopuff™) (set at a limit of 30 cmH$_2$O) and an appropriately sized mask. Use a suitable sized face mask that is big enough to cover the nose and mouth of the baby to ensure a good fit, no leak and that it does not obstruct ventilation. If no such system is available then a 500 ml self-inflating bag and a blow-off valve set at 30–40 cmH$_2$O can be used (Figure G.9). This is especially useful if compressed air or oxygen is not available. A smaller size of bag (less than 500 ml) can work but it is harder to sustain the inflation over 2–3 seconds and thus should not be used by choice unless no alternative exists. During these five breaths, it is important to remember that the chest may not be seen to move during the first few breaths as fluid is displaced and replaced by air. After the five breaths, the first reassessment should be done.

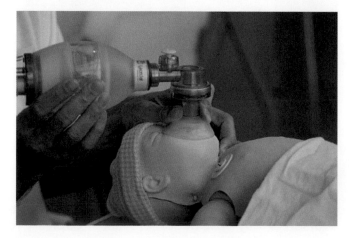

Figure G.9 Bag–mask ventilation
Children's Health Queensland / CC BY 4.0

Adequate ventilation is usually indicated by either a rapidly increasing heart rate or a heart rate that is maintained at ≥100 beats/min. It is safe to assume the chest has been inflated successfully if the heart rate responds.

Once the chest is inflated and the heart rate has increased **or** the chest has been seen to move, then ventilation should be continued at a rate of c. 30 per minute using shorter breaths (no more than 1 second inspiratory time). Continue ventilatory support until regular spontaneous breathing is established.

Where possible, start resuscitation of the newborn baby of more than 32 weeks' gestation with air. There is now good evidence for this in term babies and excessive oxygen should be avoided in premature babies. For babies under 28 weeks' start in 30% oxygen and for babies 28–32 weeks' use 21–30%. The use of supplemental oxygen should be guided by preductal pulse oximetry (see earlier), with reasonable levels listed in Table G.1 and Figure G.1 on acceptable saturations.

If the heart rate has not responded to the five inflation breaths then check that you have **seen** chest movement. Auscultation by stethoscope of fluid-filled lungs during the administration of inflation or ventilation breaths may erroneously detect 'breath' sounds even **without** effective lung inflation. Go back and check airway-opening manoeuvres and repeat the inflation breaths if you have not seen chest movement. If you have seen chest movement and the heart rate has not increased, give 30 seconds of ventilation breaths and reassess the heart rate.

Circulation

If the heart rate remains very slow (less than 60 beats/min) or absent, despite adequate lung inflation **and** subsequent ventilation for 30 seconds (with demonstrable chest movement), then chest compressions should be started.

Chest compressions in the newborn aim to move oxygenated blood from the lungs to the heart and coronary arteries; they are not intended to sustain cerebral circulation as they do in older children or adults. Once oxygenated blood reaches the coronary arteries it will usually result in a change from anaerobic energy generation to aerobic energy generation and, as a result, the heart rate will increase. This will then provide the required cardiac output to perfuse the vital organs. The blood you move using cardiac compressions **can only be oxygenated if the lungs have air in them**. Newborn cardiac compromise is almost always the result of respiratory failure and can only be effectively treated if effective ventilation is occurring.

The most efficient way of delivering chest compressions in the newborn baby is to encircle the chest with both hands, so that the fingers lie behind the baby, supporting the back, and the thumbs are overlapped, overlying over the lower third of the sternum (Figure G.10). Overlapping the thumb tips is more effective than placing the thumb tips side by side, but is more likely to cause operator

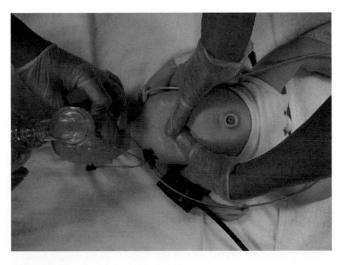

Figure G.10 Hand-encircling technique for chest compressions
Children's Health Queensland / CC BY 4.0

fatigue. Compress the chest briskly, **by one-third of the anteroposterior diameter**, and ensure that **full recoil of the anterior chest wall is allowed** after each compression, before commencing the next compression. The relaxation phase is when the blood returns to the coronary arteries and therefore is essential to effective technique. Evidence clearly supports a synchronised ratio of three compressions for each ventilation breath (3:1 ratio) as the most effective ratio in the newborn, aiming to achieve 120 events (90 compressions and 30 ventilations) per minute.

The purpose of chest compressions is to move **oxygenated** blood or drugs to the coronary arteries in order to initiate cardiac recovery. Thus there is no point in starting chest compression before effective lung inflation has been established. Similarly, compressions are ineffective unless interposed by ventilation breaths of good quality. Therefore, the emphasis must be upon **good-quality breaths**, followed by effective compressions at a ratio of one breath to three compressions. Simultaneous delivery of compressions and breaths (otherwise known as chest compression with asynchronous ventilation, as used in older children with a secure airway) should not be done even when the baby is intubated, as compressions will reduce the effectiveness of any breath if the two coincide. It is usually only necessary to continue chest compressions for about 20–30 seconds before the heart responds with an increase in heart rate, thus reassessment of the heart rate at regular 30-second intervals is recommended. If chest compressions are required in resuscitation, ensure that 100% oxygen is also being delivered to the baby by whatever ventilatory system is being used during the period of cardiopulmonary resuscitation (CPR). This can then be weaned using pulse oximetry as a guide once return of spontaneous circulation (ROSC) is established.

Once the heart rate is above 60 beats/min and rising, chest compressions may be discontinued. Ventilation breaths will need to be continued, by whichever method has been used effectively thus far, until effective spontaneous breathing commences. In the absence of breathing starting spontaneously, formal mechanical ventilation may need to be instituted.

Drugs

If adequate lung inflation and ventilation with effective cardiac compressions does not lead to the heart rate improving to above 60 beats/min, drugs should be considered. The most common reason for failure of the heart rate to respond is failure to achieve or maintain lung inflation, and there is **no point** in giving drugs unless the airway is open and the lungs have been inflated. Airway, breathing (i.e. the observed chest movement) and chest compressions must be reassessed as adequate and effective before proceeding to drug therapy. Drugs are best administered via a centrally placed umbilical venous line or, if this is not possible, an intraosseous needle is an alternative in term babies. **The outcome is likely to be poor if drugs are needed for successful resuscitation at birth**.

Adrenaline

The α-adrenergic effect of adrenaline increases coronary artery perfusion during resuscitation, enhancing oxygen delivery to the heart. In the presence of profound, unresponsive bradycardia or circulatory standstill, 20 micrograms/kg (0.2 ml/kg of 1:10 000) adrenaline may be given intravenously. This **must** be followed by a flush of 0.9% sodium chloride to ensure it reaches the circulation (3–5 ml). Further doses of adrenaline at 20 micrograms/kg (0.2 ml/kg of 1:10 000) followed by a 0.9% sodium chloride flush can be given every 3–5 minutes if there is no response to the initial bolus and resuscitation is ongoing. If intravenous or intraosseous access cannot be established, intratracheal adrenaline can be tried, although a dose of 100 micrograms/kg will be needed. This higher dose **must not** be given intravenously. If intratracheal adrenaline is given and resuscitation is ongoing then umbilical venous catheter or intraosseous access should be sought.

Glucose

Hypoglycaemia is associated with adverse neurological outcomes and worsened cerebral damage in neonatal animal models of asphyxia and resuscitation. Once the neonatal heart has consumed endogenous glycogen supplies, it also requires an exogenous energy source to continue functioning.

Therefore, during prolonged resuscitation it is appropriate to consider giving a slow bolus of 2.5 ml/kg of 10% glucose IV. Once a bolus has been given, provision of a secure intravenous glucose infusion is needed to prevent rebound hypoglycaemia (see Appendix J). A glucose bolus given during neonatal resuscitation is unlikely to cause harmful hyperglycaemia but may avoid damaging hypoglycaemia. Normoglycaemia is optimal and post-resuscitation glucose levels should be closely monitored. Many strip glucometers are not reliable in neonates and, wherever possible, should not be used for blood glucose estimation. Appropriate options include blood gas analyser, or a formal laboratory glucose measurement (unless excessive delay).

Bicarbonate

Any baby in terminal apnoea will have a significant metabolic component to the acidosis present. Acidosis depresses cardiac function. Sodium bicarbonate 1–2 mmol/kg (2–4 ml/kg of 4.2% solution) may be used to raise the pH and enhance the effects of oxygen and adrenaline in prolonged resuscitation, after adequate ventilation and circulation (with chest compressions) has been established. Bicarbonate use remains controversial and it should only be used in the absence of discernible cardiac output despite all resuscitative efforts, or in profound and unresponsive bradycardia. Its use is not recommended during short periods of CPR.

Fluid

Very occasionally hypovolaemia may be present because of known or suspected blood loss (antepartum haemorrhage, placenta/vasa praevia or bleeding from a separated but unclamped umbilical cord). Hypovolaemia secondary to loss of vascular tone following asphyxia is less common. Where a baby remains pale and shocked in appearance, or where there is a persistent bradycardia despite drug administration, intravascular volume expansion may be appropriate. Balanced crystalloids at 10 ml/kg (or 0.9% sodium chloride) can be used safely. If blood loss is likely, especially where acute and severe, uncrossmatched, cytomegalovirus-negative, group O RhD-negative blood should be given in preference. Albumin (and other plasma substitutes) cannot be recommended. However, most newborn resuscitations do not require the administration of fluid unless there has been known blood loss or septicaemic shock.

Excessive intravascular volume expansion may cause worsened cardiac function in a heart subject to prolonged hypoxia, and is associated with increased rates of (cerebral) intraventricular haemorrhage and pulmonary haemorrhage in preterm babies.

Naloxone

This is not a drug of resuscitation to be given acutely. Occasionally, a baby who has been effectively resuscitated, is pink, with a heart rate of ≥100 beats/min, may not breathe spontaneously because of the possible effects of maternal opioid medications. If respiratory-depressant effects are suspected in the baby naloxone IM (200 micrograms in a full-term baby) could be considered. Smaller doses of 10 micrograms/kg will also reverse opioid sedation but the effect will only last a short time (20 minutes compared with a few hours after IM administration). Intravenous naloxone has a half-life shorter than the opiates it is meant to reverse, and there is no evidence to recommend intratracheal administration.

Bicarbonate, glucose, fluid boluses and naloxone should **never** be given intratracheally.

G.7 Response to resuscitation

The first indication of successful progress in resuscitation will be an increase in heart rate. Recovery of respiratory drive may be delayed. Babies in terminal apnoea will tend to gasp first as they recover before starting normal respirations (see Figure G.4). Those who were in primary apnoea are likely to start with normal breaths, which may commence at any stage of resuscitation. Depending on circulatory status, skin colour may recover quickly or slowly, but universally the tone (a proxy for consciousness) of the baby is the last key metric to improve once heart function, circulation and spontaneous, effective breathing are restored.

Discontinuation of resuscitation

The outcome for a baby with no detectable heart rate at more than 10 minutes after birth outside a planned setting is likely to be very poor, but innovation in neonatal intensive care means that where there is rapid access to good neonatal intensive care this is no longer universally true. Additionally, it commonly takes longer than 10 minutes to complete all the steps in the NLS algorithm (Figure G.1).

Place of birth, likely intrauterine aetiology of the presentation and duration of events before delivery, and immediate access to treatments such as therapeutic hypothermia and good-quality neonatal intensive care, should be factored into the decision-making process when considering stopping resuscitation. Most recent studies show that if conditions exist to ensure immediate high-quality resuscitation and optimised post-resuscitation with active therapeutic hypothermia, then resuscitation can reasonably continue beyond 10 minutes without a detectable heart rate. However, particular attention to correcting reversible causes of arrest (4 Hs and 4 Ts) should be made beyond this point if not already done, and if the time without recovery of a heart rate approaches 20 minutes proactive consideration of stopping resuscitation should be made.

Resuscitation beyond 20 minutes with no detectable heart rate is most likely to end in death for the baby or severe disability in the very few survivors, regardless of the subsequent provision of NICU care.

Stopping resuscitation is a decision that lies with the most senior clinicians present, ideally with input from those experienced in resuscitation of the newborn. This may mean consulting with neonatal teams in other centres, by telephone or video-conferencing.

Where a very slow heart rate has persisted (less than 60 beats/min without improvement) during 20 minutes of continuous resuscitation, the decision to stop is much less clear. No evidence is available to recommend a universal approach beyond evaluation of the situation on a case-by-case basis by the resuscitating team and (ideally) senior clinicians. In these circumstances, availability and access to ongoing intensive care has a greater bearing on what decision may be appropriate.

A decision to limit resuscitation measures or stop before 20 minutes, or to not start resuscitation at all, may be appropriate in situations of extreme prematurity (less than 22–23 weeks), a birth weight of less than 400 g or in the presence of lethal abnormalities such as anencephaly or confirmed trisomy 13 or 18. Resuscitation is nearly always indicated in conditions with a high survival rate and acceptable morbidity. Such decisions should be taken by a senior member of the team, ideally a consultant, in consultation with the parents and other team members. When a decision has been made for discontinuation of resuscitation, the parents should be given opportunities to hold their baby.

G.8 Supraglottic airway

A supraglottic airway (SGA) may be considered as an alternative to a face mask for positive pressure ventilation among newborn babies weighing more than 2000 g or delivered at 34 weeks' or more gestation. It should be considered during resuscitation of the newborn baby if face mask ventilation is unsuccessful with a two-person technique or where there is a single rescuer. There is limited evidence evaluating its use for newborn babies weighing less than 2000 g or delivered at under 34 weeks' gestation, and none for babies who are receiving compressions.

Commonly used types of neonatal-appropriate SGA include the laryngeal mask airway (LMA) (which utilises an inflatable cuff to create a seal) and the i-gel® (which uses a soft thermoplastic that moulds itself to the shape of the baby's larynx once in place by virtue of the baby's body heat, to create a seal).

The insertion of a LMA should be undertaken only by those individuals who have been trained to use it. However, to achieve proficient use requires only short training. Due to constraints on training time and experience, it is more likely that someone can be trained to use a LMA than will have an opportunity to achieve proficiency in tracheal intubation. Evidence suggests that LMAs are not superior to face masks in trained hands and in most UK settings it will be appropriate to use face masks as the first line. If there is a need for transfer between settings and respiratory support is ongoing, a LMA may be useful to provide a secure airway. In the neonate, it is recommended that a laryngoscope or tongue depressor is used to help move the tongue out of the way before insertion of the LMA, as this creates a wider space for the LMA to pass through. It also allows examination for any potential oropharyngeal obstruction by particulate matter to be identified and resolved by use of suction before the LMA is inserted.

G.9   Tracheal intubation

Most babies can be resuscitated using a face mask or LMA. Swedish data suggest that if mask ventilation is applied effectively, only one in 500 babies actually **need** intubation. Tracheal intubation remains the gold standard in airway management but only if the tracheal tube can be correctly placed, without significantly interrupting ongoing ventilation and without causing trauma to the oropharynx and trachea. It is especially useful in prolonged resuscitations, in managing extremely preterm babies, and when a tracheal blockage is suspected. It should be considered if mask ventilation has failed, although the most common reason for this is poor positioning of the head with consequent failure to open the airway. It is, however, a common source of task fixation and can result in a significant interruption of resuscitation. It therefore needs experienced operators carefully marshalled to prevent unwarranted delay in moving along the resuscitative algorithm, **especially** if mask ventilation is effective prior to the intubation attempt (see 'Discontinuation of resuscitation' earlier in this chapter).

The technique of intubation is the same as for older infants and is described in Chapter 19. An appropriately grown, normal, term newborn baby usually needs a 3.5 mm (internal diameter) tracheal tube, but 2.5, 3.0 and 4.0 mm tubes should also be available. The smallest size available is a 2.0 mm tube and although not always available it may be needed for babies born extremely prematurely.

Tracheal tube placement must be assessed visually during intubation and in most cases will be confirmed by a rapid response in heart rate on ventilating via the tracheal tube. An exhaled carbon dioxide (CO_2) detection system (either colorimetric or quantitative, i.e. capnometry) is a rapid, and now widely available, adjunct to confirmation of correct tracheal tube placement. The detection of exhaled CO_2 should be used to confirm tracheal tube placement, but it should not be used in isolation. Listening to air entry in both axillae and seeing symmetrical chest movement may help avoid intubation of the right main bronchus, which can give a 'false positive' capnographic test. A number of other false positive reactions can occur with direct contamination of colorimetric detectors by drugs used in the newborn setting. False negatives can occur in low cardiac output states where CO_2 may not be detected despite accurate tracheal tube placement.

G.10   Preterm babies

Unexpected deliveries outside delivery suites are more likely to be preterm. Whilst moderately preterm babies (33–36 weeks' gestation) can be managed in the same way as term babies, many babies born between 32 and 33 weeks' gestation, and **all** babies born before 32 weeks' gestation, need to be carefully supported during their transition to extrauterine life. This is described as stabilisation, rather than resuscitation, and aims to prevent problems, rather than providing resuscitation from a hypoxic event.

Premature babies are more likely to get cold (because of a higher surface area to mass ratio) and are more likely to become hypoglycaemic (fewer glycogen stores). Wrapping the head and body (but not face) of all babies of less than 32 weeks' gestation in polyethylene wrap or a bag, where there is access to a radiant heater, should be done to aid maintenance of normothermia. The use of a radiant heater theoretically warms the wet baby through the plastic, trapping a warmed, humidified atmosphere around them to maintain thermal control (Box G.2). In babies of less than 32 weeks'

Box G.2 Guidelines for the use of plastic bags for preterm babies (less than 32 weeks' gestation) at birth

- Preterm babies born before 32 completed weeks of gestation may be placed in plastic bags or wrap for temperature stability during resuscitation. They should remain in the bag until they are on the NICU and the humidity within their incubator is at the desired level. It is a way of preventing evaporative heat loss and cannot replace incubators, etc. Neither should it replace all efforts to maintain a high ambient temperature around babies born outside delivery suites
- At birth the preterm baby should not be dried but should be slipped straight into the prepared plastic bag or wrapping feet first. There is no need to wrap the baby in a towel so long as this is done immediately after birth. This gives immediate humidity. The plastic bag only prevents evaporative heat loss; once in the bag the baby should be placed under a radiant heater
- Suitable plastic bags are food-grade bags designed for microwaving and roasting
- The bag should cover the baby from the shoulders to the feet. Gaps around the neck should be avoided as this allows warm humidified air out and colder air in. The head will stick out of the bag and should be dried as usual and a hat should be placed over the head to further reduce heat loss. Resuscitation/stabilisation should commence as per NLS guidelines
- A plastic bag or wrap will not interfere with standard resuscitation measures. If the umbilicus is required for vascular access then a small hole can be made in the bag to facilitate this
- The bag should not be removed unless deemed necessary by the registrar or consultant
- After transfer to a neonatal unit and stabilising ventilation, if required, the baby's temperature should be recorded. The bag is only removed when the incubator humidity is satisfactory, the baby's temperature is normal and further care provided as per nursing protocols
- This is a potentially useful technique for keeping larger babies warm when born unexpectedly outside the delivery suite or in the community. However, it should be augmented by also wrapping with warm towels and ensuring a warm environment

---

gestation other interventions may also be needed to maintain temperature such as careful use of a thermal mattress and warmed humidified respiratory gases when ventilated. Where external heat sources are used, continuous temperature monitoring is necessary to prevent hyperthermia. After 30 weeks' gestation, an alternative is to dry and wrap the baby in a dry, warm towel in a similar fashion to babies born at term.

The more premature a baby is, the less likely it is to establish adequate spontaneous respirations without assistance. Preterm babies of less than 32 weeks' gestation are likely to be deficient in surfactant especially after unexpected or precipitate delivery. Surfactant, secreted by alveolar type II pneumocytes, reduces alveolar surface tension and prevents alveolar collapse on expiration. Small amounts of surfactant can be demonstrated from about 20 weeks' gestation, but a surge in production only occurs after 30–34 weeks. Surfactant is released at birth due to aeration and distension of the alveoli. Production is reduced by hypothermia (less than 35°C), hypoxia and acidosis (pH less than 7.25). Surfactant deficiency can occur at any gestational age but is especially likely in babies born before 30 week's gestation and many units will have a policy to address this issue based on the gestation at birth. Nasal continuous positive airway pressure (CPAP) is now widely used to stabilise preterm babies with respiratory distress and may avoid the need to intubate and ventilate many of these babies. If, however, intubation and ventilation is necessary then exogenous surfactant should be given as soon as possible.

The lungs of preterm babies are more fragile than those of term babies and thus are much more susceptible to damage from overdistension. Therefore, it is appropriate to start with a lower inflation pressure of 25 cmH$_2$O (2.5 kPa), but do not be afraid to increase this to 30 cmH$_2$O (2.9 kPa) if there is no heart rate response. Using a positive end-expiratory pressure (PEEP) helps prevent collapse of the airways during expiration and is normally given using a pressure of 5 cmH$_2$O (c. 0.5 kPa). In most situations it will not be possible to measure the tidal volume of each breath given and while seeing some chest movement helps confirm aeration of the lungs, very obvious chest wall movement in premature babies of less than 28 weeks' gestation may indicate excessive and potentially damaging tidal volumes. This should be avoided and inspiratory pressures should be decreased if chest movement is excessive, the heart rate is ≥100 beats/min and there are adequate oxygen saturations.

Premature babies are more susceptible to the toxic effects of hyperoxia. Using a pulse oximeter to monitor both heart rate and oxygen saturation in these babies from birth makes stabilisation much easier. Exposing preterm babies at birth to high concentrations of oxygen can have significant long-term adverse effects. The current guidance is that for stabilisation or resuscitation of a preterm baby at less than 28 weeks start with 30% oxygen, between 28 and 32 weeks start with 21–30% oxygen, and beyond 32 weeks start in 21% oxygen (air). Inspired oxygen should be titrated to oxygen saturations and acceptable preductal saturations measured on the right arm or wrist are the same as those seen in healthy term babies:

Time from birth	Acceptable (25th centile) preductal saturation above which supplemental oxygen is not needed
2 minutes	65%
5 minutes	85%
10 minutes	90%

In preterm babies (under 28 weeks' gestation) there is association with poorer clinical outcomes if the measured oxygen saturations are less than 80% at 5 minutes of age. Inspired oxygen concentration should be increased if saturations of 85% have not been met by 5 minutes. If chest compressions are given, inspired oxygen should be increased to 100%.

CPAP via mask versus intubation

As outlined earlier, tracheal intubation to 'secure' the airway is rarely needed in term babies. In addition, it carries with it inherent risks: delaying ongoing resuscitation due to task fixation; causing traumatic injury to oropharyngeal and tracheal tissue; and, at worst, irreversibly destabilising an otherwise well baby.

In preterm babies, effective initial respiratory support of spontaneously breathing babies with respiratory distress can be given using CPAP. Therefore, CPAP should be considered a first line intervention for ongoing support in this population, especially where personnel are not skilled in, or only infrequently practice, tracheal intubation. Where a mask plus T-piece system is being used for initial resuscitation, and a PEEP valve is available on the T-piece, CPAP may be given effectively by mask. Other dedicated CPAP devices utilising small nasal masks or prongs are available.

G.11   Actions in the event of poor initial response to resuscitation

1. **Check head position, airway and breathing:**
   - Repeat five inflation breaths, does the heart rate improve or the chest rise?
   - Do you need a second pair of hands for airway control, or an airway adjunct (e.g. LM)?
2. Check for a technical fault:
   - Is mask ventilation effective? Is there a significant leak around the mask? Observe chest movement
   - Is a longer inflation time or higher inflation pressure required?
   - If the baby is intubated:
     - Is the tracheal tube in the trachea? Auscultate both axillae, listen at the mouth for a large leak and observe movement. Use an exhaled CO$_2$ detector to ensure tracheal tube position

- Is the tracheal tube in the right main bronchus? Auscultate both axillae and observe movement
- Is the tracheal tube blocked? Use an exhaled CO_2 detector to confirm tracheal position and patency of the tracheal tube. Remove it and retry mask support if there is any concern that the tracheal tube is the problem
  - If starting in air then increase the oxygen concentration. This is the least likely to be a cause of poor responsiveness, although if monitoring saturations it could be a cause for a slow increase in observed saturations
3. Does the baby have a pneumothorax? This occurs spontaneously in up to 1% of newborn babies, but pneumothoraces needing action in the delivery unit are exceptionally rare. Auscultate the chest for asymmetry of breath sounds. A cold light source can be used to transilluminate the chest – the pneumothorax may show as a hyper-illuminating area. If a tension pneumothorax is thought to be present clinically, a 21-gauge butterfly needle should be use to perform needle thoracocentesis via the second intercostal space in the mid-clavicular line. Alternatively, a 22-gauge cannula connected to a three-way tap may be used. Remember that these interventions risk causing a pneumothorax during the procedure (see Chapter 21), but can equally be life saving.
4. Does the baby remain cyanosed despite a regular breathing pattern, no increased work of breathing and a good heart rate? There may be a congenital heart malformation, which may be duct dependent (see Chapter 5), or a persistent pulmonary hypertension.
5. If, after resuscitation, the baby is pink and has a good heart rate but is not breathing effectively, and there is a history of maternal opiate administration, the baby may be suffering the effects of maternal opiates. Options include managing the airway and breathing until this effect wears off, or rarely naloxone 200 micrograms may be given intramuscularly, which should outlast the opiate effect. Naloxone is not considered a resuscitation drug.
6. Is there severe anaemia or hypovolaemia? In cases of large blood loss, 10–20 ml/kg O RhD-negative blood should be given.

G.12 Birth outside the delivery room

Whenever a baby is born unexpectedly, the greatest difficulty often lies in keeping them warm. Drying and wrapping, turning up the heating and closing windows and doors are all important in maintaining temperature. Special care must be taken when clamping the cord to prevent blood loss.

Hospitals with an emergency medicine department should have guidelines for resuscitation at birth, summoning help and post-resuscitation transfer of babies born in, or admitted to, the department.

Babies born unexpectedly outside hospital are more likely to be preterm and at risk of rapidly becoming hypothermic. However, the principles of resuscitation are identical to the hospital setting. Transport to a place of definitive care will need to be discussed according to local guidelines.

G.13 Communication with the parents

It is important that the team caring for the newborn baby informs the parents of the progress whenever possible. This is likely to be most difficult in unexpected deliveries so prior planning to cover the eventuality may be helpful. Decisions at the end of life must involve the parents whenever possible. All communication should be documented immediately after the event, ideally after a team debriefing. As it is likely to be a stressful and relatively rare occurrence to have unplanned deliveries out of hospital or in the emergency department, teams should ensure that they have mechanisms in place to facilitate timely and effective debriefing of all teams involved.

G.14 Summary

This appendix has covered the approach to newborn resuscitation, which is different to that used for children and adults, and is summarised in Figure G.1.

Drowning

Learning outcomes

After reading this appendix, you will be able to:

- Demonstrate the assessment and management of the drowned child using the structured approach

---

H.1   Introduction

The International Liaison Committee on Resuscitation (ILCOR) defines drowning as 'a process resulting in primary respiratory impairment from submersion/immersion in a liquid medium'. The terms 'near drowning' and 'wet' or 'dry' drowning are no longer official terms, mainly because they have been used differently worldwide, which has caused confusion.

Epidemiology

According to the World Health Organization (WHO) *Global Report on Drowning* (2014), 140 219 children under the age of 15 years died in 2012 as a result of drowning worldwide, which makes it a leading cause of accidental death in this age group. Male victims are more likely to die from drowning than female victims (63%, from WHO 2012 data). Infants die most commonly in bathtubs, older children die in private swimming pools, garden ponds and other inland waterways. It is estimated that up to 80% of drowning incidents are preventable. Prevention strategies such as appropriate pool fencing, teaching children to swim and reinforcing the importance of adult supervision may reduce this number.

Pathophysiology

Drowning in children usually occurs within minutes with the following sequence of events:

- Initial struggle for 20–30 seconds (often unable to call for help as breathing takes priority)
- Submersion (airway below water surface, water spat out or swallowed)
- Voluntary breath-holding (up to 60 seconds)
- Reflex inspiratory effort with aspiration of water triggering cough reflex and laryngospasm
- Respiratory impairment leads to hypoxia, hypercarbia and acidosis
- Laryngospasm abates and water is inhaled
- Pulmonary surfactant is washed out and the endothelium of the pulmonary capillaries is disrupted
- Alveoli collapse, pulmonary oedema and pulmonary hypertension develops with associated intrapulmonary shunting of blood

---

Advanced Paediatric Life Support: A Practical Approach to Emergencies, Seventh Edition. Edited by Stephanie Smith.
© 2023 John Wiley & Sons Ltd. Published 2023 by John Wiley & Sons Ltd.

- Cerebral hypoxia leads to loss of consciousness and apnoea
- Hypoxaemia leads to multiple organ damage and eventually failure
- Cardiac deterioration with bradycardia and hypotension secondary to hypoxia lead to a cardiac arrest (ventricular fibrillation is rare)

Hypoxia is thus the key pathological process that ultimately leads to death and needs to be corrected as quickly as possible.

Children who survive (because of interruption of this chain of events) not only require therapy for drowning, but also assessment and treatment of concomitant hypothermia, hypovolaemia and injury (particularly spinal). Major electrolyte abnormalities due to the amount of water swallowed seldom occur.

The type of water – freshwater or saltwater – does not predict the clinical course of drowning and should not influence treatment. However, immersion in severely contaminated water is associated with infections with unusual organisms, and aspiration of water contaminated with petroleum products can lead to severe acute respiratory distress syndrome (ARDS).

Submersion injuries are generally associated with hypothermia. The large body surface area to weight ratio in infants and children put them at particular risk. Hypothermia may have a protective effect against the neurological sequelae following hypoxia and ischaemia but is also associated with life-threatening dysrhythmias, coagulation disorders and susceptibility to infections.

The initial approach to drowning patients focuses on the correction of hypoxia, hypothermia and the treatment of associated injuries, which are common in older children and are often overlooked. Cervical spine injury should always be suspected in drowning victims for whom the mechanism of injury is unclear, although these are rare (0.5% overall, and much rarer in children under 5 years).

The following factors are associated with an increased risk of drowning in children:

- Epilepsy (4–14-fold increased risk compared with children without epilepsy)
- Cardiac arrhythmias
- Hypoglycaemia (metabolic disorders)
- Hyperventilation (can lead to syncope underwater)
- Hypothermia
- Alcohol and/or illicit drugs (consider in adolescents)

Child protection issues, whether they be physical abuse or neglect related, should always be a consideration.

H.2   Primary survey of drowning and resuscitation

The immediate priority is to remove the victim from the water as quickly as possible (without risk to the rescuer) in order to allow cardiopulmonary resuscitation and ABCDE stabilisation without delay. Immobilisation of the neck should be instigated as soon as practicable until injury is excluded, although cervical spine injury is uncommon except after diving or traffic accidents. Rescue of the victim in a vertical position may lead to cardiovascular collapse due to venous pooling. However, horizontal rescue or cervical spine immobilisation in the water should not be allowed to delay the rescue. The initiation of early and effective basic life support (BLS) reduces the mortality drastically and is the most important factor for survival. Rescue breaths must be commenced as early as possible even in shallow water (as long as this can be done without risk to the rescuer). BLS then proceeds according to the standard paediatric algorithm, even in hypothermia. The presence of cardiac arrest can be difficult to diagnose as pulses are difficult to feel. If in doubt, chest compressions should be given and continued. If an automatic external defibrillator (AED) is used, attempts should be made to quickly dry the chest before applying the electrodes.

Following a submersion episode, the stomach is usually full of swallowed water. The risk of aspiration is therefore increased and in drowning victims with severe respiratory compromise, apnoea or decreased level of consciousness (Glasgow Coma Scale (GCS) less than 13), the airway should be secured as soon as possible. This may best be done with endotracheal tube (ETT) intubation (cuffed ETT) to provide appropriate ventilation, oxygenation (aim for SpO_2 of 94–98%) and positive end-expiratory pressure (PEEP) as required. An orogastric or nasogastric tube should be inserted.

Respiratory deterioration can be delayed after submersion and even children who have initially apparently recovered should be observed for 4–8 hours. Chest X-ray changes may occur even later. Advanced life support proceeds according to the standard algorithm except for slight modifications in cases of hypothermia.

Seizures following hypoxic brain injury are common. There is no evidence for prophylactic anticonvulsant therapy after drowning but seizures should be actively managed using standard algorithms.

H.3   Hypothermia

A core temperature reading (rectal or oesophageal) should be obtained as soon as possible and further cooling prevented. Hypothermia is common following drowning and adversely affects resuscitation attempts unless treated (Figure H.1). Not only are arrhythmias more common but some, such as ventricular fibrillation, may be refractory at temperatures below 30°C. In these circumstances, defibrillation should be limited to three shocks and inotropic or antiarrhythmic drugs should not be given. The child should be warmed to above 30°C as quickly as possible, then further defibrillation may be attempted. The dose interval for resuscitation drugs is doubled between 30°C and 35°C. Resuscitation should be continued until the core temperature is at least 32°C or cannot be raised despite active measures. If a child requires endotracheal intubation, the advantages outweigh the small risk of precipitating malignant arrhythmias.

Rewarming strategies (Figure H.1) depend on the core temperature and signs of circulation. External rewarming including a warm air system is usually sufficient if the core temperature is above 30°C. Active core rewarming should be added in children with a core temperature of less than 30°C. Extracorporeal warming is the preferred method in circulatory arrest, if available locally.

The temperature is generally allowed to rise by 0.25–0.5°C per hour to reduce haemodynamic instability. Most hypothermic children are hypovolaemic. During rewarming, vasodilatation occurs, and may result in hypotension requiring large volumes of warmed intravenous fluids. Continuous haemodynamic monitoring is essential to minimise the risk of overfilling and pulmonary oedema. Strict avoidance of hyperthermia is important in the post-resuscitative care phase.

The hypothermic child in cardiac arrest

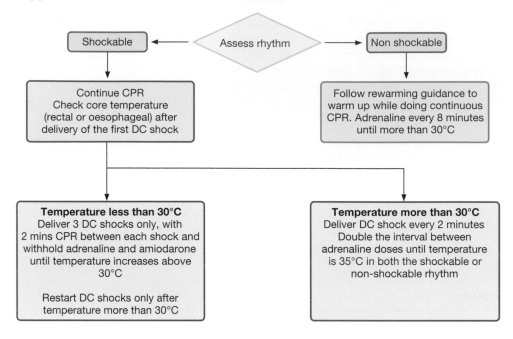

Rewarming methods

External rewarming if temperature more than 30°C
External and core rewarming if temperature less than 30°C

External rewarming	Core rewarming
• Remove cold, wet clothing • Supply warm blankets • Warm air system • Heating blanket • Infrared radiant lamp	• Warm IV fluids to 39°C • Warm ventilator gases to 42°C • Gastric/bladder lavage with saline at 42°C • Peritoneal lavage with potassium-free dialysate at 42°C, 20 ml/kg with a 15 minute cycle • Pleural or pericardial lavage • Endovascular warming • ECMO (extracorporeal blood rewarming)
Temperature to rise by 0.25–0.5°C per hour to reduce haemodynamic instability Aim for normothermia of 35–37°C	
If drowning: core temperature of less than 33°C and water temperature of less than 6°C increases chance of survival	
Resuscitate until core temperature is 32°C or cannot be raised despite resuscitation and active rewarming (Clinical decision to stop can be made despite inability to raise temperature to 32°C)	

Figure H.1 Hypothermic child in cardiac arrest algorithm
CPR, cardiopulmonary resuscitation

It is essential to monitor the vital functions closely, especially during the first couple of hours. Early suggestions of respiratory insufficiency, haemodynamic instability or hypothermia are indications for admission to the intensive care unit.

Prophylactic antibiotics have not been shown to be helpful but are often given after immersion in severely contaminated water. Fever is common during the first 24 hours but is not necessarily a sign of infection, which usually becomes manifest later. Gram-negative organisms, especially *Pseudomonas aeruginosa*, are common and *Aspergillus* species have been reported. When an infection is suspected broad-spectrum intravenous antibiotic therapy (such as cefotaxime) should be started after repeating blood and sputum cultures.

Signs of raised intracranial pressure (ICP) may develop as a result of a hypoxic brain injury, and this should be treated, although aggressive treatment to lower a raised ICP has not been shown to improve the prognosis. Other therapeutic measures, such as barbiturates, calcium channel blockers, surfactants, steroids and free-radical scavengers, have not been shown to be of benefit. Avoidance of hypo/hyperglycemia, hypoxia, hyperthermia and hypo/hypertension is important for the neurological outcome. Unless obvious, a careful search should be made for a precipitating cause of the drowning such as a channelopathy, particularly long QT syndrome.

H.6 Prognostic indicators in drowning

The clinical course of drowning is determined by the duration of hypoxic–ischaemic injury and the adequacy of initial resuscitation. It is assumed that hypoxic brain damage is reduced when the brain cools before the heart stops. No single factor can predict a good or poor outcome in drowning reliably, however the factors listed in Table H.1 may give an indication of likely outcome.

Table H.1	Prognostic indicators in drowning
Submersion time	Under 5 minutes: greater than 90% chance of mild or no neurological impairment 5–25 minutes: 90% risk of death or poor neurological outcome More than 25 minutes: almost 100% risk of death or severe neurological deficit
Time to basic life support	Under 10 minutes: 87% chance of mild or no neurological impairment 10–25 minutes: 68% risk of death or poor neurological outcome More than 25 minutes: almost 100% risk of death or severe neurological deficit
Time to first respiratory effort	If this occurs within 3 minutes after the start of basic cardiopulmonary support, the prognosis is good. If there has been no respiratory effort after 40 minutes of full cardiopulmonary resuscitation, there is little or no chance of survival unless the child's respiration has been depressed (e.g. by hypothermia, medication or alcohol)
Core temperature	Pre-existing hypothermia and rapid cooling after submersion also seems to protect vital organs and can improve the prognosis. A core temperature of less than 33°C on arrival and a water temperature of less than 6°C have been associated with increased survival. This effect is more pronounced in small children because of their large surface area to weight ratio
Persisting coma	A persistent Glasgow Coma Scale (GCS) score of under 5 indicates a bad prognosis
Arterial blood pH	If this remains under 7.0 despite treatment, the prognosis is poor
Arterial blood PO_2	If this remains under 8.0 kPa (60 mmHg) despite treatment, the prognosis is poor
Type of water	Whether the water was salt or fresh has no bearing on the prognosis

The duration of resuscitation efforts may not be a helpful prognostic factor. The decision to discontinue resuscitation attempts is particularly difficult in cases of drowning and should be taken only after all the prognostic factors discussed have been considered carefully. Resuscitation should only be discontinued out of hospital if there is clear evidence of futility such as massive trauma or rigor mortis.

H.7 Outcome of drowning

Seventy per cent of children survive drowning when BLS is provided at the scene, whereas only 40% survive without early BLS, even with maximum therapy. Of those who do survive, having required full cardiopulmonary resuscitation in hospital, around 70% will make a complete recovery and 25% will have a mild neurological deficit. The remainder will be severely disabled or remain in a vegetative state.

H.8 Summary

This appendix has described the use of the structured approach for the assessment and management of the drowned child.

Point of care ultrasound

Learning outcomes

After reading this appendix, you will be able to:

- Describe how point of care ultrasound can help the assessment of the critically ill child
- Describe how point of care ultrasound can help with practical procedures
- Discuss the limitations of point of care ultrasound in emergency situations

---

I.1   Introduction

This chapter is included in the Advanced Paediatric Life Support (APLS) course to ensure that there is awareness of when and how point of care ultrasound (POCUS) can be used in resuscitation. It is being used increasingly by practitioners caring for children from all backgrounds. Discussions are ongoing with the Royal Colleges to accredit training courses to allow it to be used even more widely and to include POCUS in competencies for training curricula.

POCUS refers to the use of ultrasound at the bedside by clinicians who are providing direct clinical care to the child. It can be used as part of primary or secondary assessment, for some procedural interventions and for clinical monitoring. POCUS is integrated with the patient clinical assessment and other investigation findings, which allows for direct correlation of signs and symptoms with the obtained images. Clinicians in acute specialties have been using POCUS to aid both diagnosis and intervention for many years. High-quality, portable, hand-held ultrasound devices are now readily available and the use of POCUS is becoming routine. POCUS does not replace any aspect of the structured APLS approach, but rather augments it.

It is important to differentiate the assessment using POCUS from traditional ultrasound and echo-cardiographic investigation as performed by radiology or cardiology services. POCUS asks binary questions and is used to rule key pathologies in or out. It is not a detailed anatomical assessment of organs. POCUS requires formal training and accreditation, which is available via several routes, including the Children's Acute Ultrasound (CACTUS) programme. This chapter aims to highlight how the use of POCUS can be integrated within the principles of APLS.

Advanced Paediatric Life Support: A Practical Approach to Emergencies, Seventh Edition. Edited by Stephanie Smith.
© 2023 John Wiley & Sons Ltd. Published 2023 by John Wiley & Sons Ltd.

I.2 Summary of the potential uses for POCUS in APLS algorithms

Point of care ultrasound can provide essential support during the resuscitation and stabilisation of any critically ill or injured person.

Primary assessment

- Identify some reversible causes of cardiac arrest

Secondary assessment

- Airway and breathing (including tracheal tube placement, pleural collections, consolidation, pneumothorax)
- Cardiac function
- Fluid status (both hypovolaemia and hypervolaemia)
- Reassessment of treated pathologies (e.g. whether a pleural effusion has been fully drained)
- Soft tissue injuries and fractures

Practical procedures

- Vascular access (centrally or peripherally inserted venous lines, arterial lines)
- Drain insertion (pleural, pericardial, abdominal)
- Nerve blocks

POCUS users should be additional to the resuscitation team and not interfere with the resuscitation efforts.

I.3 POCUS in cardiac arrest

Point of care ultrasound can be helpful for cardiac arrest management, although there are limited data demonstrating improvement in outcomes (either return of spontaneous circulation (ROSC) or survival to discharge).

POCUS in cardiac arrest can be used to:

- Rule out some of the reversible causes of cardiac arrest, namely tamponade, tension pneumothorax, thrombosis and hypovolaemia
- Identify mechanical cardiac function. Multiple adult studies have demonstrated that no mechanical activity of the heart during pulseless electrical activity (PEA) is associated with a reduced likelihood of achieving ROSC, and maybe an additional factor to consider when deciding to terminate resuscitation efforts. However, this should not be the sole factor in decision making
- Guide the effectiveness of chest compressions by evaluating the filling and emptying of the heart on ultrasound (often using transoesophageal echocardiography) and to optimise the cardiopulmonary resuscitation (CPR) provider's hand position and compression-release. This is an area currently under development

It is imperative that the use of POCUS during cardiac arrest does not interfere with chest compressions and other resuscitation measures. There is a suggested method for incorporating POCUS into the resuscitation algorithms:

- Use a POCUS experienced practitioner who is not involved in other parts of the resuscitation
- Start to obtain the views whilst CPR is ongoing (subcostal view is recommended)
- Record images during pulse checks (do not worry about image interpretation at this point)
- The team leader should direct recommencement of CPR as usual
- Interpret the recorded image POCUS images at this point and provide feedback to the team leader
- When carrying out lung ultrasound, do not stop ventilation

I.4   POCUS in the child with breathing difficulties

The use of POCUS in the management of respiratory failure is well recognised. It is very useful at ruling out key pathologies, such as a pneumothorax. It is important to apply the lung ultrasound in a systematic fashion, asking binary questions as you progress.

Lung ultrasound can be carried out with a high-frequency linear probe (traditionally used for vascular access) in smaller children, as this will give you a good image quality without the need for deep visualisation in the thorax. In older children, the use of a lower frequency curved-linear probe will allow you to see deeper into the thorax. You can also carry out lung ultrasound using a phased-array probe (traditionally used for echocardiography).

Figure I.1 demonstrates the normal locations of probe placement for lung ultrasound in a time pressured situation. This is generally where you would place your stethoscope. Ideally, you would inspect the lung in many different sites. In each of these positions the marker of the probe is orientated to the child's head, and the probe is held longitudinally at 90° to the child's skin. The probe is then held stationary to obtain the lung ultrasound images. Figure I.2a demonstrates normal lung ultrasound appearances at the anterior chest wall surface and Figure I.2b demonstrates normal lung ultrasound appearances at the lateral chest wall costophrenic angle. Lung ultrasound requires dynamic images to identify pleural sliding for true interpretation.

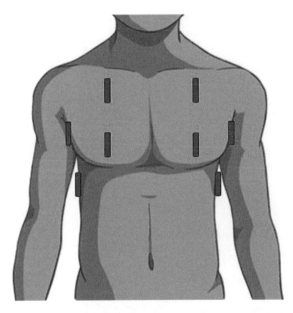

Figure I.1 Key minimum sites to place the ultrasound probe during lung ultrasound (note that the probe marker is always toward the head of the child)

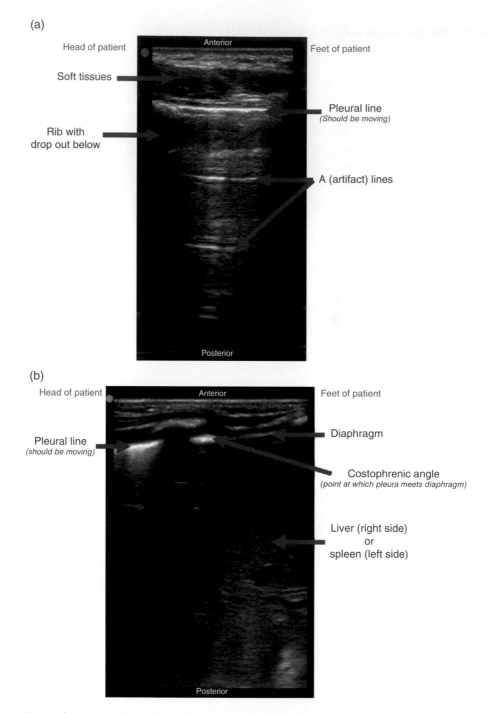

Figure I.2 {a) Normal anterior upper chest lung ultrasound anatomy, and (b) normal lateral chest costophrenic angle lung ultrasound anatomy as seen with a linear probe in a small infant

It is outside the scope of this appendix to describe how to interpret lung ultrasound findings in detail, but Table I.1 summarises some of the key findings relevant to APLS. Figure I.3 shows a modified 'BLUE' protocol, which is a structured technique to assess the respiratory system with ultrasound.

Table I.1 Introduction to features seen on lung ultrasound

Lung ultrasound finding	Description	Possible interpretation
A line	An ultrasound artifact caused by the reflection of the pleural line. A lines therefore are normal findings (Figure I.2a).	Normal finding
Absent sliding of the pleural line	The pleural line (Figure I.2a, b) normally slides forward and backward with inspiration and expiration (often described as 'marching ants'). The absence of movement suggests a pathology	Not ventilating/no respiratory effort Pneumothorax Severe consolidation
B lines	These are vertical lines arising from the pleural line and extending down through the lung parenchyma, obliterating the A lines in the process	Normal finding (if fewer than three are seen) Pulmonary oedema (always consider congenital heart disease) Consolidation Pulmonary fibrosis Chronic lung disease
Consolidation	The lung appears to have a combination of extensive localised B lines, with a disrupted/broken pleural line with air bronchograms seen and lung parenchyma that appears to look like liver tissue	Pneumonia Bronchiolitis Inadequate ventilation

(Continued)

Table I.1 *(Continued)*

Lung ultrasound finding	Description	Possible interpretation
Pleural fluid	Pleural fluid appears black on ultrasound and separates the pleural line from the subcutaneous soft tissues 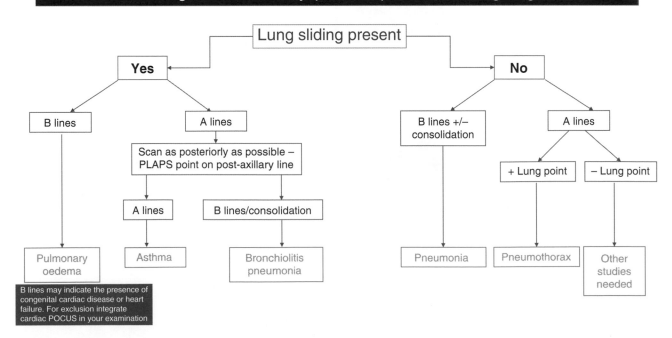 Soft tissue Pleural effusion Pleural line	Haemothorax Empyema Chylothorax Reactive serosanguinous effusion
Lung point	This describes the appearance of a moving pleura meeting a pleura that is not moving and is characteristic of the point of origin of pleural separation by air. This is a dynamic finding seen on real-time imaging. It is the only sign to confirm a pneumothorax	Pneumothorax

Differential diagnosis of acute dyspnoea in paediatrics using lung POCUS

Lung sliding present

Yes →

Yes
- B lines → Pulmonary oedema
- A lines → Scan as posteriorly as possible – PLAPS point on post-axillary line
  - A lines → Asthma
  - B lines/consolidation → Bronchiolitis pneumonia

B lines may indicate the presence of congenital cardiac disease or heart failure. For exclusion integrate cardiac POCUS in your examination

No
- B lines +/– consolidation → Pneumonia
- A lines
  - + Lung point → Pneumothorax
  - – Lung point → Other studies needed

Figure I.3 A modified BLUE protocol for using POCUS in the respiratory assessment
PLAPS, posterolateral alveolar and/or pleural syndrome

I.5   POCUS in the child with shock

The use of POCUS can help differentiate between the causes of shock (Table I.2). It is used in combination with the structured approach to assessing a child with shock (Figure I.4).

Table I.2   Components of cardiac output and how point of care ultrasound (POCUS) may identify a problem

Component of cardiac output	Potential role of POCUS
Preload	POCUS can assist with identifying volume status. It is worth noting that POCUS is better at identifying hypervolaemia rather than hypovolaemia Key findings of adequate or excessive preload include: • Distended inferior vena cava (IVC) • Volume loaded ventricles/atria • Signs of pulmonary oedema (B lines)
Contractility	A simple four-chamber view of the heart can help Identify poorly functioning ventricles. This is important as it may suggest the need for less volume resuscitation and an earlier introduction of inotropic support Key findings of reduced contractility include: • Dilated ventricles • Poor movement/reduced contractility • Loss of ventricular interdependence
Afterload	POCUS can help identify pathologies leading to an increase in afterload or tamponade physiology Key findings could include: • Pericardial effusions • Pulmonary hypertension • Pneumothorax

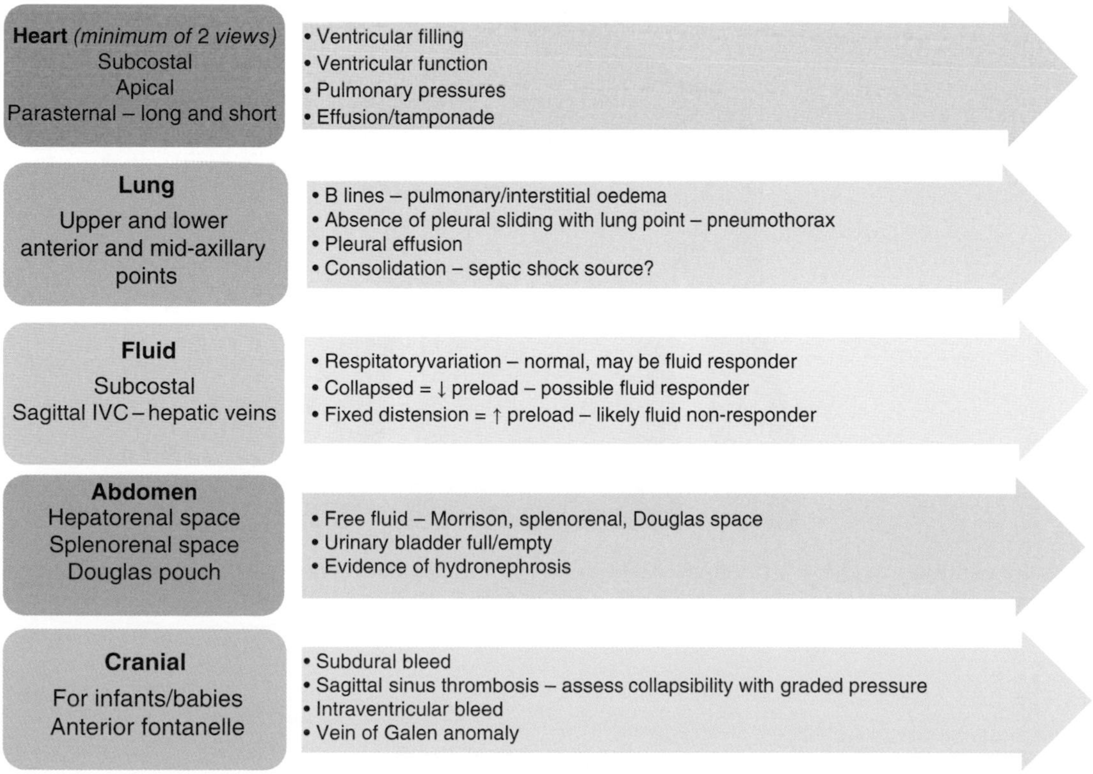

Heart *(minimum of 2 views)*
Subcostal
Apical
Parasternal – long and short
• Ventricular filling
• Ventricular function
• Pulmonary pressures
• Effusion/tamponade

Lung
Upper and lower anterior and mid-axillary points
• B lines – pulmonary/interstitial oedema
• Absence of pleural sliding with lung point – pneumothorax
• Pleural effusion
• Consolidation – septic shock source?

Fluid
Subcostal
Sagittal IVC – hepatic veins
• Respitatoryvariation – normal, may be fluid responder
• Collapsed = ↓ preload – possible fluid responder
• Fixed distension = ↑ preload – likely fluid non-responder

Abdomen
Hepatorenal space
Splenorenal space
Douglas pouch
• Free fluid – Morrison, splenorenal, Douglas space
• Urinary bladder full/empty
• Evidence of hydronephrosis

Cranial
For infants/babies
Anterior fontanelle
• Subdural bleed
• Sagittal sinus thrombosis – assess collapsibility with graded pressure
• Intraventricular bleed
• Vein of Galen anomaly

Figure I.4 POCUS algorithm for assessing paediatric undifferentiated shock
IVC, inferior vena cava

POCUS should never delay resuscitation. Cardiac POCUS does not exclude congenital cardiac disease and, if this is suspected, formal echocardiography is mandated. A child with extensive B lines may also have congenital heart disease, so the lung ultrasound should be integrated with cardiac POCUS.

It is very helpful to be able to identify the left and right ventricles when examining ventricular function. A dilated and/or poorly functioning left ventricle may require earlier inotropic support, with less volume resuscitation. A dilated and/or poorly functioning right ventricle might indicate pulmonary hypertension, especially in the newborn.

Whilst any recognised echocardiographic view is suitable to identify the left ventricle, it is often easier to use a traditional four-chamber view for the beginner. To identify the four-chamber view use either a view from the subcostal area (ideal in neonates/infants and smaller children) or the apical area (ideal in older children). These windows are shown in Figure I.5.

In both situations the probe marker is pointed towards the left, and the probe directed towards the expected location of the heart. The probe is then tilted up and down to find the maximum size of the left ventricle, along with the other chambers. It does not matter which up–down orientation of the ventricles is used (Figure I.6). This is personal preference. It is important that any finding in a cardiac POCUS view is confirmed in a second alternative window, to ensure the accuracy of the finding.

To assess function grossly look for:

- Size of the left ventricle
- Walls moving together
- Volume of the ventricle reducing with each contraction

Cardiac POCUS is only good for identifying a significant reduction in function. If there is any doubt about cardiac function or structural heart disease, obtain a formal echocardiograph.

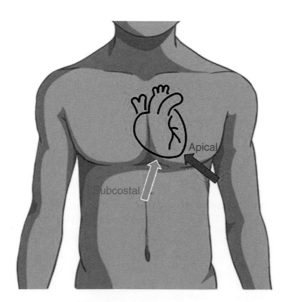

Figure I.5 Possible windows to identify the four-chamber view (note the arrows represent the direction on the ultrasound probe, with the probe marker always angled towards the left-hand side)

(a)   (b)

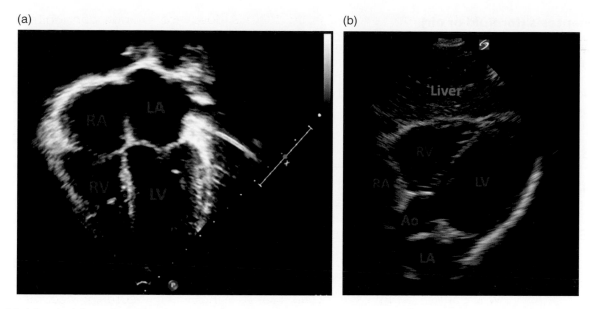

Figure I.6 **(a) Apical four-chamber view (traditional paediatric orientation), and (b) subcostal view (traditional adult orientation)**
Ao, aortic outlet; LA, left atria; LV, left ventricle; RA, right atria; RV, right ventricle

I.6   POCUS in trauma

The first use of POCUS was in trauma patients as part of the focused assessment with sonography for trauma (FAST) scan. This was used as a tool to look for free fluid in the abdomen to help triage adult patients to the operating theatre or computed tomography (CT) scan. There are currently no data to support using the FAST scan in paediatric practice, although in the hands of an experienced paediatric radiologist, true abdominal ultrasound is sometimes an alternative to abdominal CT to reduce radiation exposure to children. Each trauma network will have local guidance on this.

The main roles of POCUS in modern paediatric trauma managements are as part of the structured approach to ABCDE, as described earlier to identify key pathologies, and for supporting practical procedures.

I.7   Ultrasound-guided procedures

Ultrasound can be used efficiently to guide various practical procedures. The techniques required for performing such procedures are beyond the scope of this chapter.

Vascular access

- Establishing venous access is critically important but can be technically challenging, especially in a child presenting with haemodynamic compromise
- In the child presenting in cardiac arrest, successful venous cannulation in the first minutes is directly correlated with successful resuscitation
- The use of ultrasound to guide intravascular line placement reduces the number of attempts and complications. Dynamic real-time ultrasound guidance during needle placement is recommended
- There may be a role for the most experienced ultrasound practitioner to be in charge of acute vascular access in an acutely deteriorating child

Thoracentesis (for fluid or air)

- Identification of both pleural fluid and air using thoracic sonography compares favourably with CT and may be superior to chest radiography when performed by experienced clinicians
- Landmark techniques for pleural drain insertion have proven to be unreliable. Ultrasound guidance reduces complications such as visceral pleural injury, which can result in a bronchopleural fistula

I.8 Summary

This appendix has emphasised the importance of point of care ultrasound which is a rapidly developing clinical tool that can aid diagnosis, management and interventions during the resuscitation of a critically ill or injured child. Users should have appropriate training and use of POCUS must not delay or compromise resuscitation.

Formulary

This appendix contains drugs mentioned elsewhere in the book, set out alphabetically, along with their routes of administration, dosage and some notes on their use.

J.1   General guidance on the use of the formulary

- When dosage is calculated on a basis of per kilogram and a maximum dose is not stated, then the dose given should not exceed that for a 40 kg child based on the World Health Organization (WHO) 50th centile of a 12-year-old (WHO growth charts)
- The exact dose calculated on a basis of per kilogram may be difficult to administer because of the make up of the formulations available. If this is the case the dose may be rounded up or down to a more manageable figure
- Doses in other formularies are sometimes written as µg or ng. When prescribing such doses, all terms apart from milligrams (abbreviated mg) should be written in full (micrograms or nanograms, respectively) in order to avoid confusion
- Although every effort has been made to ensure accuracy, the writers, editors, publishers and printers cannot accept liability for errors or omissions
- More detailed information about individual drugs is available from the manufacturers, from product datasheets (also called Summary of Product Characteristics), from the British National Formulary for Children, from hospital drug information centres and from the pharmacy departments of children's hospitals

Abbreviations

The following abbreviations to indicate administration route are used:

ET	Endotracheal
IM	Intramuscular
IO	Intraosseous
IV	Intravenous
SC	Subcutaneous

The final responsibility for the delivery of the correct dose remains that of the physician prescribing and administering the drug.

J.2 *N*-acetylcysteine doses <40 kg

Bag 1 Dose: 100 mg/kg acetylcysteine in 0.9% saline or 5% glucose. Volume: 2 ml/kg (gives a concentration of 50 mg/ml) over 2 hours

Bag 2 Dose: 200 mg/kg acetylcysteine in 0.9% saline or 5% glucose. Volume: 20 ml/kg (gives a concentration 10 mg/ml) over 10 hours

Acetylcysteine prescription for children weighing 39 kg or less				
12-hour regimen	**First infusion**		**Second infusion**	
Drug	Acetylcysteine 200 mg/ml for infusion, 10 ml ampoule			
Infusion fluid	0.9% saline or 5% glucose			
Duration of infusion	2 hours		10 hours	
Drug dose	100 mg/kg acetylcysteine		200 mg/kg acetylcysteine	
Concentration of infusion	50 mg/ml		10 mg/ml	
Patient weight	**Total infusion volume**	**Infusion rate**	**Total infusion volume**	**Infusion rate**
kg	ml	ml/h	ml	ml/h
1	2	1	20	2
2	4	2	40	4
3	6	3	60	6
4	8	4	80	8
5	10	5	100	10
6	12	6	120	12
7	14	7	140	14
8	16	8	160	16
9	18	9	180	18
10–14	24	12	240	24
15–19	34	17	340	34
20–24	44	22	440	44
25–29	54	27	540	54
30–34	64	32	640	64
35–39	74	37	740	74

This is an example of the SNAP (Scottish and Newcastle Anti-emetic Pre-treatment for Paracetamol Poisoning) regimen which is now widely used in the UK, however please check with local protocols.

J.3 Drugs

INDICATION	ROUTE	AGE/WEIGHT				FREQUENCY
ACICLOVIR		**Neonate**	**1–2 months**	**3 months to 11 years**	**12–18 years**	
Herpes simplex virus treatment Normal immunity and immuno-compromised	IV infusion	20 mg/kg every 8 hours for 14 days (at least 21 days in CNS involvement)	10 mg/kg every 8 hours for 14 days (at least 21 days in CNS involvement)	250 mg/m² every 8 hours for 5 days. Double to 500 mg/m² in immuno-compromise or in simplex encephalitis	5 mg/kg every 8 hours usually for 5 days. Double to 10 mg/kg in immuno-compromise or in simplex encephalitis (at least 14 days in encephalitis and at least 21 days in immunocompromise and encephalitis)	

Notes:
In cases of central nervous system (CNS) involvement, confirm cerebrospinal fluid is negative for herpes simplex virus before stopping treatment
Reconstitute to 25 mg/ml with water for injections or sodium chloride 0.9% then dilute to a concentration of 5 mg/ml with sodium chloride 0.9% or sodium chloride and glucose and give over 1 hour. Alternatively, may be administered in a concentration of 25 mg/ml using a suitable infusion pump and central venous access and given over 1 hour
To avoid excessive dose in obese patients, parenteral dose should be calculated on the basis of ideal weight for height
Reduce dosage frequency to 12-hourly if estimated glomerular filtration rate is 25–50 ml/min/1.73 m² and to once daily if it is 10–25 ml/min/1.73 m²
Maintain adequate hydration

INDICATION	ROUTE	AGE/WEIGHT				FREQUENCY
ADENOSINE		**Neonates**	**1–11 months**	**1–11 years**	**12–18 years**	
Antiarrhythmic to terminate supraventricular tachycardia and to elucidate mechanism of tachycardia	Rapid IV injection	150 micrograms/kg If necessary repeat every 1–2 minutes increasing the dose by 50–100 micrograms/kg until tachycardia terminated or max. single dose of 300 micrograms/kg given	150 micrograms/kg If necessary repeat every 1–2 minutes increasing the dose by 50–100 micrograms/kg until tachycardia terminated or max. single dose of 500 micrograms/kg given	100 micrograms/kg If necessary repeat every 1–2 minutes increasing the dose by 100 micrograms/kg to a max. of 12 mg	Initially 3 mg; if necessary followed by 6 mg after 1–2 minutes and then by 12 mg after a further 1–2 minutes In some children over 12 years a 3 mg dose is ineffective (e.g. if small peripheral vein used) and higher initial dose may be used	Single dose
		Notes: Drug should be given rapidly over 2 seconds followed by rapid sodium chloride 0.9% flush. A large vein is required Caution should be executed when considering adenosine in the asthmatic child Children who have had a heart transplant are very sensitive to the effects of adenosine Children receiving dipyridamole should receive a quarter (1/4) of the usual dose of adenosine				

INDICATION	ROUTE	AGE/WEIGHT				FREQUENCY
ADRENALINE (EPINEPHRINE)		**Neonates**	**<6 years**	**6–12 years**	**12–18 years**	
Anaphylaxis treatment by health professionals	Deep IM	150 micrograms	150 micrograms	300 micrograms	500 micrograms	Single dose
		Notes: Repeat the dose at 5–15-minute intervals as clinically needed Children taking β-blockers may not respond to adrenaline therapy, consider bronchodilator therapy Children taking non-cardioselective β-blockers may experience severe hypertension and bradycardia with adrenaline				

INDICATION	ROUTE	AGE/WEIGHT			FREQUENCY
ADRENALINE (EPINEPHRINE)		**<6 years**	**6–11 years**	**12–18 years**	
Anaphylaxis treatment by autoinjector	Deep IM	150 micrograms	300 micrograms	300 or 500 micrograms	Single dose
		Notes: As above for adrenaline Depending on autoinjector prescribed, the dose for 12–18-year-olds may be 300 or 500 micrograms			

INDICATION	ROUTE	AGE/WEIGHT	FREQUENCY
ADRENALINE (EPINEPHRINE)		**Neonates to 18 years**	
Cardiopulmonary resuscitation	IV/IO	10 micrograms/kg (max. 1 mg) of 1:10 000 (100 micrograms/ml) repeated every 3–5 minutes if necessary	Single dose
		Notes: In neonates, a higher dose of up to 30 micrograms/kg may be used if the first doses are ineffective Outside the neonatal period, doses over 10 micrograms/kg may be disadvantageous except in the rare circumstances of cardiac arrest following β-blocker overdose	
Management of hypotension	IV/IO	Infusion concentration: 0.3 mg/kg in 50 ml of 5% glucose or 0.9% sodium chloride will give 0.1 micrograms/kg/min if run at a rate of 1 ml/h. Use 1:1000 (1 mg/ml) adrenaline concentrate. The infusion may be run via a central intravenous line at 0.1–10 ml/h in order to deliver 0.01–1 micrograms/kg/min. To safely administer via a peripheral IV cannula or IO needle, use 1/10th dilution: add 0.03 mg/kg in 50 ml or 0.3 mg/kg in 500 ml of 5% glucose or 0.9% sodium chloride, which will give 0.1 micrograms if run at a rate of 10 ml/h The infusion should be started at 0.1 micrograms/kg/min and titrated to response, increasing to 1 micrograms/kg/min (or on rare occasions even higher) depending on clinical response	Infusion
Prevention of allergic reaction with antivenom in envenomation	SC	5–10 micrograms/kg (max. 1 g)	Single dose
Management of croup	Nebuliser	400 micrograms/kg (0.4 ml/kg of 1:1000 adrenaline 1 mg/ml solution) made up to 5 ml total with normal saline	Single dose
		Notes: May be repeated after 30 minutes if necessary Effects last for 2–3 hours, monitor carefully	

INDICATION	ROUTE	AGE/WEIGHT	FREQUENCY
ALPROSTADIL		**Birth to 1 month**	
Duct-dependent congenital heart defects in neonates	IV infusion	Start at 5 nanograms/kg/min increasing in increments of 5 nanograms/kg/min to 20 nanograms/kg/min Then decrease to lowest effective dose	Single dose
		Notes: If intensive support required: max. doses of 100 nanograms/kg/min have been used	

INDICATION	ROUTE	AGE/WEIGHT				FREQUENCY
AMINOPHYLLINE		**Neonates**	**1 month to 1 year**	**1–12 years**	**12–18 years**	
Severe acute asthma	IV loading dose over 20–30 minutes, followed by IV infusion	–		5 mg/kg (max. 500 mg)	Single loading dose over 20–30 minutes	
			1 month to 11 years		**12–17 years**	
	IV infusion		1 mg/kg/h, adjusted according to plasma theophylline concentration		500–700 micrograms/kg/h, adjusted according to plasma theophylline concentration	
		Notes: Loading dose only used if no theophylline or aminophylline has been given in the last 24 hours Aminophylline requires therapeutic drug monitoring				

AMIODARONE		**Neonates**	**1 month to 18 years**		
Resistant supraventricular and ventricular arrhythmias	IV	5 mg/kg every 12–24 hours, dose to be given over 30 minutes	Initially 5–10 mg/kg, dose to be given over at least 20 minutes to 2 hours, then (by continuous infusion) 300 micrograms/kg/h, dose to be adjusted according to response, increased if necessary up to 1.5 mg/kg/h Maximum 1.2 g per day		Single dose
		Notes: Administration by a central line recommended if possible Dilute to a concentration of not less than 600 micrograms/ml with glucose 5% Incompatible with sodium chloride solution Avoid bolus injection in: cardiomyopathy, congestive heart failure, circulatory collapse (except in cardiac arrest), severe arterial hypotension and severe respiratory failure				
In cardiac arrest: ventricular fibrillation and pulseless ventricular tachycardia refractory to defibrillation	Rapid IV bolus	N/A	5 mg/kg (max. 300 mg) over 3 minutes		Single dose
		Notes: Should be given over at least 3 minutes Administration by central line recommended if possible			

INDICATION	ROUTE	AGE/WEIGHT				FREQUENCY
ATROPINE SULPHATE		**Neonate**	**1 month to 11 years**	**12–18 years**		
Immediately before induction of anaesthesia	IV injection	10 micrograms/kg	20 micrograms/kg (min. 100 micrograms, max. 600 micrograms)	300–600 micrograms		Single dose
Intraoperative bradycardia	IV injection	10–20 micrograms/kg	10–20 micrograms/kg	300–600 micrograms (larger doses in emergencies)		Single dose

INDICATION	ROUTE	AGE/WEIGHT		FREQUENCY
BUDESONIDE		**Neonate**	**1 month to 18 years**	
Croup	Nebuliser sus-pension	N/A	2 mg	Single dose
		Notes: May be repeated 12-hourly until clinical improvement		

INDICATION	ROUTE	AGE/WEIGHT		FREQUENCY
BUPIVACAINE 0.25% (2.5 mg/ml)		**Birth to 12 years**	**12–18 years**	
Long-acting local anaesthetic for nerve blocks	Local infiltration	Maximum 0.8 ml/kg	0.8 ml/kg up to a max. of 60 ml	Single dose
		Notes: To avoid toxicity in obese patients, use ideal weight Takes 30 minutes for onset Not to be repeated within 8 hours		

INDICATION	ROUTE	AGE/WEIGHT	FREQUENCY
CALCIUM GLUCONATE 10%		**Birth to 18 years**	
For acute hypocalcaemia and hyperkalaemia	Slow injection	0.5 ml/kg (max. 20 ml)	Single dose
		Notes: Slow IV injection over 5–10 minutes Ensure there is no extravasation into tissues	

INDICATION	ROUTE	AGE/WEIGHT			FREQUENCY
CALCIUM RESONIUM		**Neonate (by rectum)**	**1 month to 18 years (by mouth)**		
Hyperkalaemia associated with anuria or oliguria, or in dialysis patients	See route next to age	0.5–1 g/kg daily (irrigate colon to remove resin after 8–12 hours)	0.5–1 g/kg (max. 60 g) daily in divided doses		Single dose
		Notes: Administer rectally in water or 10% glucose Administer orally in water, not juice/squash which has a high potassium content			

INDICATION	ROUTE	AGE/WEIGHT				FREQUENCY
CEFOTAXIME		**Neonate <7 days**	**Neonate 7–21 days**	**Neonate >21 days**	**1 month to 18 years**	
Severe infections, including meningitis	IV injection or infusion or IM	50 mg/kg every 12 hours	50 mg/kg every 8 hours	50 mg/kg every 6–8 hours	50 mg/kg every 6 hours (max. 12 g daily)	Single dose

INDICATION	ROUTE	AGE/WEIGHT			FREQUENCY
CEFTRIAXONE		**Neonate (IV infusion over 60 minutes)**	**1 month to 12 years (IV infusion)**	**12–18 years (and younger if >50 kg) (IV infusion or IM injection divided between 2–4 sites)**	
Severe infections, including meningitis	See route with age	20–50 mg/kg	80 mg/kg (if <50 kg)	2–4 g daily (max. IV 2 g and max. IM 4 g daily)	Once daily

INDICATION	ROUTE	AGE/WEIGHT		FREQUENCY
CODEINE PHOSPHATE		**Birth to 12 years**	**12–18 years**	
Moderate pain, short-term use	Oral or IM	Not indicated	30–60 mg every 6 hours where necessary (max. daily dose 240 mg; max. use 3 days)	Single dose
		Notes: Use only if paracetamol or ibuprofen ineffective Significant risk of serious and life-threatening adverse effects in children who undergo tonsillectomy or adenoidectomy for obstructive sleep apnoea Contraindicated in any patient known to be an ultrarapid metaboliser of codeine (CYP2D6 ultrarapid metaboliser). Will be ineffective in a patient who is a CYP2D6 poor metaboliser Not recommended in children in whom breathing may be compromised, including those with neuromuscular disorders, severe cardiac or respiratory disorders, respiratory infections, multiple trauma or extensive surgical procedures		

INDICATION	ROUTE	AGE/WEIGHT	FREQUENCY
DANTROLENE		**1 month to 18 years**	
Malignant hyperthermia	IV bolus	2–3 mg/kg initially	Single dose
		Notes: Discontinue trigger agent NB: needs reconstituting from powder, and is slow to dissolve Repeat with 1 mg/kg as required at 5–10-minute intervals to a max. cumulative dose of 10 mg/kg	

INDICATION	ROUTE	AGE/WEIGHT	FREQUENCY
DESFERRIOXAMINE MESILATE		**1 month to 18 years**	
Acute iron poisoning	IV infusion	Initially up to 15 mg/kg/h Reduce after 4–6 hours as indicated	Continuous
		Notes: If shocked, hypotensive or seriously ill, administer IV Decrease rate of administration after 4–6 hours to ensure that total maximum dose does not exceed 80 mg/kg/day, seek expert help Continue until serum iron is less than total iron-binding capacity Use with caution in patients with renal impairment	

INDICATION	ROUTE	AGE/WEIGHT		FREQUENCY
DEXAMETHASONE		**1 month to 2 years**		
Croup	Oral	150 micrograms/kg		Twice daily
		Notes: No definitive standard dose has been agreed in the UK Suggested maximum single dose of 12 mg		
Short course to relieve symptoms of brain tumour	IV or oral	Under 35 kg, initial dose 16.6 mg Over 35 kg, initial dose 20.8 mg		Twice daily
		Notes: Can also be used to reduce oedema around tumours compressing nerves		

INDICATION	ROUTE	AGE/WEIGHT		FREQUENCY
DIAMORPHINE		**Birth to 1 month**	**1 month to 18 years**	
Control of severe pain	Intranasal	Not recommended	0.1 mg/kg	Single dose
		Notes: Dilute with saline to volume of 0.2 ml Monitor closely for at least 30 minutes and repeat if needed; may repeat 6-hourly Avoid in acute respiratory depression Naloxone is an antidote Use with caution in head injury		

INDICATION	ROUTE	AGE/WEIGHT	FREQUENCY
DIAZEPAM		**Birth to 18 years**	
Treatment of status epilepticus	Rectal	0.5 mg/kg	Single dose
		Notes: If needed, repeat after 5 minutes Maximum per dose 20 mg Parenteral and rectal use can depress respiration Caution with other central nervous system depressants	
In place of lorazepam where this is not available	IV or IO	0.25 mg/kg	

INDICATION	ROUTE	AGE/WEIGHT		FREQUENCY
DICLOFENAC		**1 month to 2 years**	**2–18 years**	
Non-steroidal anti-inflammatory drug (NSAID)	Oral or rectal	<6 months: not recommended	300 micrograms to 2 mg/kg	3 times daily
		>6 months: 300 micrograms to 2 mg/kg		
		Notes: Up to a maximum of 150 mg per day Caution where there is a history of hypersensitivity and in dehydration (risk of renal failure)		

INDICATION	ROUTE	AGE/WEIGHT					FREQUENCY

DOBUTAMINE		**Birth to 18 years**		
Provides inotropic support in the treatment of low-output cardiac failure, e.g. in septicaemia	IV infusion	5–20 micrograms/kg/min		Continuous
		Notes: Dose can be increased up to a maximum of 40 micrograms/kg/min in older children if necessary (20 micrograms/kg/min in newborn infants) but side effects are more likely at this higher dose		

DOPAMINE HYDROCHLORIDE		**Birth to 1 month**	**1 month to 18 years**	
Treatment of low-output cardiac states	IV infusion	Start at 3 micrograms/kg/min, increasing as clinically indicated to a max. of 20 micrograms/kg/min	5–20 micrograms/kg/min	Continuous
		Notes: Direct inotropic effect but vasoconstriction may occur at higher doses		

ERYTHROMYCIN		**Neonate**	**1 month to 2 years**	**2–12 years**	**12–18 years**	
Upper and lower respiratory tract infections	Oral or IV	10–12.5 mg	12.5 mg/kg (max. 1 g)			4 times daily
	Oral		125 mg	2–8 years: 250 mg	500 mg	4 times daily
				9–12 years: 500 mg		
		Notes: Doses can be doubled in severe infections Maximum single dose 1 g				

FENTANYL		**From 7 kg to 18 years**	
Acute management of pain	IN	1.5 micrograms /kg	Single dose
		Notes: Prepare using 100 micrograms/2 ml (Minimum of 0.2 ml due to atomiser)	
Induction of anaesthesia	IV	1 microgram/kg repeated as necessary	

FLECAINIDE ACETATE		**Birth to 18 years**	
Treatment of resistant re-entry supraventricular tachycardia, ventricular ectopics or ventricular tachycardia	Slow IV bolus	2 mg/kg	Single dose
		Notes: Give over at least 10 minutes with ECG monitoring Avoid in patients with pre-existing heart block Maximum dose 150 mg Only use with expert cardiological input	

INDICATION	ROUTE	AGE/WEIGHT				FREQUENCY

FLUCLOXACILLIN		**Birth to 1 month**	**1 month to 2 years**	**2–12 years**	**12–18 years**	
Treatment of infections due to Gram-positive organisms (anti-staphylococcal)	Oral or IV	<7 days: 25–50 mg/kg	–	–	–	Twice daily
		7–21 days: 25–50 mg/kg	–	–	–	3 times daily
		>21 days: 25–50 mg/kg	–	–	–	4 times daily
		Notes: Dose may be increased to 100 mg/kg per dose IV in severe infection (meningitis, cerebral abscess, staphylococcal osteitis) Oral route only recommended for minor infection				
	IV bolus or IM	–	12.5–25 mg/kg			4 times daily
		Notes: Maximum single dose 1 g Dose may be doubled in severe infection, max. single dose 2 g				
	Oral	–	<1 year: 62.5 mg >1 year: 125 mg	<5 years: 125 mg >5 years: 250 mg	250 mg	4 times daily
		Notes: Doses may be doubled in severe infection				

FLUMAZENIL		**Birth to 1 month**	**1 month to 2 years**	**2–12 years**	**12–18 years**	
Reversal of acute benzodiazepine overdosage	IV bolus over 15 seconds	10 micrograms/kg (max. dose 50 micrograms/kg)	10 micrograms/kg (max. dose 50 micrograms/kg)		200 micrograms (max. dose 1 mg)	Single dose
		Notes: Initial dose as shown If the desired effect is not achieved, repeat at 1-minute intervals to a max. total dose of 40 micrograms/kg (2 mg max. dose in 12–18-year-olds)				
	IV infusion	2–10 micrograms/kg/h (max. dose 400 micrograms/h)			100–400 micrograms/h	Continuous
		Notes: This should be individually adjusted to achieve the desired level of arousal There is limited experience of the use of flumazenil in children				

FUROSEMIDE		**Birth to 12 years**	**12–18 years**	
To induce diuresis in cardiac or renal failure or fluid overload; hypertension	IV bolus	500 micrograms to 1 mg/kg	20–40 mg	Single dose
		Notes: Single doses up to 4 mg/kg have been used. Dose can be repeated every 8 hours		

INDICATION	ROUTE	AGE/WEIGHT			FREQUENCY

GLUCAGON

Indication	Route	Birth to 1 month	1 month to 2 years	2–18 years	Frequency
Severe insulin-induced hypoglycaemia in treatment of diabetes	IM, SC	Not recommended	500 micrograms	500 micrograms to 1 mg (<25 kg: 500 micrograms; >25 kg: 1 mg)	Single dose
		Notes: Should be effective within 10 minutes Only use when IV glucose is difficult or impossible to administer. If not, give IV glucose 5–10% instead			

IBUPROFEN

Indication	Route	1 month to 2 years	2–12 years	12–18 years	Frequency
Pyrexia, mild to moderate pain	Oral dose by weight	5 mg/kg		–	3–4 times daily
	Oral dose by age	1–2 years: 50 mg	3–7 years: 100 mg	200–600 mg	3–4 times daily
			8–12 years: 200 mg		
		Notes: Maximum of 20 mg/kg/day up to 2.4 g/day Avoid where there is a history of hypersensitivity and in dehydration (risk of renal failure)			

INSULIN

Indication	Route	Birth to 18 years	Frequency
Primary treatment for patients with type 1 and 2 diabetes uncontrolled by other means	IV infusion in keto-acidosis	0.05–0.1 units/kg/h	Continuous
		Notes: Adjust dose according to blood glucose level	

IPRATROPIUM

Indication	Route	Birth to 1 month	1 month to 2 years	2–12 years	12–18 years	Frequency
Treatment of chronic reversible airways obstruction. May be used with a β₂-agonist in the treatment of severe, acute asthma	Nebulised	25 micrograms/kg	125 micrograms	250 micrograms	500 micrograms	Single dose
		Notes: Can be repeated every 20–30 minutes in the first 2 hours in acute severe asthma Reduce dose frequency as clinical improvement occurs				

INDICATION	ROUTE	AGE/WEIGHT			FREQUENCY

LABETALOL		**Birth to 1 month**	**1 month to 11 years**	**12–18 years**	
Hypertension and hypertensive crises	IV bolus	–	250–500 micrograms/kg	50 mg	Single dose
		Notes: Loading dose			
	IV infusion	500 micrograms/kg/h up to a max. of 4 mg/kg/h	1–3 mg/kg/h	30–120 mg/h	Continuous
		Notes: Start at low dose and titrate according to response, until blood pressure has been reduced to acceptable level Avoid in asthma, heart failure and heart block			

LEVETIRACETAM		**Birth to 18 years**	
Status epilepticus	IV or IO	40 mg/kg over 5 minutes	
		Notes: Can be given if already taking Maximum single dose 4.5 g	

LIGNOCAINE (LIDOCAINE)		**Birth to 11 years**	**12–18 years**	
Antiarrhythmic ventricular fibrillation or pulseless tachycardia Local anaesthetic	IV/IO	1 mg/kg (max. dose 100 mg)	50–100 mg	Single dose
		Notes: Repeat every 5 minutes if needed to a total maximum of 3 mg/kg In the 12–18-year age group give 50 mg in lighter patients or those whose circulation is impaired		
	IV infusion	600 micrograms/kg to 3 mg/kg/h	4 mg/min for 30 minutes, then 2 mg/min for 2 hours, then 1 mg/min	Continuous
		Notes: In the 12–18-year group: reduce concentration further if infusion is continued beyond 24 hours Maintenance dosing: ECG monitoring with infusion		
	Local infiltration	Up to 3 mg/kg	Up to 200 mg	Single dose
		Notes: No more often than every 4 hours Use fine needles (27–29 gauge) It is less painful if buffered before use with 8.4% sodium bicarbonate 1 ml to every 10 ml lidocaine 1%		
	Intraurethral	3–4 mg/kg	–	Single dose
		Notes: Use Instillagel® (2% gel with chlorhexidine 0.25%) solution prior to urinary catheterisation. Warm the solution to body temperature and inject it very slowly to reduce local stinging		

INDICATION	ROUTE	AGE/WEIGHT			FREQUENCY

LORAZEPAM		**Birth to 12 years**	**12–18 years**	
Status epilepticus	IV, rectal or sublingual	100 micrograms/kg (max. dose 4 mg)	4 mg	Single dose
		Notes: Generally given as a single dose; may be repeated once if initial dose is ineffective Limited experience in neonates May cause apnoea Flumazenil is an antidote		

MAGNESIUM SULFATE		**Birth to 1 month**	**1 month to 2 years**	**2–18 years**	
Hypomagnesaemia in septicaemia	IV		0.2 ml/kg 50% mgSO$_4$ over 30 minutes (max. 10 ml)		Single dose
		Notes: Repeat later if serum magnesium remains low			
Treatment of asthma	IV	Not recommended	Limited experience	40 mg/kg	Single dose over 20 minutes
		Notes: Has been used in infants but experience is limited Maximum of 2 g			
Treatment of torsades de pointes	IV	Not recommended	25–50 mg/kg	25–50 mg/kg	Single dose
		Notes: Maximum of 2 g			

MANNITOL		**Birth to 18 years**	
Treatment of oedematous states, including ascites and treatment of raised intracranial pressure	IV infusion over 30 minutes	250–500 mg/kg (1.25–2.5 ml/kg of 20% solution)	Single dose
		Notes: Cerebral and ocular oedema May be repeated once or twice after an interval of 4–8 hours if necessary (if serum osmolality <310 mOsm/l)	

MIDAZOLAM		**3-11 months**	**1–2 years**	**2–12 years**	**12–18 years**	
Status epilepticus	Buccal/intranasal	0.3 mg/kg	0.3 mg/kg	0.3 mg/kg	0.3 mg/kg	Single dose
		2.5 mg	2.5 mg	1–4 years: 5 mg 5–9 years: 7.5 mg >10 years: 10 mg	10 mg	Single dose
		Notes: Buccal administration is the preferred route over intranasal administration. The parenteral preparation can be used for this route The dose by weight for the buccal route is 0.3 mg/kg from 6 months; max. dose 10 mg Use of prefilled age/weight-dependent syringes are suitable				

INDICATION	ROUTE	AGE/WEIGHT				FREQUENCY
MORPHINE		**Birth to 1 month**	**1 month to 2 years**	**2–12 years**	**12–18 years**	
Control of severe pain	IV infusion	Preterm: 25–50 micrograms/kg	–	–	–	Single dose Loading dose
		Then: 5 micrograms/kg/h	–	–	–	Continuous
		Term: 50 micrograms/kg	–	–	–	Single dose Loading dose
		Then: 10–20 micrograms/kg/h	–	–	–	Continuous
	IV bolus	–	100 micrograms/kg		5 mg every 4 hours adjusted according to response	<6 months: up to 4 times in 24 hours >6 months: up to 6 times in 24 hours
		Notes: Respiratory monitoring is mandatory Give IV over at least 5–10 minutes <1 year: use the lower stated dose and consider oxygen saturation monitoring				
	IV infusion	–	10–30 micrograms/kg/h			Continuous
			<6 months: initial rate is 10 micrograms/kg/h			
			>6 months: initial rate is 20 micrograms/kg/h			
		Notes: Use IV bolus as starting dose first 1 mg/kg body weight in 50 ml saline, infused at 1 ml/h = 20 micrograms/kg/h				
	Oral	–	1–3 months: 50–100 micrograms/kg every 4 hours adjusted according to response 3–6 months: 100–150 micrograms/kg every 4 hours adjusted according to response 6–12 months: 200 micrograms/kg every 4 hours adjusted according to response 1–2 years: 200–300 micrograms/kg every 4 hours adjusted according to response	200–500 micrograms/kg (max. 10 mg)	5–10 mg	Up to 6 times in 24 hours
		Notes: Doses should be reviewed regularly and adjusted according to the patient's response				

INDICATION	ROUTE	AGE/WEIGHT				FREQUENCY
NALOXONE		**Birth to 1 month**	**1 month to 2 years**	**2–12 years**	**12–18 years**	
Reversal of opioid-induced central and respiratory depression	IV infusion	10 micrograms/kg	–	–	–	Continuous
		Notes: Use 400 micrograms/ml naloxone preparation Gradual onset of action (3–4 minutes) but the effect is prolonged				
	IV bolus	–	100 micrograms/kg (max. dose 2 mg)		400 micrograms	Single dose
		–	Then, if no response: 100 micrograms/kg at 1-minute intervals to max. of 2 mg		Then, if no response after 1 minute: 800 micrograms Then, if no response after a further 1 minute: 800 micrograms Then, if no response after a further 1 minute: 2 mg (4 mg may be required in a seriously poisoned child)	Single dose
		Notes: Then review diagnosis; further doses may be required if respiratory function deteriorates Due to short half-life of naloxone, repeat doses as necessary to maintain opioid reversal Observe for recurrence of central nervous system and respiratory depression If IV not possible use IM or SC				
	IV infusion	–	5–20 micrograms/kg/h		Infuse a solution of 4 micrograms/ml at a rate adjusted according to response	Continuous

Notes:
Specifically indicated for the reversal of respiratory depression in a newborn infant whose mother has received narcotics within 4 hours of delivery. It is generally preferred to give an IM injection for a prolonged effect
Do not administer to newborns whose mothers are suspected of narcotic abuse, as a withdrawal syndrome may be precipitated
Always establish and maintain adequate ventilation before administration of naloxone

INDICATION	ROUTE	AGE/WEIGHT		FREQUENCY
NIFEDIPINE		**Birth to 1 month**	**1 month to 18 years**	
Hypertensive crisis	Oral	–	250–500 micrograms/kg	Single dose
		Notes: Administration for rapid effect in hypertensive crisis or acute angina: bite capsules and swallow liquid, or use liquid preparation if 5 or 10 mg dose inappropriate If liquid form is unavailable, extract contents of capsule via a syringe and use immediately – cover syringe with foil to protect contents from light; capsule contents may be diluted with water if necessary Modified-release tablets may be crushed although this may alter the release profile; crushed tablets should be administered within 30–60 seconds to avoid significant loss of potency of drug		

INDICATION	ROUTE	AGE/WEIGHT	FREQUENCY
NORADRENALINE (NOREPINEPHRINE)		**Neonates to 18 years**	
Management of hypotension	IV/IO	Infusion concentration: 0.3 mg/kg in 50 ml of 5% glucose or 0.9% sodium chloride will give 0.1 micrograms/kg/min if run at a rate of 1 ml/h. Use 1:1000 (1 mg/ml) adrenaline concentrate. The infusion may be run via a central intravenous line at 0.1–10 ml/h in order to deliver 0.01–1 micrograms/kg/min. To safely administer via a peripheral IV cannula or IO needle, use 1/10th dilution: add 0.03 mg/kg in 50 ml or 0.3 mg/kg in 500 ml of 5% glucose or 0.9% sodium chloride, which will give 0.1 micrograms if run at a rate of 10 ml/h The infusion should be started at 0.1 micrograms/kg/min and titrated to response, increasing to 1 micrograms/kg/min (or on rare occasions even higher) depending on clinical response	Infusion

INDICATION	ROUTE	AGE/WEIGHT				FREQUENCY
PARACETAMOL		**Birth to 1 month**	**1 month to 2 years**	**2–12 years**	**12–18 years**	
Analgesic/ antipyretic	Oral loading dose	15 mg/kg	15 mg/kg	15 mg/kg	1 g	Single dose
	Oral maintenance dose	15 mg/kg	15 mg/kg	15 mg/kg	500 mg to max. 1 g	4–6-hourly, max. 4 doses per day <32 weeks' gestation: 8–12-hourly (max. 60 mg) 32 weeks' gestation to 1 month: 8-hourly (max. 30 mg)
		Notes: Maximum daily dose 60 mg/kg (total 4 g) Preterm 28–32 weeks: max. daily dose 30 mg/kg				
	Rectal loading dose		1–2 months: 30 mg 3–11 months: 60–125 mg 1–2 years: 125 mg	125–500 mg/kg	1 g	Single dose
		Notes: Maximum daily dose 60 mg/kg (total 4 g) Preterm 28–32 weeks: max. daily dose 30 mg/kg				
	IV	7.5 mg/kg 32 weeks' gestation to term: 8-hourly Term infants: 4–6 hourly, give over 15 minutes	10–50 kg: 15 mg/kg	15 mg/kg	>50 kg: 1 g (15 mg/kg)	4–6-hourly <32 weeks' gestation: 12-hourly 32 weeks' gestation to 1 month: 8-hourly
		Notes: <10 kg: max. daily dose 30 mg/kg 10–50 kg: max. daily dose 60 mg/kg >50 kg: max. daily dose 4 g				

PARALDEHYDE		Birth to 18 years	
Status epilepticus	Rectal	0.8 ml/kg to max. 20 ml	Single dose
		Notes: Doses are stated in ml/kg or as ml of paraldehyde Dilute with an equal volume of olive oil before administration, or if using a ready-prepared 'special', remember that it is already diluted and dose accordingly	

INDICATION	ROUTE	AGE/WEIGHT			FREQUENCY
PHENOBARBITAL (PHENOBARBITONE)		**Birth to 12 years**	**12–18 years**		
Status epilepticus Respiratory depression especially when used with benzodiazepines	IV slow bolus	20 mg/kg	20 mg/kg		Single
		Notes: Loading dose at 1 mg/kg/min, i.e. over 20 minutes			
		Then: 2.5–5 mg/kg	Then: 300 mg dose		Once to twice daily (once daily in neonatal period)
		Notes: Maintenance at 1 mg/kg/min, i.e. over 20 minutes			

PHENYTOIN		**Birth to 1 month**	**1 month to 12 years**	**12–18 years**	
Antiepileptic	IV	20 mg/kg	20 mg/kg	20 mg/kg	Single dose
		Notes: Maximum dose 2 g Loading dose over 20 minutes Monitor ECG and blood pressure Therapeutic drug monitoring recommended			

POTASSIUM CHLORIDE		**Birth to 1 month**	**1 month to 18 years**	
Acute hypokalaemia	IV infusion		0.1–0.25 mmol/kg/h	Continuous
		Notes: Always check the dose carefully, as an overdose can be rapidly fatal; dilute with at least 50 times its volume and mix well Restrict to critical care areas, store in a locked cupboard and document as for controlled drugs Recheck the potassium level after 3 hours		

PREDNISOLONE		**Birth to 1 month**	**1 month to 12 years**	**12–18 years**	
Acute asthma	Oral	–	1 mg/kg (max. dose 40 mg)	40–50 mg	Once daily
		Notes: Treat for 1–5 days and then stop (no need to taper doses)			
Croup requiring intubation	Oral	–	1 mg/kg	40–50 mg	Twice daily

INDICATION	ROUTE	AGE/WEIGHT		FREQUENCY
PROPRANOLOL		**Birth to 12 years**	**12–18 years**	
Dysrhythmias	IV bolus	25–50 micrograms/kg (max. dose 1 mg)	1 mg	Single dose
		Notes: Repeat injection as needed up to 4 times daily Give slowly over at least 3–5 minutes; rate of administration should not exceed 1 mg/min ECG monitoring required		

INDICATION	ROUTE	AGE/WEIGHT	FREQUENCY
QUININE		**Birth to 18 years**	
Treatment of *Plasmodium falciparum* malaria	IV infusion over 4 hours at least	20 mg/kg (max. 1.4 g)	Single loading dose
		Notes: For seriously ill patients or those unable to take tablets	
		Then: 10 mg/kg (max. 700 mg)	Then after 8 hours maintenance dose
		Notes: Maintenance dose can be repeated 3 times daily but change to oral therapy as soon as possible	

Notes:
Risk of arrhythmias with amiodarone and flecainide
Side effects are common: tinnitus, headache, visual disturbance and hypoglycaemia
Use glucose 5% to dilute to a concentration of 2 mg/ml (max. 30 mg/ml in fluid restriction)
Monitor ECG and blood sugar

INDICATION	ROUTE	AGE/WEIGHT			FREQUENCY
SALBUTAMOL		**Birth to 1 month**	**1 month to 2 years**	**2–18 years**	
Treatment of asthma	Aerosol inhaler	–	Up to 1 mg		Single dose
		Notes: Asthma reliever given as required; 1–2-hourly initially, then reduce frequency to 4–6-hourly 1000 micrograms = 10 sprays (each of 100 micrograms)			
	Nebuliser solution		2.5 mg	<5 years: 2.5 mg >5 years: 5 mg	Single dose
		Notes: Asthma reliever given as required according to severity and response			
	IV bolus over 5 minutes	5 micrograms/kg	5 micrograms/kg	15 micrograms/kg (max. 250 micrograms)	Single dose
		Notes: Status asthmaticus: maximum concentration 50 micrograms in 1 ml			
	IV infusion	1–5 micrograms/kg/min	1–5 micrograms/kg/min	1–5 micrograms/kg/min	Continuous
		Notes: Status asthmaticus: doses up to 10 micrograms/kg/min have been used Solution compatible with potassium but not with aminophylline			
Renal hyperkalaemia	IV bolus (over 5 mins)	4 micrograms/kg	4 micrograms/kg	4 micrograms/kg	Single dose
		Notes: Repeat if necessary			
	Nebuliser	2.5–5 mg	2.5–5 mg	2.5–5 mg	Single dose
		Notes: Repeat if necessary			

SODIUM BICARBONATE		**Birth to 18 years**	
Cardiac arrest	Slow IV	1 ml/kg of 8.4% initially if indicated	
		Followed by 0.5 ml/kg of 8.4% if needed	
Renal hyperkalaemia	Slow IV	1 mmol/kg	Single dose
		Notes: Dose adjusted according to plasma bicarbonate level	

SODIUM CHLORIDE 3%		**Birth to 18 years**	
Management of raised intracranial pressure	IV	3–5 ml/kg IV over 15 minutes	Single dose

INDICATION	ROUTE	AGE/WEIGHT				FREQUENCY
SODIUM NITROPRUSSIDE		**Birth to 18 years**				
Hypertensive crisis	IV infusion	0.5 micrograms/kg/min				Continuous
		Notes: Initial dose: increase in increments of 100–200 nanograms/kg/min as necessary to a maximum of 8 micrograms/kg/min Maximum dose after 24 hours: 4 micrograms/kg/min Use only with expert advice				

INDICATION	ROUTE	**Birth to 1 month**	**1 month to 2 years**	**2–12 years**	**12–18 years**	FREQUENCY
TERBUTALINE						
Relief of bronchospasm in bronchial asthma	Nebulised	–	2.5–5 mg	<5 years: 2.5–5 mg >5 years: 5–10 mg	10 mg	Single dose
		Notes: Reliever doses are repeated as required				

INDICATION	ROUTE	**Birth to 12 months**	**1–2 years**	**2–12 years**	**12–18 years**	FREQUENCY
VERAPAMIL						
Treatment for supraventricular tachycardia (adenosine first line)	Slow IV bolus	–	100–300 micrograms/kg (max. 5 mg)	100–300 micrograms/kg (max. 5 mg)	5 mg	Single dose over 2–3 minutes
		Notes: ECG and blood pressure monitoring required Dose may be repeated after 30 minutes if necessary Many cases are controlled by doses at the lower end of the range Caution in liver disease. Do not use with β-blockers Use only with expert advice				

List of algorithms

Advanced Paediatric Life Support: A Practical Approach to Emergencies, Seventh Edition. Edited by Stephanie Smith.
© 2023 John Wiley & Sons Ltd. Published 2023 by John Wiley & Sons Ltd.

Working group for seventh edition

Working group

Jason Acworth MBBS FRACP (PEM), Paediatric Emergency Physician, Queensland Children's Hospital; Clinical Professor, Faculty of Medicine, University of Queensland, Australia

Andrew C. Argent MBBCh MMed(Paediatrics) MD(Paediatrics) DCH(SA) FCPaeds(SA) FRCPCH, Professor Emeritus, Department of Paediatrics and Child Health, University of Cape Town, Cape Town, South Africa

Pete Arrowsmith Resuscitation Manager, Hamad International Training Centre, Doha, Qatar

Andrew Baldock FRCA FFICM, Consultant Paediatric Anaesthetist and Intensivist, Southampton Children's Hospital, Southampton

Alan Charters Consultant Practitioner, Paediatric Emergency Care, Portsmouth

Jonathan Davies MB BChir MA DCH FRCA, Consultant Paediatric Anaesthetist, Nottingham University Hospitals NHS Trust, Nottingham

Peter Davis MRCP(UK) FRCPCH FFICM, Consultant in Paediatric Critical Care Medicine, Bristol Royal Hospital for Children, University Hospitals Bristol and Weston NHS Foundation Trust, Bristol

Els Duval MD PhD, Clinical Head Pediatric Intensive Care Unit, University Hospital Antwerp, Edegem, Belgium

Julie Grice MRCPCH, Consultant in Paediatric Emergency Medicine, Alder Hey Children's Hospital NHS Foundation Trust, Liverpool

Richard Hollander MD, Consultant in Pediatric Critical Care, Beatrix Children's Hospital, University Medical Centre Groningen, the Netherlands

Despoina Iordanidou MD MSc PhD, Pediatric Anesthetist, Senior Consultant in Anesthesia, Anesthesia Department, Hippokrateio General Hospital of Thessaloniki – Greece, Hellenic National Health System, Greece

Maria Janson Pediatric Surgeon and Senior Consultant, Medical Dispatch Centre of Southern Sweden, Sweden

Bimal Mehta MBChB BSc FRCPCH FRCEM, Consultant in Paediatric Emergency Medicine, Alder Hey Children's Hospital NHS Foundation Trust, Liverpool

Julije Meštrović MD PhD, Consultant in Paediatrics, Subspecialist in Paediatric Intensive Care and Emergency Medicine, Head of the Reference Center for Paediatric Emergency Medicine, Head of Department of Clinal Skills, University Hospital of Split, School of Medicine Split, Split, Croatia

Phuc Huu Phan MD PhD, Pediatric Intensive Care Unit, Vietnam National Children's Hospital, Hanoi, Vietnam

Thomas Rajka Consultant in Paediatrics, Akershus University Hospital, Oslo, Norway

Tanya Ralph RSCN BSc, Resuscitation Training Officer, Sheffield Children's NHS Foundation Trust, Sheffield

Paul Reavley MBChB FRCEM FRCS (A&E)Ed MRCGP DipMedTox, Paediatric Emergency Medicine Consultant, Bristol Royal Hospital for Children, Bristol

Julian Sandell MB BS MRCPI FRCPCH FRCEM, Consultant in Paediatric Emergency Medicine

Advanced Paediatric Life Support: A Practical Approach to Emergencies, Seventh Edition. Edited by Stephanie Smith.
© 2023 John Wiley & Sons Ltd. Published 2023 by John Wiley & Sons Ltd.

References and further reading

Chapter 2

Bromiley, M. *Just a Routine Operation*. https/vimeo.com/970665. Clinical Human Factors Group, www.chfg.co.uk (last accessed January 2023).

Flin R, O'Connor P, Crichton M. *Safety at the Sharp End: A Guide to Non technical Skill*. Abingdon: CRC Press, 2008.

Kohn LT, Corrigan JM, Donaldson MS (eds); Institute of Medicine; Committee on Quality of Health Care in America (eds) *To Err is Human: Building a Safer Health System*. Washington, DC: National Academies Press, 2000.

Kohn LT, Corrigan JM, Donaldson MS (eds); Institute of Medicine (US) Committee on Quality of Health Care in American. *To Err is Human: Building a Safer Health System*. Washington DC: National Academies Press, 2010.

Chapter 4

Scottish Intercollegiate Guidelines Network (SIGN). *British Guideline on the Management of Asthma*. SIGN No. 158. Edinburgh: SIGN, 2019. https://www.sign.ac.uk/media/1773/sign158-updated.pdf (last accessed January 2023).

World Health Organization (WHO). *Pneumonia in Children*. 2022. https://www.who.int/news-room/fact-sheets/detail/pneumonia (last accessed March 2023).

Chapter 5

FEAST Trial Group. FEAST: mortality after fluid bolus in African children with severe infection. *N Engl J Med* 2011; 364(26): 2483–95.

Flin R, O'Connor P, Crichton M. *Safety at the Sharp End: A Guide to Non-technical Skill*. Abingdon: CRC Press, 2008.

Singer M, Deutschman CS, Seymour CW, et al. The Third International Consensus definitions for sepsis and septic shock (Sepsis-3). *JAMA* 2016; 315(8): 801–10.

World Health Organization (WHO). *Dengue and Severe Dengue*. 2022. https://www.who.int/news-room/fact-sheets/detail/dengue-and-severe-dengue (last accessed March 2023).

Chapter 6

Paediatric National Institute of Health Stroke Scale (PedNIHSS). *Pediatric NIH Stroke Scale (NIHSS)*. https://www.mdcalc.com/calc/10270/pediatric-nih-stroke-scale-nihss (last accessed March 2023).

Royal College or Paediatrics and Child Health (RCPCH). *The Management of Children and Young People with an Acute Decrease in Conscious Level (DECON).* https://www.rcpch.ac.uk/sites/default/files/2019-04/RCPCH%20DeCon%20Poster_R9%20A1%20updated%20April%202019.pdf (last accessed January 2023).

Chapter 7

National Institute for Health and Care Excellence (NICE). *NICE Traffic Light System for Identifying Risk of Serious Illness in under 5s.* https://www.nice.org.uk/guidance/ng143/resources/support-for-education-and-learning-educational-resource-traffic-light-table-pdf-6960664333 (last accessed February 2023).

Society for Paediatric Anaesthesia in New Zealand and Australia (SPANZA). *EPIC website.* https://www.spanza.org.au/epic (last accessed January 2023).

Chapter 8

Eastern Associaton for the Surgery of Trauma (EAST). *Pediatric Trauma.* https://www.east.org/education-career-development/publications/landmark-papers-in-trauma-and-acute-care-surgery/pediatric-trauma (last accessed May 2023).

King RB, Filips D, Blitz S, et al. Evaluation of a possible tourniquet system for use in the Canadian Forces. *J Trauma* 2006; 60: 1061–71.

Lee C, Porter KM, Hodgetts TJ. Tourniquet use in the civilian prehospital setting. *Emerg Med J* 2007; 24(8): 584–7.

National Institute for Health and Care Excellence (NICE). *Clinical Guidelines for Major Incidents and Mass Casualty Events.* London: NICE, 2018 (updated 2020).

NHS England. *Clinical Guidelines for Major Incidents and Mass Casualty Events.* 2018 (last updated 2020). https://www.england.nhs.uk/publication/clinical-guidelines-for-major-incidents-and-mass-casualty-events/ (last accessed January 2023).

Royal College of Surgeons of Edinburgh (RCSEd). *Position statement on the application of tourniquets.* Edinburgh: RCSEd, 2017. https://fphc.rcsed.ac.uk/media/2876/position-statement-on-the-application-of-tourniquets-july-2017.pdf (last accessed January 2023).

Trauma Audit and Research Network (TARN) *Severe Injury in Children January 2019–December 2020.* https://user-lfb0jbt.cld.bz/Severe-Injury-In-Children-Report-2019-20 (last accessed May 2023).

Wakai A, Winter DC, Street JT, et al. Pneumatic tourniquets in extremity surgery. *J Am Acad Orthop Surg* 2001; 9(5): 345–51.

Chapter 9

Office for National Statistics (ONS). *Homicide in England and Wales: Year Ending March 2020.* London: ONS, 2022 https://www.ons.gov.uk/peoplepopulationandcommunity/crimeandjustice/articles/homicideinenglandandwales/march2022 (last accessed January 2023).

Pallet JR, Sutherland E, Glucksman E, Tunnicliff M, Keep JW. A cross-sectional study of knife injuries at a London major trauma centre. *Ann R Coll Surg Engl* 2014; 96(1): 23–6.

Chapter 10

Cotton BA, Nance ML. Penetrating trauma in children. *Semin Pediatr Surg* 2004; 13(2): 87–97.

Holcomb GW, Murphy JP, St Peter SD. *Holcomb and Ashcraft's Paediatric Surgery, 7e.* Amsterdam: Elsevier, 2019.

Saha M. Abdominal and thoracic impalement injuries in children due to fall from height: our experience. *Ind J Surg* 2019; 81: 439–44.

Sinha CK, Lander A. Trauma in children: abdomen and thorax. *Paed Surg* 2013; 31(3): 123–9.

Chapter 11

Abdelmasih M, Kayssi A, Roche-Nagle G. Penetrating paediatric neck trauma. *BMJ Case Rep* 2019; 12: e226436.

Anon. Antiseizure prophylaxis for penetrating brain injury. *J Trauma* 2001; 51 (Suppl. 2): S41–3.

Anon. Part 1: Guidelines for the management of penetrating brain injury. Introduction and methodology. *J Trauma* 2001; 51 (Suppl. 2): S3–6.

Brain Trauma Foundation. *Guidelines for the Management of Pediatric Severe TBI*, 3rd edn. https://braintrauma.org/coma/guidelines/pediatric (last accessed May 2023).

CRASH 3 Collaborators. Effects of tranexamic acid on death, disability, vascular occlusive events and other morbidities in patients with acute traumatic brain injury (CRASH-3): a randomised, placebo-controlled trial. *Lancet* 2019; 394: 1713–23.

Evans C, Chaplain T, Zelt D. Management of major vascular neck injuries: neck, extremities and other things that bleed. *Emerg Med Clin North Am* 2018; 36(1): 181–202.

Kazim SF, Sharmim MS, Tahir MZ, Enam SA, Wheed S. Management of penetrating brain injury. *J Emerg Trauma Shock* 2011; 4: 395–402.

Mikhael M, Frost E, Cristancho M. Perioperative care for pediatric patients with penetratng brain injury. *J Neurosurg Anesthesiol* 2018; 30(4): 290–8.

National Institute for Health and Care Excellence (NICE). *Head Injury: Assessment and Early Management*. CG176. London: NICE, 2014 (last updated 2019).

Nowicki JL, Stew B, Ooi E. Penetrating neck injuries: a guide to evaluation and management. *Ann R Coll Surg Engl* 2018; 100: 6–11.

Chapter 12

British Orthopaedic Association (BOA). *BOA Standards for Trauma and Orthopaedics (BOASTs)*. https://www.boa.ac.uk/standards-guidance/boasts.html (last accessed May 2023).

National Institute for Health and Care Excellence (NICE). *Spinal Injury Assessment and Initial Management. NG41*. London: NICE, 2016.

Chapter 13

International Best Practice Guidelines. *Effective Skin and Wound Management of Non-complex Burns*. London: Wounds International, 2014. https://www.woundsinternational.com/uploads/resources/5ebace6c70d4ea53a5d3e28ca65f1b74.pdf (last accessed May 2023).

Mersey Burns app: www.merseyburns.com.

World Health Organization (WHO). *Burns*. 2018. https://www.who.int/news-room/fact-sheets/detail/burns (last accessed January 2023).

Chapter 15

King RB, Filips D, Blitz S, et al. Evaluation of a possible tourniquet system for use in the Canadian Forces. *J Trauma* 2006; 60: 1061–71.

Lee C, Porter KM, Hodgetts TJ. Tourniquet use in the civilian prehospital setting. *Emerg Med J* 2007; 24(8): 584–7.

Royal College of Surgeons of Edinburgh (RCSEd). *Position statement on the application of tourniquets*. Edinburgh: RCSEd, 2017. https://fphc.rcsed.ac.uk/media/2876/position-statement-on-the-application-of-tourniquets-july-2017.pdf (last accessed January 2023).

Vassallo J, Nutbeam T, Rickard AC, et al. Paediatric traumatic cardiac arrest: the development of an algorithm to guide recognition, management and decisions to terminate resuscitation. *Emerg Med J* 2018; 35(11): 669–74.

Wakai A, Winter DC, Street JT, et al. Pneumatic tourniquets in extremity surgery. *J Am Acad Orthop Surg* 2001; 9(5): 345–51.

Wolf SJ, Bebarta VS, Bonnett CJ, Pons PT, Cantrill SV. Blast injuries. *Lancet* 2009; 374: 405–15.

Chapter 16

Maconochie IK, Aickin R, Hazinski MF, et al. Pediatric Life Support: 2020 International Consensus on Cardiopulmonary Resuscitation and Emergency Cardiovascular Care Science With Treatment Recommendations. *Resuscitation* 2020; 156: A120–55.

Chapter 17

Association of Anaesthetists of Great Britain and Ireland (AAGBI). Recommendations for standards of monitoring during anaesthesia and recovery 2015. *Anaesthesia* 2016; 71: 85–93.

Cook TM, Woodall N, Frerk C. Major complications of airway management in the UK: results of the 4th National Audit Project of the Royal College of Anaesthetists and the Difficult Airway Society. Part 1 Anaesthesia. *Br J Anaesth* 2011a; 106: 617–31.

Cook TM, Woodall N, Harper J, Benger J. Major complications of airway management in the UK: results of the 4th National Audit Project of the Royal College of Anaesthetists and the Difficult Airway Society. Part 2 Intensive care and emergency department. *Br J Anaesth* 2011b; 106: 632–42.

Van de Voorde P, Turner NM, Djakow J, et al. European Resuscitation Council guidelines 2021: paediatric life support. *Resuscitation* 2021; 161: 327–87.

Chapter 18

Maconochie IK, Aickin R, Hazinski MF, et al. Pediatric Life Support: 2020 International Consensus on Cardiopulmonary Resuscitation and Emergency Cardiovascular Care Science With Treatment Recommendations. *Resuscitation* 2020; 156: A120–55.

Chapter 21

King RB, Filips D, Blitz S, et al. Evaluation of a possible tourniquet system for use in the Canadian Forces. *J Trauma* 2006; 60: 1061–71.

Lee C, Porter KM, Hodgetts TJ. Tourniquet use in the civilian prehospital setting. *Emerg Med J* 2007; 24(8): 584–7.

Royal College of Surgeons of Edinburgh (RCSEd); Faculty of Pre-Hospital Care. Position statement on the application of tourniquets. 2017. https://fphc.rcsed.ac.uk/media/2876/position-statement-on-the-application-of-tourniquets-july-2017.pdf (last accessed March 2023).

Wakai A, Winter DC, Street JT, et al. Pneumatic tourniquets in extremity surgery. *J Am Acad Orthop Surg* 2001; 9: 345–51.

Chapter 22

National Institute for Health and Care Excellence (NICE). *Head injury: Assessment and Early Management*. CG176. London: NICE, 2014 (last updated 2019).

National Institute for Health and Care Excellence (NICE). *Major Trauma: Assessment and Initial Management*. NG39. London: NICE, 2016.

National Institute for Health and Care Excellence (NICE). *Spinal Injury: Assessment and Initial Management*. NG41. London: NICE, 2016.

Royal College of Radiologists (RCR). *Paediatric Trauma Protocols* London: RCR, 2014 (last updated 2017). https://www.rcr.ac.uk/publication/paediatric-trauma-protocols (last accessed January 2023).

Chapter 23

Advanced Life Support Group (ALSG) *Neonatal, Adult and Paediatric Safe Transfer and Retrieval: the Practical Approach (NAPSTaR)*. Manchester: ALSG, 2016.

Appendix A

Stewart PA. Independent and dependent variables of acid-base control. *Respir Physiol* 1978; 33: 9–26.

Appendix B

Holliday MA, Segar WE. The maintenance need for water in parenteral fluid therapy. *Pediatrics* 1957; 19: 823–32.

Appendix C

May L, Kelly A, Wyse M, Thies K, Newton T. *FTC Manual*. https://www.europeantraumacourse.com/on-line-resources (last accessed March 2023).

Appendix D

Royal College of Radiologists (RCR)/Society and College of Radiographers (SCoR). *The Radiological Investigation of Suspected Physical Abuse in a Child,* revised 1e. London: RCR/SCoR, 2018.

Appendix E

Association for Paediatric Palliative Medicine (APPM). *Master Formulary*. https://www.appm.org.uk/guidelines-resources/appm-master-formulary/ (last accessed March 2023).

Child and Young Person's Advance Care Plan Collaborative (CYPACP). *Policy. Child and Young Person's Advance Care Plan*. http://cypacp.uk/wp-content/uploads/2020/02/CYPACP-Policy-Final-V-1.6.pdf (last accessed January 2023).

General Medical Council (GMC) *0–18 Years: Guidance for all Doctors*. London: GMC. https://www.gmc-uk.org/ethical-guidance/ethical-guidance-for-doctors/0-18-years (last accessed March 2023).

HM Government. *Child Death Review – Statutory and Operational Guidance (England)*. London: HM Government, 2018. https://assets.publishing.service.gov.uk/government/uploads/system/uploads/attachment_data/file/859302/child-death-review-statutory-and-operational-guidance-england.pdf (last accessed January 2023).

Larcher V, Craig F, Bhogal K et al. Making decisions to limit treatment in life-limiting and life-threatening conditions in children: a framework for practice. *Arch Dis Child* 2015; 100 (Suppl. 2): s3–23.

Paediatric FOAMed. *The 'Hot' Debrief*. https://www.paediatricfoam.com/2017/01/hot-debrief/ (last accessed January 2023).

Appendix F

Bauman B, McEachron K, Goldman D, et al. Emergency management of the ingested magnet: an algorithmic approach. *Pediatr Emerg Care* 2019; 35(8): e141–4.

Daly FS, Fountain JS, Murray L, Graudins A, Buckley NA; Panel of Australian New Zealand Clinical Toxicologists. Guidelines for the management of paracetomol poisoning in Australia and New Zealand: explanation and elaboration. A consensus statement from clinical toxicologists consulting to the Australasian poisons information centres. *Med J Aust* 2008; 188(5): 296–301.

Hussain SZ, Bousvaros A, Gilger M, et al. Management of ingested magnets in children. *J Pediatr Gastroenterol Nutr* 2012; 55(3): 239–42.

Kramer RE, Lerner DG, Lin T, et al. Management of ingested foreign bodies in children: a clinical report of the NASPGHAN Endoscopy Committee. *J Pediatr Gastroenterol Nutr* 2015; 60(4): 562–74.

Litovitz T, Whitaker N, Clark L, et al. Emerging battery-ingestion hazard: clinical implications. *Paediatrics* 2010; 125: 1168–77.

National Poisons Information Service. *Toxbase*. https://www.toxbase.org/poisons-index-a-z/b-products/button-battery/.

Royal College of Emergency Medicine (RCEM). *Ingestion of Super Strong Magnets in Children. Best Practice Guideline*. London: RECEM, 2021. https://rcem.ac.uk/wp-content/uploads/2021/10/RCEM_BPC_Ingestion_of_Super_Strong_Magnets_in_Children_170521.pdf (last accessed January 2023).

Russell R, Griffin R, Weinstein E, Billmire DF. Esophageal button battery ingestions: decreasing time to operative intervention by level 1 trauma activation. *J Pediatr Surg* 2014; 49: 1360–2.

Tavarez MM, Saladino RA, Gaines BA, Manole MD. Prevalence, clinical features and management of pediatric magnetic foreign body ingestions. *J Emerg Med*; 2013; 44(1): 261–8.

Wright K, Parkins K, Haiko J, Rowlands R, Davies F. Catastrophic haemorrhage from button battery ingestion in children: a growing problem. *Acta Paediatr* 2017; 106: 1391–3.

Appendix G

Laptook AR, Salhab W, Bhaskar B, et al. Admission temperature of low birth weight infants: predictors and associated morbidities. *Pediatrics* 2007; 119: e643–9.

Appendix H

Tipton MJ, Golden FStC. A proposed decision-making guide for the search, rescue and resuscitation of submersion (head under) victims based on expert opinion. *Resuscitation* 2011; 82: 819–24.

World Health Organization (WHO). *Global Report on Drowning: Preventing a Leading Killer*. Geneva: WHO, 2014.

Appendix I

American Academy of Pediatrics. Recognition and management of cardiac arrest. In: Chameides L, Samson RA, Schexnayder SM, Hazinski MF (eds). *Pediatric Advanced Life Support Provider Manual*. Dallas: American Heart Association, 2012: p. 141.

Blanco P, Martínez Buendía C. Point-of-care ultrasound in cardiopulmonary resuscitation: a concise review. *J Ultrasound* 2017; 20(3): 193–8.

Hardwick JA, Griksaitis MJ. Fifteen-minute consultation: point of care ultrasound in the management of paediatric shock. *Arch Dis Child Educ Pract Ed* 2021: 106(3): 136–41.

Lichtenstein DA. Lung ultrasound in the critically ill. *Ann Intensive Care* 2014; 4(1): 1.

Ord HL, Griksaitis MJ. Fifteen-minute consultation: using point of care ultrasound to assess children with respiratory failure. *Arch Dis Child Educ Pract Ed* 2019; 104(1): 2–10.

Rosetti VA, Thompson BM, Aprahamian C, et al. Difficulty and delay in intravascular access in pediatric arrests. *Ann Emerg Med* 1984; 13: 406.

General

European Resuscitation Council: https://www.erc.edu/.

ILCOR 2021 Resus Guidelines: https://ilcor.org/.

Resuscitation Council: https://www.resus.org.uk/.

Wolters Kluwer: https://www.wolterskluwer.com/en/solutions/uptodate.

Index

Page references in *italics* refer to figures; those in **bold** refer to tables

---

How to use your textbook

The anytime, anywhere textbook

Wiley E-Text

Your textbook comes with free access to a **Wiley E-Text: Powered by VitalSource** version – a digital version of this textbook which you own as soon as you download it.

Your **Wiley E-Text** allows you to:

Search: Save time by finding terms and topics instantly in your book, your notes, even your whole library (once you've downloaded more textbooks)

Note and highlight: Colour code, highlight and make digital notes right in the text so you can find them quickly and easily

Organize: Keep books, notes and class materials organized in folders inside the application

Share: Exchange notes and highlights with others

Upgrade: Your textbook can be transferred when you need to change or upgrade computers

The **Wiley E-Text** version will also allow you to copy and paste any photograph or illustration into assignments, presentations and your own notes.

To access your Wiley E-Text:

- Find the redemption code on the inside back cover of this book and carefully scratch away the top coating of the label. Visit **http://www.vitalsource.com/downloads** to download the Bookshelf application to your computer, laptop, tablet or mobile device.
- If you have purchased this title as an e-book, access to your **Wiley E-Text** is available with proof of purchase within 90 days. Visit **http://support.wiley.com** and click on the 'Contact Support' tab.
- Open the Bookshelf application on your computer and register for an account.
- Follow the registration process and enter your redemption code to download your digital book.

The VitalSource Bookshelf can now be used to view your Wiley E-Text on iOS, Android and Kindle Fire!

- **For iOS:** Visit the app store to download the VitalSource Bookshelf: **http://bit.ly/17ib3XS**
- **For Android and Kindle Fire:** Visit the Google Play Market to download the VitalSource Bookshelf: **http://bit.ly/BSAAGP**

You can now sign in with the email address and password you used when you created your VitalSource Bookshelf Account

Full E-Text support for mobile devices is available at: **http://support.vitalsource.com**
